Obika L.

CONTRIBUTORS

Sheryl Sommer, PhD, RN, CNE
VP Nursing Education & Strategy

Janean Johnson, MSN, RN
Nursing Education Strategist

Sherry L. Roper, PhD, RN
Nursing Education Strategist

Karin Roberts, PhD, MSN, RN, CNE
Nursing Education Coordinator

Mendy G. McMichael, DNP, RN
Nursing Education Specialist and Content Project Coordinator

Marsha S. Barlow, MSN, RN
Nursing Education Specialist

Judy Drumm, DNS, RN, CPN
Nursing Education Specialist

Carrie B. Elkins, DHSc, MSN, RN
Nursing Education Specialist

Audrey Knippa, MS, MPH, RN, CNE
Nursing Education Coordinator

EDITORIAL AND PUBLISHING

Derek Prater
Spring Lenox
Michelle Renner
Mandy Tallmadge
Kelly Von Lunen

CONSULTANTS

Nancy Bailey, MSN, BSN, RN
Christi Blair, MSN, RN
Mary Kay Smid, EdD, MSN, RN, CNE

Intellectual Property Notice

ATI Nursing is a division of Assessment Technologies Institute®, LLC

Important Notice to the Reader

User's Guide

Welcome to the Assessment Technologies Institute® PN Nursing Care of Children Review Module Edition 9.0. The mission of ATI's Content Mastery Series® review modules is to provide user-friendly compendiums of nursing knowledge that will:

- Help you locate important information quickly.

- Assist in your learning efforts.

- Provide exercises for applying your nursing knowledge.

- Facilitate your entry into the nursing profession as a newly licensed PN.

Organization

This review module is organized into units covering the foundations of nursing care of children, nursing care of children with systems disorders, and nursing care of children with special needs. Chapters within these units conform to one of four organizing principles for presenting the content:

- Nursing concepts

- Growth and development

- Procedures

- Systems disorders

Nursing concepts chapters begin with an overview describing the central concept and its relevance to nursing. Subordinate themes are covered in outline form to demonstrate relationships and present the information in a clear, succinct manner.

Procedures chapters include an overview describing the procedure(s) covered in the chapter. These chapters will provide you with nursing knowledge relevant to each procedure, including indications, interpretations of findings, nursing actions, and complications.

Systems disorders chapters include an overview describing the disorder(s) and/or disease process. These chapters may provide information on health promotion and disease prevention before addressing data collection, including risk factors, subjective data, and objective data. Next, you will focus on patient-centered care, including nursing care, medications, teamwork and collaboration, therapeutic procedures, surgical interventions, and care after discharge. Finally, you will find complications related to the disorder, along with nursing actions in response to those complications.

Application Exercises

Questions are provided at the end of each chapter so you can practice applying your knowledge. The Application Exercises include NCLEX-style questions, such as multiple-choice and multiple-select items, and questions that ask you to apply your knowledge in other formats, such as by using an ATI Active Learning Template. After the Application Exercises, an answer key is provided, along with rationales for the answers.

NCLEX® Connections

To prepare for the NCLEX-PN, it is important for you to understand how the content in this review module is connected to the NCLEX-PN test plan. You can find information on the detailed test plan at the National Council of State Boards of Nursing's Web site: https://www.ncsbn.org/. When reviewing content in this review module, regularly ask yourself, "How does this content fit into the test plan, and what types of questions related to this content should I expect?"

To help you in this process, we've included NCLEX Connections at the beginning of each unit and with each question in the Application Exercises Answer Keys. The NCLEX Connections at the beginning of each unit will point out areas of the detailed test plan that relate to the content within the section or unit. The NCLEX Connections attached to the Application Exercises Answer Keys will demonstrate how each exercise fits within the detailed content outline.

These NCLEX Connections will help you understand how the detailed content outline is organized, starting with major client needs categories and subcategories and followed by related content areas and tasks. The major client needs categories are:

- Safe and Effective Care Environment
  - Coordinated Care
  - Safety and Infection Control
- Health Promotion and Maintenance
- Psychosocial Integrity
- Physiological Integrity
  - Basic Care and Comfort
  - Pharmacological Therapies
  - Reduction of Risk Potential
  - Physiological Adaptation

An NCLEX Connection might, for example, alert you that content within a unit is related to:

- Physiological Adaptation
  - Alterations in Body Systems
    - Identify clinical manifestations and incubation periods of infectious diseases.

QSEN Competencies

As you use the review modules, you will note the integration of the Quality and Safety Education for Nurses (QSEN) competencies throughout the chapters. These competencies are integral components of the curriculum of many nursing programs in the United States and prepare you to provide safe, high-quality care as a newly licensed PN. Icons appear to draw your attention to the six QSEN competencies:

- Safety: The minimization of risk factors that could cause injury or harm while promoting quality care and maintaining a secure environment for clients, self, and others.

- Patient-Centered Care: The provision of caring and compassionate, culturally sensitive care that addresses clients' physiological, psychological, sociological, spiritual, and cultural needs, preferences, and values.

- Evidence-Based Practice: The use of current knowledge from research and other credible sources, on which to base clinical judgment and client care.

- Informatics: The use of information technology as a communication and information-gathering tool that supports clinical decision-making and scientifically based nursing practice.

- Quality Improvement: Care related and organizational processes that involve the development and implementation of a plan to improve health care services and better meet clients' needs.

- Teamwork and Collaboration: The delivery of client care in partnership with multidisciplinary members of the health care team to achieve continuity of care and positive client outcomes.

Icons

Icons are used throughout the review module to draw your attention to particular areas. Keep an eye out for these icons:

 This icon is used for NCLEX connections.

 This icon is used for content related to safety and is a QSEN competency. When you see this icon, take note of safety concerns or steps that nurses can take to ensure client safety and a safe environment.

This icon is a QSEN competency that indicates the importance of a holistic approach to providing care.

 This icon, a QSEN competency, points out the integration of research into clinical practice.

 This icon is a QSEN competency and highlights the use of information technology to support nursing practice.

 This icon is used to focus on the QSEN competency of integrating planning processes to meet clients' needs.

This icon highlights the QSEN competency of care delivery using an interprofessional approach.

This icon indicates that a media supplement, such as a graphic, animation, or video, is available. If you have an electronic copy of the review module, this icon will appear alongside clickable links to media supplements. If you have a hardcopy version of the review module, visit www.atitesting.com for details on how to access these features.

Feedback

ATI welcomes feedback regarding this review module. Please provide comments to: comments@atitesting.com.

TABLE OF CONTENTS

UNIT 1   Foundations of Nursing Care of Children

SECTION   Perspectives of Nursing Care of Children

NCLEX® CONNECTIONS 1

1   Family-Centered Nursing Care 2

2   Physical Assessment Findings..8

3   Health Promotion of Infants (1 Month to 1 Year) 23

4   Health Promotion of Toddlers (1 to 3 Years) 34

5   Health Promotion of Preschoolers (3 to 6 Years).......................................43

6   Health Promotion of School-Age Children (6 to 12 Years) 51

7   Health Promotion of Adolescents (12 to 20 Years)..60

SECTION   Special Considerations of Nursing Care of CHildren

NCLEX® CONNECTIONS 68

8   Safe Administration of Medication 69

9   Pain Management...78

10   Hospitalization, Illness, and Play 89

11   Death and Dying 98

UNIT 2   Nursing Care of Children with System Disorders

SECTION   Neurosensory Disorders

NCLEX® CONNECTIONS 107

12   Acute Neurological Disorders 108

13   Seizures..124

SECTION   Respiratory Disorders

NCLEX® CONNECTIONS 134

14   Oxygen and Inhalation Therapy 135

15   Acute and Infectious Respiratory Illnesses 148

16   Asthma...163

17   Cystic Fibrosis 172

SECTION Cardiovascular and Hematologic Disorders

  NCLEX® CONNECTIONS 181

  18 Cardiovascular Disorders 182

  19 Hematologic Disorders 203

SECTION Gastrointestinal Disorders

  NCLEX® CONNECTIONS 219

  20 Acute Infectious Gastrointestinal Disorders...................................220

  21 Gastrointestinal Structural and Inflammatory Disorders.............230

SECTION Genitourinary and Reproductive Disorders

  NCLEX® CONNECTIONS 248

  22 Enuresis and Urinary Tract Infections..249

  23 Structural Disorders of the Genitourinary Tract
      and Reproductive System 260

  24 Renal Disorders 269

SECTION Musculoskeletal Disorders

  NCLEX® CONNECTIONS 280

  25 Fractures..281

  26 Musculoskeletal Congenital Disorders 292

  27 Chronic Neuromusculoskeletal Disorders.......................................307

SECTION Integumentary Disorders

  NCLEX® CONNECTIONS 329

  28 Skin Infections and Infestations..330

  29 Dermatitis and Acne 344

  30 Burns...358

SECTION Endocrine Disorders

  NCLEX® CONNECTIONS 371

  31 Diabetes Mellitus 372

  32 Growth Hormone Deficiency 384

SECTION Immune and Infectious Disorders

NCLEX® CONNECTIONS 392

33 Immunizations 393

34 Communicable Diseases 402

35 Acute Otitis Media 412

36 HIV/AIDS 421

SECTION Neoplastic Disorders

NCLEX® CONNECTIONS 430

37 Pediatric Cancers 431

UNIT 3 Nursing Care of Children with Special Needs

NCLEX® CONNECTIONS 450

38 Pediatric Emergencies 451

39 Psychosocial Issues of Infants, Children, and Adolescents 465

References 483

APPENDIX Active Learning Templates

Basic Concept A1

Diagnostic Procedure A2

System Disorder A3

Growth and Development A4

Medication A5

Nursing Skill A6

Therapeutic Procedure A7

UNIT 1 ## Foundations of Nursing Care of Children

SECTION: PERSPECTIVES OF NURSING CARE OF CHILDREN

› Family-Centered Nursing Care
› Physical Assessment Findings
› Health Promotion of Infants (1 Month to 1 Year)
› Health Promotion of Toddlers (1 to 3 Years)
› Health Promotion of Preschoolers (3 to 6 Years)
› Health Promotion of School-Age Children (6 to 12 Years)
› Health Promotion of Adolescents (12 to 20 Years)

NCLEX® CONNECTIONS

When reviewing the chapters in this section, keep in mind the relevant sections of the NCLEX® outline, in particular:

Client Needs: Safety and Infection Control

› Relevant topics/tasks include:
  » Accident/Injury Prevention
    › Assist in or reinforce education to client about safety precautions.

Client Needs: Basic Care and Comfort

› Relevant topics/tasks include:
  » Nutrition and Oral Hydration
    › Monitor and provide for nutritional needs of client.
  » Rest and Sleep
    › Provide measures to promote sleep/rest.

Client Needs: Health Promotion and Maintenance

› Relevant topics/tasks include:
  » Aging Process
    › Provide care and education for the newborn less than 1 month old through the infant or toddler client through 2 years.
    › Provide care that meets the needs of the preschool, school age and adolescent client ages 3 through 17 years.
  » Data Collection Techniques
    › Collect data for health history
    › Collect baseline physical data
    › Report physical examination results to health care provider.
  » Developmental Stages and Transitions
    › Identify occurrence of expected body image changes.
    › Compare client development to norms.
    › Modify approaches to care in accordance with client development stage.
  » Health Promotion/Disease Prevention
    › Identify clients in need of immunizations.
    › Identify precautions and contraindications to immunizations.
    › Provide assistance for screening examinations.
    › Monitor incorporation of healthy behaviors into lifestyle by client.
    › Reinforce teaching with client about health risks and health promotion.

chapter 1

Overview

- Families are groups that should remain constant in children's lives.

- Family is defined by what an individual considers it to be.

- Families often include individuals with a biological, marital, or adoptive relationship. In the absence of these characteristics, families also consist of individuals who have a strong emotional bond and commitment to one another.

- Due to the expanding concepts of family, the term household is sometimes used.

- Positive family relationships are characterized by parent-child interactions that show mutual warmth and respect.

- Family-centered nursing care includes the following:

  o Agreed-upon partnerships between families of children, nurses, and providers, in which the families and children benefit.

  o Respecting cultural diversity, and incorporating cultural views in the plan of care.

  o Understanding growth and developmental needs of children and their families.

  o Treating children and their families as clients.

  o Working with all types of families.

  o Collaborating with families regarding hospitalization, home, and community resources.

  o Allowing families to serve as experts regarding their children's health conditions, usual behaviors in different situations, and routine needs.

- Promoting family-centered care

  o Nurses should collect data to identify strengths and weaknesses.

    ▪ Characteristics of healthy families

      □ Members communicate well and listen to each other.

      □ Members teach respect for others, and share responsibilities, traditions, and rituals.

  o Nurses should pay close attention when family members state that a child "isn't acting right" or has other concerns.

  o Nurses should consider children's opinions when providing care.

Family Composition

TYPE	MEMBERS
Traditional nuclear family	› Married couple and their biologic children (only full brothers and sisters)
Nuclear family	› Two parents and their children (biologic, adoptive, step, foster)
Single-parent family	› One parent and one or more children
Blended family (also called reconstituted)	› At least one stepparent, stepsibling, or half-sibling
Extended family	› At least one parent, one child, and other individuals – either related or not
Gay/lesbian family	› Two members of the same sex who have children and a legal or common-law tie
Foster family	› A child or children who have been placed in an approved living environment away from the family of origin – usually with one or two parents
Binuclear family	› Parents who have terminated spousal roles but continue their parenting roles
Communal family	› Individuals who share common ownership of property and goods and exchange services without monetary consideration

- Changes that occur with the birth (or adoption) of the first child
  - Parents' sense of self as they transition to the new parental role
  - Division of labor and roles within the relationships of couples
  - Relationships with grandparents
  - Work relationships
  - Increased financial responsibilities and possible loss of income
  - Necessary sleep habit changes

Parenting Styles

TYPE	DESCRIPTION	EXAMPLE
Dictatorial or authoritarian	› Parents try to control the child's behaviors and attitudes through unquestioned rules and expectations.	› The child is never allowed to watch television on school nights.
Permissive	› Parents exert little or no control over the child's behaviors and consult the child when making decisions.	› The child assists with deciding whether he will watch television.
Democratic or authoritative	› Parents direct the child's behavior by setting rules and explaining the reason for each rule setting. › Parents negatively reinforce deviations from the rules.	› The child can watch television for 1 hr on school nights after completing all of his homework and chores. › The privilege is taken away but later reinstated based on new guidelines.
Passive	› Parents are uninvolved, indifferent, and emotionally removed.	› The child may watch television whenever he wants.

- Positive parental influences
  - Parents have good mental health.
  - Structure and routine are maintained in the household.
  - Parents engage in activities with the child.
  - There is communication that validates the child's feelings.
  - The child is monitored for safety with special consideration for her developmental needs.

- Guidelines for promoting acceptable behavior in children
  - Set clear and realistic limits and expectations based on the developmental level of the child.
  - Validate the child's feelings, and offer sympathetic explanations.
  - Provide role modeling and reinforcement for appropriate behavior.
  - Focus on the child's behavior when disciplining the child.

Family Data Collection

- History – Medical history for parents, siblings, and grandparents
- Structure – Family members (mother, father, son), roles/position within the family, and occupation and education of family members
- Developmental tasks – Tasks a family works on as the child grows (parents with a school-age child helping the child to develop peer relations)
- Family characteristics – Cultural, religious, and economic influences on behavior, attitudes, and actions
- Family stressors – Expected (birth of a child) and unexpected (illness of a child, divorce, disability, or death of a family member) events that cause stress
- Environment – Availability of and family interactions with community resources
- Family support systems – Availability of extended family, work and peer relationships, as well as social systems and community resources to assist the family in meeting needs or adapting to a stressor

APPLICATION EXERCISES

1. A 9-year-old child who has sickle cell anemia lives with her father, stepmother, and half-sibling. Which of the following describes this family's composition?

    A. Nuclear family

    B. Blended family

    C. Extended family

    D. Binuclear family

2. A nurse is assisting a group of parents of adolescents to develop skills that will improve communication within the family. The nurse hears one parent state, "My son knows he better do what I say." Which of the following parenting styles is the parent exhibiting?

    A. Authoritarian

    B. Permissive

    C. Authoritative

    D. Passive

3. A nurse is collecting data from the parents of two school-age children. Which of the following should the nurse include? (Select all that apply.)

    _____ A. Grandparents' health status

    _____ B. Parents' education level

    _____ C. Children's physical growth

    _____ D. Support systems

    _____ E. Children's nutritional intake

4. A nurse is reinforcing anticipatory guidance to the mother of a toddler. The nurse learns that the household includes the mother, the toddler, an older brother, and a grandmother. Use the ATI Active Learning Template: Basic Concept to complete this item to include the following:

    A. Related Content: Describe the composition of this family.

    B. Underlying Principles:
        • Two methods the parent can use to positively influence the child.
        • Two ways the parent can promote acceptable behavior in the child.

    C. Nursing Interventions: Data collection the nurse should perform.

APPLICATION EXERCISES KEY

1. A. INCORRECT: A nuclear family includes two parents and their children.

    B. **CORRECT:** A blended family includes at least one stepparent, stepsibling, and/or half-sibling.

    C. INCORRECT: An extended family includes one or more parents, one or more children, and other family members such as a grandmother.

    D. INCORRECT: A binuclear family includes parents who have terminated spousal roles but continue their parenting roles.

    Ⓝ NCLEX® Connection: Health Promotion and Maintenance, Developmental Stages and Transitions

2. A. **CORRECT:** This parent is exhibiting an authoritarian parenting style. Using this style, the parent controls the adolescent's behaviors and attitudes through unquestioned rules and expectations.

    B. INCORRECT: This parent is not exhibiting a permissive parenting style. Using this style, the parent exerts little or no control over the adolescent's behaviors, and consults the adolescent when making decisions.

    C. INCORRECT: This parent is not exhibiting an authoritative parenting style. Using this style, the parent directs the adolescent's behavior by setting rules and explaining the reason for each rule setting.

    D. INCORRECT: This parent is not exhibiting a passive parenting style. Using this style, the parent is uninvolved, indifferent, and emotionally removed.

    Ⓝ NCLEX® Connection: Health Promotion and Maintenance, Developmental Stages and Transitions

3. A. **CORRECT:** The nurse should include a medical history on the parents, siblings, and grandparents when performing a family assessment.

    B. **CORRECT:** The nurse should include the family structure, which includes family members, roles/positions within the family, and occupation and education of family members, when performing a family assessment.

    C. INCORRECT: The nurse should include the child's physical growth when performing an individual assessment on the child.

    D. **CORRECT:** The nurse should include support systems to determine the availability of extended family, work and peer relationships, and social systems and community resources to assist the family in meeting needs when performing a family assessment.

    E. INCORRECT: The nurse should include the children's nutritional intake when performing individual assessments on each child.

    Ⓝ NCLEX® Connection: Health Promotion and Maintenance, Developmental Stages and Transitions

4. *Using the ATI Active Learning Template: Basic Concept*

    A. Related Content
        *   Family composition: This is an extended family, which includes at least one parent, one or more children, and other individuals who are either related or not related.

    B. Underlying Principles
        *   Positive parental influences
            ○ Have good mental health.
            ○ Maintain structure and routine in the household.
            ○ Engage in activities with the child.
            ○ Validate the child's feelings when communicating.
            ○ Monitor for safety concerns with special consideration for the child's developmental needs.
        *   Promoting acceptable behavior
            ○ Validate the child's feelings, and offer sympathetic explanations.
            ○ Provide role modeling and reinforcement for acceptable behavior.
            ○ Set clear and realistic limits and expectations based on the child's developmental level.
            ○ Focus on the behavior when implementing discipline.

    C. Nursing Interventions
        *   Family data collection
            ○ Medical history on parents, siblings, and grandparents
            ○ Family structure for roles/position within the family, as well as occupation and education of family members
            ○ Developmental tasks a family works on as the child grows
            ○ Family characteristics, such as cultural, religious, and economic influences on behavior, attitudes, and actions
            ○ Family stressors, such as expected (birth of a child) and unexpected (illness of a child, divorce, disability or death of a family member) events that cause stress
            ○ Availability of and family interactions with community resources
            ○ Family support systems, such as availability of extended family, work and peer relationships, as well as social systems and community resources to assist the family in meeting needs or adapting to a stressor

    Ⓝ NCLEX® Connection: Health Promotion and Maintenance, Developmental Stages and Transitions

chapter 2

Overview

- Perform examinations in nonthreatening environments.
- Alter exams to accommodate developmental needs.
- Observe behaviors that signal the child's readiness to cooperate.
- If the child is uncooperative, determine reasons, be firm and direct about expected behavior, complete the assessment quickly, and use a calm voice.
- Involve children and family members in examinations.
- Praise children for cooperation during exams.

Nursing Considerations

- Keep the room warm and well lit.
- Keep medical equipment out of sight.
- Provide privacy. Determine whether older school-age children and adolescents prefer a caregiver to remain during examination.
- Explain each step of the examination to the child.
  - Use age-appropriate language.
  - Demonstrate what will happen using dolls, puppets, or paper drawings.
  - Allow child manipulate and handle equipment.
  - Encourage child to use equipment on others.
- Examine the child in a secure, comfortable position. For example, a toddler may sit on a parent's lap if desired.
- Proceed to examine the child in an organized sequence when possible.
- Encourage the child and/or family to ask questions during physical exams.

Expected Vital Signs

- Temperature

AGE	EXPECTED LEVEL	RECOMMENDED ROUTES
3 months	37.5° C (99.5° F)	› Axillary › Rectal (if exact measurement necessary)
6 months	37.5° C (99.5° F)	
1 year	37.7° C (99.9° F)	
3 years	37.2° C (99.0° F)	› Axillary › Tympanic › Oral (if child cooperative) › Rectal (if exact measurement necessary)
5 years	37.0° C (98.6° F)	
7 years	36.8° C (98.2° F)	› Oral › Axillary › Tympanic › Oral
9 years	36.7° C (98.1° F)	
11 years	36.7° C (98.1° F)	
13 years	36.6° C (97.9° F)	

- Pulse Rate
    - Newborn – 80 to 180/min (depending on activity)
    - 1 week to 3 months – 80 to 220/min (depending on activity)
    - 3 months to 2 years – 70 to 150/min (depending on activity)
    - 2 to 10 years – 60 to 110/min (depending on activity)
    - 10 years and older – 50 to 90/min (depending on activity)
- Respirations
    - Newborn to 1 year – 30 to 35/min
    - 1 to 2 years – 25 to 30/min
    - 2 to 6 years – 21 to 25/min
    - 6 to 12 years – 19 to 21/min
    - 12 years and older – 16 to 19/min

Q
EBP

- Blood Pressure

  - Age, height, and gender all influence blood pressure readings. Readings should be compared with standard measurements (National High Blood Pressure Education Program Working Group on High Blood Pressure in Children and Adolescents).

  - Infants – 65 to 80 mm Hg systolic and 40 to 50 mm Hg diastolic

  - The following chart provides examples of expected ranges of blood pressure by age and gender.

	GIRLS		BOYS	
	Systolic (mm Hg)	Diastolic (mm Hg)	Systolic (mm Hg)	Diastolic (mm Hg)
1 year	83 to 114	38 to 67	80 to 114	34 to 66
3 years	86 to 117	47 to 76	86 to 120	44 to 75
6 years	91 to 122	54 to 83	91 to 125	53 to 84
10 years	98 to 129	59 to 88	97 to 130	58 to 90
16 years	108 to 138	64 to 93	111 to 145	63 to 94

Expected Physical Assessment Findings

- General Appearance

  - Appears undistressed.

  - Appears clean and well-kept.

  - Muscle tone – Erect head posture is expected in infants after 4 months of age.

  - Has no body odors.

  - Makes eye contact when addressed (except infants).

  - Follows simple commands as age appropriate.

  - Uses speech, language, and motor skills spontaneously.

Q
EBP

  - Growth – Growth can be evaluated using weight, height, body mass index (BMI), and head circumference. Growth charts are tools that can be used to assess the overall health of a child. To see growth charts by age and gender, visit the website for the Centers for Disease Control and Prevention (www.cdc.gov).

- Skin, Hair, and Nails

  - Skin

    - Variations in skin color are expected based on race and ethnicity.

    - Temperature should be warm or slightly cool to the touch.

    - Skin turgor exhibits brisk elasticity with adequate hydration.

    - Skin texture should be smooth and slightly dry, not oily.

    - Lesions are not expected findings.

    - Skin folds should be symmetric.

- Hair and Scalp
  - Hair should be evenly distributed, smooth, and strong.
    - Manifestations of nutritional deficiencies include hair that is stringy, dull, brittle, and dry.
    - Hair loss or balding spots on infants may indicate he is spending too much time in the same position.
  - Observe children approaching adolescence for the presence of secondary hair growth.
  - Scalp should be clean and absent from any scaliness, infestations, and trauma.
- Nails
  - Pink over the nail bed and white at the tips
  - Smooth and firm (but slightly flexible in infants)
  - No clubbing
- Lymph nodes should be nonpalpable. Lymph nodes that are small, palpable, nontender, and mobile may be an expected finding in children.
- Head and Neck
  - Head
    - The shape of the head should be symmetric.
    - Fontanels should be flat. The posterior fontanel usually closes between 6 and 8 weeks of age, and the anterior fontanel usually closes between 12 and 18 months of age.
  - Face
    - Symmetric appearance and movement
    - Proportional features
  - Neck
    - Short in infants
    - No palpable masses
    - Midline trachea
    - Full range of motion present whether assessed actively or passively
- Eyes
  - Visual acuity – May be difficult to check in children younger than 3 years of age
    - Check visual acuity in infants by holding an object in front of the eyes and checking to see whether the infant is able to fix on the object and follow it.
    - Use the tumbling E or HOTV test to check visual acuity of children who are unable to read letters and numbers.
    - Older children should be tested using a Snellen chart or symbol chart.
  - Check color vision using the Ishihara color test or the Hardy-Rand-Rittler test. The child should be able to correctly identify shapes, symbols, or numbers.

- Peripheral visual fields should be
  - Upward 50°
  - Downward 70°
  - Nasally 60°
  - Temporally 90°
- Extraocular movements may not be symmetric in newborns.
  - Corneal light reflex should be symmetric.
  - Cover/uncover test should demonstrate equal movement of the eyes.
  - Six cardinal fields of gaze should demonstrate no nystagmus.
- Eyebrows should be symmetric and evenly distributed from the inner to the outer canthus.
- Eyelids should close completely and open to allow the lower border and most of the upper portion of the iris to be seen.
- Eyelashes should curve outward and be evenly distributed with no inflammation around any of the hair follicles.
- Conjunctiva
  - Palpebral is pink.
  - Bulbar is transparent.
- Lacrimal apparatus is without excessive tearing, redness, or discharge.
- Sclera should be white.
- Corneas should be clear.
- Pupils should be
  - Round
  - Equal in size
  - Reactive to light
  - Accommodating
- Irises should be round with the permanent color manifesting around 6 to 12 months of age.
- Internal Exam
  - Red reflex should be present in infants.
  - Arteries, veins, optic discs, and maculas may be visualized in older children and adolescents.
- Ears
  - Alignment
    - The top of the auricles should meet in an imaginary horizontal line that extends from the outer canthus of the eye.
  - External Ear
    - The external ear should be free of lesions and nontender.
    - The ear canal should be free of foreign bodies or discharge.
    - Cerumen is an expected finding.

- Internal Ear
  - In infants and toddlers, pull the pinna down and back to visualize the tympanic membrane.
  - In children older than 3 years of age, pull the pinna up and back to visualize.
  - The ear canal should be pink with fine hairs.
  - The tympanic membrane should be pearly pink, or gray.
  - The light reflex should be visible.
  - Umbo (tip of the malleolus) and manubrium (long process or handle) are the bony landmarks that should be visible.
- Hearing
  - Newborns should have intact acoustic blink reflexes to sudden sounds.
  - Infants should turn toward sounds.
  - Older children can be screened by whispering a word from behind to see whether they can identify the word.

- Nose
  - The position should be midline.
  - Patency should be present for each nostril without excessive flaring.
  - Internal structures
    - The septum is midline and intact.
    - The mucosa is deep pink and moist with no discharge.
  - Smell can be checked in older children.
- Mouth and Throat
  - Lips
    - Darker pigmented than facial skin
    - Smooth, soft, moist, and symmetric
  - Gums
    - Coral pink
    - Tight against the teeth
  - Mucous membranes
    - Without lesions
    - Moist, pink, smooth, and glistening
  - Tongue
    - Infants may have white coatings on their tongues from milk that can be easily removed. Oral candidiasis coating is not easily removed.
    - Children and adolescents should have pink, symmetric tongues that they are able to move beyond their lips.
  - Teeth
    - Infants should have six to eight teeth by 1 year of age.
    - Children and adolescents should have teeth that are white and smooth, and begin replacing the 20 deciduous teeth with 32 permanent teeth.

- ○ Hard and soft palates – Intact, firm, and concave
- ○ Uvula – Intact and moves with vocalization
- ○ Tonsils
    - Infants – May not be able to visualize
    - Children – Barely visible to prominent, same color as surrounding mucosa, deep crevices that hold food particles
- ○ Speech
    - Infants – Strong cry
    - Children and adolescents – Clear and articulate
- Thorax and Lungs
    - ○ Chest shape
        - Infants – Shape is almost circular with anteroposterior diameter equaling the transverse or lateral diameter.
        - Children and adolescents – The transverse diameter to anteroposterior diameter changes to 2:1.
    - ○ Ribs and sternum – More soft and flexible in infants; symmetric and smooth, with no protrusions or bulges
    - ○ Movement – Symmetric, no retractions
        - Infants – Irregular rhythms are common.
        - Children younger than 7 – More abdominal movement is seen during respirations.
    - ○ Breath sounds
        - Inspiration is longer and louder than expiration.
        - Vesicular, or soft, swishing sounds, are heard over most of the lungs.
    - ○ Breasts
        - Newborns – Breasts may be enlarged during the first few days.
        - Children and adolescents – Nipples and areolas are darker pigmented and symmetric.
            - □ Females – Breasts typically develop between 10 to 14 years of age. The breasts should appear asymmetric, have no masses, and be palpable.
            - □ Males may develop gynecomastia, which is unilateral or bilateral breast enlargement that occurs during puberty.
- Circulatory System
    - ○ Heart sounds – S_1 and S_2 heart sounds should be clear and crisp. S_1 is louder at the apex of the heart. S_2 is louder near the base of the heart. Sinus arrhythmias that are associated with respirations are common. Physiologic splitting of S_2 and S_3 heart sounds are expected findings in some children.
    - ○ Pulses
        - Infants – Brachial, temporal, and femoral pulses should be palpable, full, and localized.
        - Children and adolescents – Pulse locations and expected findings are the same as those in adults.

- Abdomen – Without tenderness, no guarding. Peristaltic waves may be visible in thinner children.
  - Shape – Symmetric and without protrusions around the umbilicus
    - Infants and toddlers have rounded abdomens.
    - Children and adolescents should have flat abdomens.
  - Bowel sounds should be heard every 5 to 30 seconds.
- Genitalia
  - Male
    - Hair distribution is diamond shaped after puberty in adolescent males. No pubic hair is noted in infants and small children.
    - Penis
      - Penis should appear straight.
      - Urethral meatus should be at the tip of the penis.
      - Foreskin may not be retractable in infants and small children.
      - Enlargement of the penis occurs during adolescence.
      - The penis may look abnormally small in males who are obese due to skin folds partially covering the base.
    - Scrotum
      - The scrotum hangs separately from the penis.
      - The skin on the scrotum has a rugated appearance and is loose.
      - The left testicle hangs slighter lower than the right.
      - The inguinal canal should be absent of swelling.
      - During puberty, the testes and scrotum enlarge with darker scrotal skin.
  - Female
    - Hair distribution over the mons pubis should be documented in terms of amount and location during puberty. Hair should appear in an inverted triangle. No pubic hair should be noted in infants or small children.
    - Labia – Symmetric, without lesions, moist on the inner aspects.
    - Clitoris – Small, without bruising or edema.
    - Urethral meatus – Slit-like in appearance with no discharge.
    - Vaginal orifice – The hymen may be absent, or it may completely or partially cover the vaginal opening prior to sexual intercourse.
  - Anus – Surrounding skin should be intact with sphincter tightening noted if the anus is touched. Routine rectal exams are not done with the pediatric population.
- Musculoskeletal System
  - Length, position, and size are symmetric.
  - Joints are stable and symmetric with full range of motion and no crepitus or redness.

- Spine
  - Infants' spines should be without dimples or tufts of hair. They should be midline with an overall C-shaped lateral curve.
  - Toddlers appear squat with short legs and protuberant abdomens.
  - Preschoolers appear more erect than toddlers.
  - Children should develop the cervical, thoracic, and lumbar curvatures like that of adults.
  - Adolescents should remain midline (no scoliosis noted).
- Gait
  - Toddlers and young children – A bowlegged or knock-knee appearance is a common finding. Feet should face forward while walking.
  - Older children and adolescents – A steady gait should be noted, with even wear on the soles of shoes.
- Neurologic System
  - Infant Reflexes

REFLEX	EXPECTED FINDING	EXPECTED AGE
Sucking and rooting reflexes	› Elicited by stroking an infant's cheek or the edge of an infant's mouth » The infant turns her head toward the side that is touched and starts to suck.	Birth to 4 months
Palmar grasp	› Elicited by placing an object in an infant's palm » The infant grasps the object.	Birth to 3 months
Plantar grasp	› Elicited by touching the sole of an infant's foot » The infant's toes curl downward.	Birth to 8 months
Moro reflex	› Elicited by allowing the head and trunk of an infant in a semi-sitting position to fall backward to an angle of at least 30° » The infant's arms and legs symmetrically extend and then abduct while her fingers spread to form a C shape.	Birth to 4 months
Startle reflex	› Elicited by clapping hands or by a loud noise. The newborn will abduct arms at the elbows, and the hands will remain clenched.	Birth to 4 months
Tonic neck reflex (fencer position)	› Elicited by turning an infant's head to one side » The infant extends the arm and leg on that side and flexes the arm and leg on the opposite side.	Birth to 3 to 4 months
Babinski reflex	› Elicited by stroking the outer edge of the sole of an infant's foot up toward the toes » The infant's toes fan upward and out.	Birth to 1 year
Stepping	› Elicited by holding an infant upright with his feet touching a flat surface » The infant makes stepping movements.	Birth to 4 weeks

○ Cranial Nerves

CRANIAL NERVE	EXPECTED FINDINGS INFANTS	EXPECTED FINDINGS CHILDREN/ADOLESCENTS
I Olfactory	› Difficult to test	› Identifies smells through each nostril individually
II Optic	› Looks at face and tracks with eyes	› Has intact visual acuity, peripheral vision, and color vision
III Oculomotor	› Blinks in response to light › Has pupils that are reactive to light	› Has no nystagmus and PERRLA is intact
IV Trochlear	› Looks at face and tracks with eyes	› Has the ability to look down and in with eyes
V Trigeminal	› Has rooting and sucking reflexes	› Is able to clench teeth together › Detects touch on face with eyes closed
VI Abducens	› Looks at face and tracks with eyes	› Is able to see laterally with eyes
VII Facial	› Has symmetric facial movements	› Has the ability to differentiate between salty and sweet on tongue › Has symmetric facial movements
VIII Acoustic	› Tracks a sound › Blinks in response to a loud noise	› Does not experience vertigo › Has intact hearing
IX Glossopharyngeal	› Has an intact gag reflex	› Has an intact gag reflex › Is able to taste sour sensations on back of tongue
X Vagus	› Has no difficulties swallowing	› Speech clear, no difficulties swallowing › Uvula is midline
XI Spinal Accessory	› Moves shoulders symmetrically	› Has equal strength of shoulder shrug against examiner's hands
XII Hypoglossal	› Has no difficulties swallowing › Opens mouth when nares are occluded	› Has a tongue that is midline › Is able to move tongue in all directions with equal strength against tongue blade resistance

○ Deep tendon reflexes should demonstrate the following:
- Partial flexion of the lower arm at the biceps tendon
- Partial extension of the lower arm at the triceps tendon
- Partial extension of the lower leg at the patellar tendon
- Plantar flexion of the foot at the Achilles tendon

○ Cerebellar function (children and adolescents)
- Finger to nose test – Rapid coordinated movements
- Heel to shin test – Able to run the heel of one foot down the shin of the other leg while standing
- Romberg test – Able to stand with slight swaying while eyes are closed

○ Language, cognition, and fine and gross motor development can be screened using a standardized tool such as the Denver Developmental Screening Test – Revised (Denver II). A combination of data collected from psychosocial and medical histories and a physical examination is used to determine need and make a referral for further evaluation.

APPLICATION EXERCISES

1. A nurse is preparing to collect data from a preschool-age child. Which of the following is an appropriate action by the nurse to prepare the child?

    A. Allow the child to role-play using miniature equipment.

    B. Use medical terminology to describe what will happen.

    C. Separate the child from her parent during the examination.

    D. Keep medical equipment visible to the child.

2. A nurse is checking the vital signs of a 3-year-old child during a well-child visit. Which of the following findings should the nurse report to the provider?

    A. Temperature 37.2° C (99.0° F)

    B. Pulse 104/min

    C. Respirations 30/min

    D. Blood pressure 90/52 mm Hg

3. When collecting data from a toddler, which of the following characteristics should the nurse expect to find? (Select all that apply.)

    _____ A. Bowlegged gait

    _____ B. Abdominal breathing

    _____ C. Established eye color

    _____ D. Absent red reflex

    _____ E. Bowel sounds heard every 2 to 3 min on auscultation

4. When collecting data from an infant, which of the following techniques should the nurse use to elicit the stepping reflex?

    A. Hold the infant upright with his feet touching a flat surface.

    B. Strike a flat surface on which the infant is lying.

    C. Place an object in the infant's palm.

    D. Stroke the outer edge of the sole of the infant's foot up toward the toes.

5. A nurse is collecting neurological data on an adolescent. Which of the following is an appropriate reaction by the adolescent when the nurse checks the trigeminal cranial nerve? (Select all that apply.)

_____ A. Clenching teeth together tightly

_____ B. Recognizing sour tastes on the back of the tongue

_____ C. Identifying smells through each nostril

_____ D. Detecting facial touches with eyes closed

_____ E. Looking down and in with the eyes

6. A nurse is preparing to examine a preschool-age child. Use the ATI Active Learning Template: Basic Concept to complete this item to include the following:

A. Underlying Principles: Two behaviors that indicate the child is ready to cooperate.

B. Nursing Interventions:

- Two actions to take if child is uncooperative.

- Three actions to promote the child's comfort during the examination.

APPLICATION EXERCISES KEY

1. A. **CORRECT:** The nurse should allow the child to role-play or manipulate actual or miniature equipment to reduce the anxiety and fear related to the examination.

   B. INCORRECT: The nurse should use neutral words and avoid overestimating the child's understanding of words when describing what will happen.

   C. INCORRECT: The nurse should encourage parental presence during the examination.

   D. INCORRECT: The nurse should keep medical equipment out of sight unless showing or using it on the child.

   (N) NCLEX® Connection: Health Promotion and Maintenance, Developmental Stages and Transitions

2. A. INCORRECT: A temperature of 37.2° C (99.0° F) is within the expected reference range for a 3-year-old child and should not be reported to the provider.

   B. INCORRECT: A pulse of 104/min is within the expected reference range for a 3-year-old child and should not be reported to the provider.

   C. **CORRECT:** Respirations of 30/min is above the expected reference range for a 3-year-old child and should be reported to the provider.

   D. INCORRECT: A blood pressure of 90/52 mm Hg is within the expected reference range for a 3-year-old child and should not be reported to the provider.

   (N) NCLEX® Connection: Health Promotion and Maintenance, Data Collection Techniques

3. A. **CORRECT:** The toddler should appear bowlegged or have a knock-knee appearance.

   B. **CORRECT:** The toddler should show abdominal breathing.

   C. **CORRECT:** The toddler should have established permanent eye color by 6 to 12 months of age.

   D. INCORRECT: It is an expected finding to have the red reflex present.

   E. INCORRECT: The nurse should auscultate bowel sounds every 5 to 30 seconds.

   (N) NCLEX® Connection: Health Promotion and Maintenance, Data Collection Techniques

4. A. **CORRECT:** Holding the infant upright with his feet touching a flat surface will elicit the stepping reflex. The infant will make stepping movements.

    B. INCORRECT: Striking a flat surface on which the infant is lying will elicit the Moro reflex. The infant's arms and legs extend symmetrically and then abduct while her fingers spread to form a C shape.

    C. INCORRECT: Placing an object in the infant's palm will elicit the grasp reflex. The infant will grasp the object.

    D. INCORRECT: Lightly stroking the outer edge of the infant's sole up toward the toes will elicit the Babinski reflex. The infant's toes should fan upward and out.

     NCLEX® Connection: Health Promotion and Maintenance, Data Collection Techniques

5. A. **CORRECT:** Clenching teeth together tightly is an appropriate reaction by the adolescent when checking the trigeminal cranial nerve.

    B. INCORRECT: Recognizing sour tastes on the back of the tongue is an appropriate reaction by the adolescent when checking the glossopharyngeal cranial nerve.

    C. INCORRECT: Identifying smells through each nostril is an appropriate reaction by the adolescent when checking the olfactory cranial nerve.

    D. **CORRECT:** Detecting facial touches with eyes closed is an appropriate reaction by the adolescent when checking the trigeminal cranial nerve.

    E. INCORRECT: Looking down and in with the eyes is an appropriate reaction by the adolescent when checking the trochlear cranial nerve.

     NCLEX® Connection: Health Promotion and Maintenance, Data Collection Techniques

6. *Using the ATI Active Learning Template: Basic Concept*

A. Underlying Principles
- Child is ready to cooperate
  - Interacting with nurse
  - Making eye contact
  - Permitting physical touch
  - Willingly sitting on examination table
  - Accepting and handling equipment

B. Nursing Interventions
- Actions to take if child is uncooperative
  - Engage both the child and parent.
  - Be firm and direct about expected behavior.
  - Complete data collection as quickly as possible.
  - Use a calm voice.
  - Reduce environmental stimuli.
  - Limit the people in the room.
- Actions to enhance child's comfort
  - Perform examination in nonthreatening environment.
  - Take time to play and develop rapport prior to beginning the examination.
  - Keep the room warm and well lit.
  - Keep medical equipment out of sight until needed.
  - Provide privacy.
  - Explain each step of the examination to the child.
  - Examine the child in a secure, comfortable position.
  - Examine the child in an organized sequence when possible.
  - Encourage the child and family to ask questions during the examination.

(N) NCLEX® Connection: Health Promotion and Maintenance, Developmental Stages and Transitions

chapter 3

Expected Growth and Development

- Physical Development
  - The infant's posterior fontanel closes by 6 to 8 weeks of age.
  - The infant's anterior fontanel closes by 12 to 18 months of age.
  - Weight, height, and head circumference measurements are used to track the size of infants.
    - Weight – Infants gain approximately 150 to 210 g (about 5 to 7 oz) per week the first 6 months of life. Birth weight is at least doubled by the age of 6 months, and tripled by the age of 12 months.
    - Height – Infants grow approximately 2.5 cm (1 in) per month the first 6 months of life. Growth occurs in spurts after the age of 6 months, and the birth length increases by 50% by the age of 12 months.
    - Head circumference – The circumference of infants' heads increases approximately 1.5 cm (0.6 in) per month for the first 6 months of life, and then approximately 0.5 cm (0.2 in) between 6 and 12 months of age.
  - Dentition – Six to eight teeth should erupt in infants' mouths by the end of the first year of age. The first teeth typically erupt between the ages of 6 and 10 months.
    - Teething pain can be eased using cold teething rings and over-the-counter teething gels. Acetaminophen (Tylenol) or ibuprofen (Advil) is appropriate if irritability interferes with sleeping and feeding, but should not be used for more than 3 days. Ibuprofen should be used only in infants older than 6 months.
    - Clean infants' teeth using cool, wet washcloths.
    - Bottles should not be given to infants when they are falling asleep because prolonged exposure to milk or juice can cause early childhood caries.

AGE	GROSS MOTOR SKILLS	FINE MOTOR SKILLS
1 month	› Demonstrates head lag	› Has a grasp reflex
2 months	› Lifts head off mattress when prone	› Holds hands in an open position
3 months	› Raises head and shoulders off mattress when prone › Only slight head lag	› No longer has a grasp reflex › Keeps hands loosely open
4 months	› Rolls from back to side	› Places objects in mouth
5 months	› Rolls from front to back	› Uses palmar grasp dominantly
6 months	› Rolls from back to front	› Holds bottle
7 months	› Bears full weight on feet	› Moves objects from hand to hand

AGE	GROSS MOTOR SKILLS	FINE MOTOR SKILLS
8 months	› Sits unsupported	› Begins using pincer grasp
9 months	› Pulls to a standing position › Creeps on hands and knees instead of crawling	› Has a crude pincer grasp
10 months	› Changes from a prone to a sitting position	› Grasps rattle by its handle
11 months	› Walks while holding onto something	› Places objects into a container › Neat pincer grasp
12 months	› Sits down from a standing position without assistance	› Tries to build a two-block tower without success

M View Video: Fine and Gross Motor Development

- Cognitive Development
  - Piaget – Sensorimotor stage (birth to 24 months)
    - Separation, object permanence, and mental representation are the three important tasks accomplished in this stage.
      - Separation – Infants learn to separate themselves from other objects in the environment.
      - Object permanence – Knowing that an object still exists when it is out of view. This occurs at approximately 9 months of age.
      - Mental representation – The recognition of symbols.
  - Language Development
    - Crying is the first form of verbal communication.
    - Vocalizes with cooing noises.
    - Responds to noises.
    - Turns head to the sound of a rattle.
    - Laughs and squeals.
    - Pronounces single-syllable words.
    - Begins speaking two-word phrases and progresses to speaking three-word phrases.
    - Says three to five words and comprehends "no" by the age of 1 year.
- Psychosocial Development
  - Erikson – Trust vs. Mistrust (birth to 1 year)
    - Achieving this task is based on the quality of the caregiver-infant relationship and the care received.
    - The infant begins to learn delayed gratification.
    - Trust is developed by meeting comfort, feeding, stimulation, and caring needs.
    - Mistrust develops if needs are inadequately or inconsistently met, or if needs are continuously met before being vocalized by the infant.

○ Social Development

- Social development is initially influenced by infants' reflexive behaviors and includes attachment, separation, recognition/anxiety, and stranger fear.

- Attachment is seen when infants begin to bond with their parents. This development is seen within the first month, but it actually begins before birth. The process is enhanced when infants and parents are in good health, have positive feeding experiences, and receive adequate rest.

- Separation-individuation occurs during the first year of life as infants first distinguish themselves and their primary caregivers as separate individuals, and then develop object permanence.

- Separation anxiety begins around 4 to 8 months of age. Infants will protest when separated from parents, which can cause considerable anxiety for parents.

- Stranger fear becomes evident between 6 and 8 months of age, when infants are less likely to accept strangers.

○ Body-Image Changes

- Infants discover that mouths are pleasure producers.

- Hands and feet are seen as objects of play.

- Infants discover that smiling causes others to react.

Q
PCC • Age-Appropriate Activities

○ Play should provide interpersonal contact and educational stimulation.

○ Infants have short attention spans and will not interact with other children during play (solitary play). Appropriate toys and activities that stimulate the senses and encourage development include the following.

- Rattles

- Teething toys

- Nesting toys

- Playing pat-a-cake

- Playing with balls

- Reading books

- Mirrors

- Brightly colored toys

- Playing with blocks

Health Promotion

- Immunizations

○ The Centers for Disease Control and Prevention (CDC) immunization recommendations for healthy infants less than 12 months of age (www.cdc.gov)

- Birth – Hepatitis B (Hep B)

- 2 months – Diphtheria and tetanus toxoids and pertussis (DTaP), rotavirus vaccine (RV), inactivated poliovirus (IPV), Haemophilus influenzae type B (Hib), pneumococcal vaccine (PCV), and Hep B

- 4 months – DTaP, RV, IPV, Hib, PCV
- 6 months – DTaP, IPV (6 to 18 months), PCV, and Hep B (6 to 12 months); RV; Hib
- 6 to 12 months – Seasonal influenza vaccination yearly (the trivalent inactivated influenza vaccine (TIV) is available as an intramuscular injection)

- Nutrition
  - Feeding alternatives
    - Breastfeeding provides a complete diet for infants during the first 6 months.
    - Iron-fortified formula is an acceptable alternative to breast milk. Cow's milk is not recommended.
    - It is recommended to begin vitamin D supplements within the first few days of life.
    - Iron supplements are recommended for infants who are being exclusively breastfed after the age of 4 months.
    - Alternative sources of fluids, such as juice or water, are not needed during the first 4 months of life.
    - After the age of 6 months, 100% fruit juice should be limited to 4 to 6 oz per day.
  - Solids are introduced around 4 to 6 months of age.
    - Indicators for readiness include interest in solid foods, voluntary control of the head and trunk, and disappearance of the extrusion reflex.
    - Iron-fortified cereal is typically introduced first due to its high iron content.
    - New foods should be introduced one at a time, over a 4- to 7-day period, to observe for signs of allergy or intolerance, which can include fussiness, rash, vomiting, diarrhea, and constipation.
    - Vegetables or fruits are started first between 6 and 8 months of age. After both have been introduced, meats can be added.
    - Citrus fruits, meat, and eggs are not started until after 6 months of age.
    - Breast milk/formula should be decreased as intake of solid foods increases, but should remain the primary source of nutrition through the first year.
    - Table foods that are cooked, chopped, and unseasoned are appropriate by 9 months of age.
    - Appropriate finger foods include ripe bananas; toast strips; graham crackers; cheese cubes; noodles; and peeled chunks of apples, pears, or peaches.
  - Weaning can be accomplished when infants show signs of readiness, and are able to drink from a cup (sometime in the second 6 months).
    - One meal can be replaced with breast milk or formula in a cup with handles.
    - Bedtime feedings are the last to be stopped.
- Sleep Patterns
  - Nocturnal sleep pattern is established by 3 to 4 months of age.
  - Infant sleeps 14 to 15 hr daily and 9 to 11 hr at night around the age of 4 months.
  - Infant sleeps through the night and takes one to two naps during the day by the age of 12 months.

- Injury Prevention
  - Aspiration of foreign objects
    - Small objects that can become lodged in the throat (grapes, coins, candy) should be avoided.
    - Age-appropriate toys should be provided.
    - Clothing should be checked for safety hazards (loose buttons).
  - Bodily harm
    - Sharp objects should be kept out of reach.
    - Anchor heavy objects and furniture so they cannot be overturned on top of infant.
    - Infants should not be left unattended with any animals present.
  - Burns
    - The temperature of bath water should be checked.
    - Hot water thermostats should be set at or below 49° C (120° F).
    - Working smoke detectors should be kept in the home.
    - Handles of pots and pans should be kept turned to the back of stoves.
    - Sunscreen should be used when infants are exposed to the sun.
    - Electrical outlets should be covered.
  - Drowning
    - Infants should not be left unattended in bathtubs or around water sources such as toilets, cleaning buckets, or drainage areas.
    - Secure fencing around swimming pools.
  - Falls
    - Crib mattresses should be kept in the lowest position possible with the rails all the way up.
    - Restraints should be used in infant seats.
    - Infant seats should be placed on the ground or floor if used outside of the car, and they should not be left unattended or on elevated surfaces.
    - Place safety gates at the top and bottom of stairs.
  - Poisoning
    - Exposure to lead paint should be avoided.
    - Toxins and plants should be kept out of reach.
    - Safety locks should be kept on cabinets that contain cleaners and other household chemicals.
    - The phone number for a poison control center should be kept near the phone.
    - Medications should be kept in childproof containers, away from the reach of infants.
    - A working carbon monoxide detector should be kept in the home.

- ○ Motor-vehicle injuries
  - Infant-only and convertible infant-toddler car seats are available.
  - Infants and toddlers remain in a rear-facing car seat until the age of 2 years or the height recommended by the manufacturer.
  - Safest area for infants and children is the backseat of the car.
  - Do not place rear-facing car seats in the front seat of vehicles with passenger air bags.
- ○ Suffocation
  - Plastic bags should be avoided.
  - Balloons should be kept away from infants.
  - Crib mattresses should fit snugly.
  - Crib slats should be no farther apart than 6 cm (2.36 in).
  - Crib mobiles or crib gyms should be removed by 4 to 5 months of age.
  - Pillows should be kept out of the crib.
  - Infants should be placed on their backs for sleep.
  - Toys with small parts should be kept out of reach.

APPLICATION EXERCISES

1. A nurse is checking a 6-month-old infant prior to administering the diphtheria, tetanus, and acellular pertussis (DTaP) vaccine. For which of the following findings should the nurse delay administering the vaccine?

    A. Family history of sudden infant death syndrome (SIDS)

    B. Temperature of 38.5° C (101.3° F) following the 4 month vaccinations

    C. Acute bilateral ear infection

    D. Living with a family member who is immunocompromised

2. A nurse is speaking with the mother of a 1-month-old during a well-baby visit. The mother asks the nurse if her infant is developing normally. Which of the following developmental milestones should the nurse expect the infant to perform?

    A. Smiles and laughs out loud

    B. Rolls from back to side

    C. Visually searches to locate sounds

    D. Turns head from side to side

3. A nurse is assisting with a well-baby visit with a 4-month-old infant. Which of the following immunizations should the nurse administer to the infant? (Select all that apply.)

    _____ A. Measles, mumps, rubella (MMR)

    _____ B. Polio (IPV)

    _____ C. Pneumococcal vaccine (PCV)

    _____ D. Varicella

    _____ E. Rotavirus vaccine (RV)

4. A nurse is reinforcing teaching about introducing new foods to the parents of a 4-month-old. Which of the following foods should the nurse recommend the parents introduce first?

    A. Strained yellow vegetables

    B. Iron-fortified cereals

    C. Pureed fruits

    D. Whole milk

5. A nurse is reinforcing teaching about dental care and teething to the parent of a 9-month-old infant. Which of the following statements by the parent indicates an understanding of the teaching?

    A. "I can give my baby a frozen, fluid-filled teething ring to relieve discomfort."

    B. "I should clean my baby's teeth with a cool, wet wash cloth."

    C. "I can give Advil for up to 5 days while my baby is teething."

    D. "I should dilute juice with water in the bottle my baby drinks while falling asleep."

6. A nurse is assisting with an educational program for a group of parents of infants. Use the ATI Active Learning Template: Growth and Development to complete this item to include the following:

    A. Developmental Stage: Identify the infant's developmental stage according to Piaget and Erikson.

    B. Cognitive Development: List two cognitive developmental tasks the infant should accomplish in the first year of life.

    C. Age-Appropriate Activities: List five activities appropriate for infants.

    D. Injury Prevention: Identify two injury prevention methods in each of the following categories.
- Aspiration
- Drowning
- Suffocation
- Poisoning

APPLICATION EXERCISES KEY

1. A. INCORRECT: There is no evidence that suggests vaccines raise the risk of SIDS.

    B. INCORRECT: A mild temperature is expected up to 48 hr after administration of scheduled vaccines.

    C. **CORRECT:** The nurse should delay administering the DTaP vaccine in the presence of an acute infection, with or without fever, because this decreases the infant's ability to develop good immunity.

    D. INCORRECT: The DTaP is not a live vaccine. Therefore, there is no contraindication for the infant to receive the vaccine if there are immunosuppressed family members.

    Ⓝ NCLEX® Connection: Health Promotion and Maintenance, Health Promotion/Disease Prevention

2. A. INCORRECT: Smiling and laughing aloud is expected behavior of a 2- to 3-month-old infant.

    B. INCORRECT: Rolling from the back to the side is expected behavior of a 4-month-old infant.

    C. INCORRECT: Visually searching to locate sounds is expected behavior of a 3-month-old infant.

    D. **CORRECT:** From birth, an infant is able to lift the head and turn it from side to side when lying prone.

    Ⓝ NCLEX® Connection: Health Promotion and Maintenance, Developmental Stages and Transitions

3. A. INCORRECT: The first MMR vaccine is given between the ages of 12 and 15 months.

    B. **CORRECT:** The nurse should administer an IPV vaccine to a 4-month-old infant.

    C. **CORRECT:** The nurse should administer a PCV vaccine to a 4 month-old infant.

    D. INCORRECT: The first varicella vaccine is given at a minimum age of 12 months.

    E. **CORRECT:** The nurse should administer an RV vaccine to a 4-month-old infant.

    Ⓝ NCLEX® Connection: Health Promotion and Maintenance, Health Promotion/Disease Prevention

4.   A. INCORRECT: The parents should not introduce strained yellow vegetables first because they are not a good source of needed nutrients.

B. **CORRECT:** The parents should first introduce iron-fortified cereals because of their high iron content. The order of introducing solid foods after this is variable.

C. INCORRECT: The parents should not introduce pureed fruits first because they are not a good source of needed nutrients.

D. INCORRECT: The parents should not introduce whole milk until the child is 1 year of age.

(N) NCLEX® Connection: Basic Care and Comfort, Nutrition and Oral Hydration

5.   A. INCORRECT: If fluid-filled, the teething ring is kept cold, not frozen.

B. **CORRECT:** It is appropriate to use a cool, wet wash cloth for cleaning the infant's teeth.

C. INCORRECT: Ibuprofen (Advil) should not be used for more than 3 days.

D. INCORRECT: To prevent early childhood caries, infants should not be given bottles while falling asleep.

(N) NCLEX® Connection: Health Promotion and Maintenance, Health Promotion/Disease Prevention

6. *Using the ATI Active Learning Template: Growth and Development*

A. Developmental Stage
   - Piaget: Sensorimotor stage
   - Erikson: Trust vs. mistrust

B. Cognitive Development
   - Separation: Learning to separate themselves from other objects in the environment.
   - Object permanence: Understanding that an object still exists when it is out of view.
   - Mental representation: Ability to recognize symbols.

C. Age-Appropriate Activities
   - Rattles
   - Teething toys
   - Nesting toys
   - Playing pat-a-cake
   - Playing with balls
   - Reading books
   - Mirrors
   - Brightly colored toys
   - Playing with blocks

D. Injury Prevention
   - Aspiration
     - Avoid small objects.
     - Provide age-appropriate toys.
     - Check clothing for hazards such as loose buttons.
   - Poisoning
     - Keep toxins and plants out of reach.
     - Place safety locks on cabinets where cleaners/chemicals are stored.
     - Use a carbon monoxide detector in the home.
     - Keep medications in childproof containers and out of reach.
   - Drowning
     - Do not leave unattended around any water source.
     - Secure fencing around swimming pool.
   - Suffocation
     - Avoid plastic bags.
     - Ensure crib mattress fits snugly.
     - Remove crib mobiles by 4 to 5 months of age.
     - Keep pillows out of the crib.
     - Back to sleep

Ⓝ NCLEX® Connection: Health Promotion and Maintenance, Developmental Stages and Transitions

chapter 4

Expected Growth and Development

- Physical Development
  - Anterior fontanels close by 18 months of age.
  - Weight – At 30 months of age, toddlers should weigh four times their birth weights.
  - Height – Toddlers grow about 7.5 cm (3 in) per year.
  - Head circumference and chest circumference are usually equal by 1 to 2 years of age.

AGE	GROSS MOTOR SKILLS	FINE MOTOR SKILLS
15 months	› Walks without help › Creeps up stairs	› Uses a cup well › Builds a tower of two blocks
18 months	› Assumes a standing position › Throws a ball overhand	› Manages a spoon without rotation › Turns pages in a book, two or three at a time
2 years	› Walks up and down stairs by placing both feet on each step	› Builds a tower of six or seven blocks
2.5 years	› Jumps in place with both feet › Stands on one foot momentarily	› Draws circles › Has good hand-finger coordination

- Cognitive Development
  - Piaget – The sensorimotor stage transitions to the preoperational stage around the age of 19 to 24 months.
    - The concept of object permanence becomes fully developed.
    - Toddlers have and demonstrate memories of events that relate to them.
    - Domestic mimicry (playing house) is evident.
    - Preoperational thought does not allow for toddlers to understand other viewpoints, but it does allow them to symbolize objects and people to imitate previously seen activities.
  - Language
    - Language increases to about 300 words by the age of 2 years.

- Psychosocial Development
  - Erikson – autonomy vs. shame and doubt
    - Independence is paramount for toddlers, who are attempting to do everything for themselves.
  - Moral Development
    - Moral development is closely associated with cognitive development.
    - Egocentric – Toddlers are unable to see things from the perspectives of others. They can only view things from their personal points of view.
    - Punishment and obedience orientation begin with a sense that good behavior is rewarded and bad behavior is punished.
  - Self-Concept Development
    - Toddlers progressively see themselves as separate from their parents and increase their explorations away from them.
  - Body-Image Changes
    - Toddlers appreciate the usefulness of various body parts.
    - Toddlers develop gender identity by 3 years of age.
- Age-Appropriate Activities
  - Solitary play evolves into parallel play, in which toddlers observe other children and then can engage in activities nearby.
  - Appropriate activities
    - Filling and emptying containers
    - Playing with blocks
    - Looking at books
    - Push-pull toys
    - Tossing balls
    - Finger paints
    - Large-piece puzzles
    - Thick crayons
  - Temper tantrums result when toddlers are frustrated with restrictions on independence. Providing consistent, age-appropriate expectations helps toddlers to work through frustration.
  - Toilet training can begin when toddlers have the sensation of needing to urinate or defecate. Parents should demonstrate patience and consistency in toilet training. Nighttime control can develop last.
  - Discipline should be consistent with well-defined boundaries that are established to develop appropriate social behavior.

Health Promotion

- Immunizations
  - The Centers for Disease Control and Prevention (CDC) immunization recommendations for healthy toddlers 12 months to 3 years of age (www.cdc.gov) include:
    - 12 to 15 months – Inactivated poliovirus (IPV) (third dose between 6 to 18 months); *Haemophilus influenzae* type B (Hib); pneumococcal vaccine (PCV); measles, mumps, and rubella (MMR); and varicella.
    - 12 to 23 months – Hepatitis A (Hep A) second dose should be given 6 to 8 months later.
    - 15 to 18 months – Diphtheria and tetanus toxoids and pertussis (DTaP).
    - 12 to 36 months – Yearly seasonal trivalent inactivated influenza vaccine (TIV); two doses given at least 4 weeks apart are recommended for children age 6 months through 8 years of age who are getting a flu vaccine for the first time.

- Nutrition
  - Children can establish lifetime eating habits during early childhood.
  - Toddlers begin developing taste preferences, and are generally picky eaters who repeatedly request their favorite foods.
  - Toddlers should consume 24 to 30 oz of milk per day, and can switch from drinking whole milk to low-fat milk after 2 years of age.
  - Juice consumption should be limited to 4 to 6 oz per day.
  - Diet should include 1 cup of fruit daily.
  - Food serving size should be 1 tbsp for each year of age, or 1/4 to 1/3 of an adult portion.
  - Toddlers generally prefer finger foods because of increasing autonomy.
  - Regular meal times and nutritious snacks best meet nutrient needs.
  - Snacks or desserts that are high in sugar, fat, or sodium should be avoided.
  - Foods that are potential choking hazards (nuts, grapes, hot dogs, peanut butter, raw carrots, tough meats, popcorn) should be avoided.
  - Adult supervision should always be provided during snack and mealtimes.
  - Toddlers should not be allowed to engage in drinking or eating during play activities or while lying down.
  - Parents should follow the U.S. Department of Agriculture's guidelines (www.choosemyplate.gov).

- Sleep and Rest
  - Toddlers typically average 11 to 12 hr of sleep per day, including one nap.
  - Naps often are eliminated in older toddlerhood.
  - Resistance to bedtime and expression of fears are common in this age group.
  - Maintaining a regular bedtime and bedtime routines are helpful to promote sleep.

- Dental Health
  - Children should have an established dental home by the age of 1 year.
  - Flossing and brushing should be performed by the adult caregiver, and is the best method of removing plaque.
  - Brushing should occur after meals and at bedtime. Nothing to eat or drink, except water, is given to the child after the bedtime cleaning.
  - Early childhood caries is a form a tooth decay that develops in toddlers, and is more common in children who are put to bed with a bottle of juice or milk.
- Injury Prevention
  - Aspiration of foreign objects
    - Small objects (grapes, coins, candy) that can become lodged in the throat should be avoided.
    - Toys that have small parts should be kept out of reach.
    - Age-appropriate toys should be provided.
    - Clothing should be checked for safety hazards (loose buttons).
    - Balloons should be kept away from toddlers.
    - Parents should know emergency procedures for choking.
  - Bodily harm
    - Sharp objects should be kept out of reach.
    - Firearms should be kept in locked boxes or cabinets.
    - Toddlers should not be left unattended with any animals present.
    - Toddlers should be taught stranger safety.
  - Burns
    - The temperature of bath water should be checked.
    - Thermostats on hot water heaters should be turned down to 49° C (120° F) or below.
    - Working smoke detectors should be kept in the home.
    - Pot handles should be turned toward the back of the stove.
    - Electrical outlets should be covered.
    - Toddlers should wear sunscreen when outside.
  - Drowning
    - Toddlers should not be left unattended in bathtubs.
    - Toilet lids should be kept closed.
    - Toddlers should be closely supervised when near pools or any other body of water.
    - Toddlers should be taught to swim.
  - Falls
    - Doors and windows should be kept locked.
    - Crib mattresses should be kept in the lowest position with the rails all the way up.
    - Safety gates should be used across the top and bottom of stairs.

- ○ Motor-vehicle injuries
  - ▪ Infants and toddlers remain in a rear-facing car seat until the age of 2 years or the height recommended by the manufacturer.
  - ▪ Toddlers over the age of 2 years, or who exceed the height recommendations for rear-facing car seats, are moved to a forward-facing car seat.
  - ▪ The safest area for infants and children is the back seat of the car.
  - ▪ Do not place rear-facing car seats in the front seat of vehicles with deployable passenger air bags.
- ○ Poisoning
  - ▪ Exposure to lead paint should be avoided.
  - ▪ Safety locks should be placed on cabinets that contain cleaners and other chemicals.
  - ▪ The phone number for a poison control center should be kept near the phone.
  - ▪ Medications should be kept in childproof containers, away from the reach of toddlers.
  - ▪ A working carbon monoxide detector should be placed in the home.
- ○ Suffocation
  - ▪ Plastic bags should be avoided.
  - ▪ Crib mattresses should fit tightly.
  - ▪ Crib slats should be no farther apart than 6 cm (2.36 in).
  - ▪ Pillows should be kept out of cribs.
  - ▪ Drawstrings should be removed from jackets and other clothing.

APPLICATION EXERCISES

1. A nurse is checking a 2½-year-old toddler at a well-child visit. Which of the following findings should the nurse report to the provider?

    A. Height increased by 7.5 cm (3 in) in the past year.

    B. Head circumference exceeds chest circumference.

    C. Anterior and posterior fontanels closed.

    D. Current weight equals four times the birth weight.

2. A nurse is assisting with a developmental screening on an 18-month-old. Which of the following skills should the toddler be able to perform? (Select all that apply.)

    _____ A. Build a tower with six blocks

    _____ B. Throw a ball overhand

    _____ C. Walk up and down stairs

    _____ D. Draw circles

    _____ E. Use a spoon without rotation

3. A nurse is observing a 2-year-old child during a routine visit to the clinic for a check-up. Which of the following activities should the nurse expect the child to do?

    A. Tie his shoelaces

    B. Ride a tricycle

    C. Kick a ball forward

    D. Use blunt scissors

4. A nurse is providing anticipatory guidance to the parents of a toddler. Which of the following should the nurse include? (Select all that apply.)

    _____ A. Develop food habits that will prevent dental caries.

    _____ B. Meeting caloric needs results in an increased appetite.

    _____ C. Expression of bedtime fears is common.

    _____ D. Behaviors associated with negativism and ritualism.

    _____ E. Importance of annual screenings for phenylketonuria.

5. A nurse is assisting with a well-child visit with a 2-year-old. Use the ATI Active Learning Template: Growth and Development to complete this item to include the following:

A. Developmental Stage: Identify the toddler's developmental stage according to Piaget and Erikson.

B. Nutrition: List three concepts to include in teaching with the family.

C. Injury Prevention: Identify two injury prevention methods to include in teaching with the family for each of the following categories.
- Bodily harm
- Drowning
- Burns
- Falls

APPLICATION EXERCISES KEY

1. A. INCORRECT: Toddler height should increase by 7.5 cm (3 in) each year. The nurse should not report this finding to the provider.

    B. **CORRECT:** The head and chest circumference should be equal by 1 to 2 years of age, with the chest circumference continuing to increase in size until it exceeds the head circumference. The nurse should report this finding to the provider.

    C. INCORRECT: The posterior fontanel closes by the age of 6 to 8 weeks, and the anterior fontanel closes by 12 to 18 months. The nurse should not report this finding to the provider.

    D. INCORRECT: The current weight should be four times the birth weight at the age of 2½ years. The nurse should not report this finding to the provider.

    Ⓝ NCLEX® Connection: Health Promotion and Maintenance, Data Collection Techniques

2. A. INCORRECT: The toddler should build a tower with six blocks at the age of 2 years.

    B. **CORRECT:** An 18-month-old should be able to throw a ball overhand.

    C. INCORRECT: The toddler should be able to walk up and down stairs by placing both feet on each step at the age of 2 years.

    D. INCORRECT: The toddler should be able to draw circles at the age of 2½ years.

    E. **CORRECT:** An 18-month-old should be able to use a spoon without rotation.

    Ⓝ NCLEX® Connection: Health Promotion and Maintenance, Health Promotion/Disease Prevention

3. A. INCORRECT: Tying shoelaces is typical behavior of a 5-year-old child.

    B. INCORRECT: Riding a tricycle is typical behavior of a 3-year-old child.

    C. **CORRECT:** Kicking a ball forward is typical behavior of a 2-year-old child.

    D. INCORRECT: Using blunt scissors to cut out objects is typical behavior of a 3-year-old child.

    Ⓝ NCLEX® Connection: Health Promotion and Maintenance, Developmental Stages and Transitions

4. A. **CORRECT:** Because the toddler is developing taste preferences, the development of food habits that will prevent dental caries should be included in the anticipatory guidance.

B. INCORRECT: Toddlers often experience physiologic anorexia and become fussy eaters because of a decreased appetite.

C. **CORRECT:** Expression of bedtime fears is common for toddlers and should be included in the anticipatory guidance.

D. **CORRECT:** Negativism and ritualism are exhibited by toddlers as they seek autonomy. Associated behaviors should be included in the anticipatory guidance.

E. INCORRECT: Screening for phenylketonuria occurs in the newborn, not the toddler.

Ⓝ NCLEX® Connection: Health Promotion and Maintenance, Aging Process

5. *Using the ATI Active Learning Template: Growth and Development*
   A. Developmental Stage
      - Piaget: Preoperational stage
      - Erikson: Autonomy vs. shame and doubt
   B. Nutrition
      - Can switch from whole milk to low-fat milk after the age of 2 years.
      - Trans fatty acids and saturated fats should be avoided.
      - Diet should include 1 cup of fruit daily.
      - Limit fruit juice to 4 to 6 oz per day.
      - Cut food into small, bite-size pieces to prevent choking.
      - Do not allow drinking or eating during play activities or while lying down.
   C. Injury Prevention
      - Bodily harm
        - Keep sharp objects out of reach.
        - Lock firearms in a cabinet or box.
        - Teach toddler stranger safety.
        - Do not leave toddler unattended with animals.
      - Drowning
        - Do not leave toddler unattended in bathtub.
        - Keep toilet lids closed.
        - Begin teaching toddler water safety and to swim.
        - Keep bathroom doors closed.
      - Burns
        - Check bath water temperature prior to toddler contact with water.
        - Set hot water heaters to 49° C (120° F) or below.
        - Keep pot handles pointed to back of stove when cooking.
        - Cover electrical outlets.
        - Keep working smoke detectors in the home.
        - Apply sunscreen when toddler will be outside.
      - Falls
        - Keep doors and windows locked.
        - Place crib mattresses in lowest position with rails all the way up.
        - Use safety gates at the top and bottom of stairs.

Ⓝ NCLEX® Connection: Health Promotion and Maintenance, Health Promotion/Disease Prevention

UNIT 1   FOUNDATIONS OF NURSING CARE OF CHILDREN
SECTION: PERSPECTIVES OF NURSING CARE OF CHILDREN

CHAPTER 5   **Health Promotion of Preschoolers (3 to 6 Years)**

Expected Growth and Development

- Physical Development
  - Weight – Preschoolers should gain about 2 to 3 kg (4.4 to 6.6 lb) per year.
  - Height – Preschoolers should grow about 6.5 to 9 cm (2.6 to 3.5 in) per year.
  - Preschoolers' bodies evolve away from the characteristically unsteady wide stances and protruding abdomens of toddlers, into a more graceful, posturally erect, and sturdy physicality.
  - Fine and gross motor skills
    - Preschoolers should show improvement in fine motor skills, which are displayed by activities like copying figures on paper and dressing independently.

GROSS MOTOR SKILLS BY AGE		
3-year-old	4-year-old	5-year-old
› Rides a tricycle	› Skips and hops on one foot	› Jumps rope
› Jumps off bottom step	› Throws ball overhead	› Walks backward with heel to toe
› Stands on one foot for a few seconds		› Throws and catches a ball with ease

- Cognitive Development
  - Piaget – The preconceptual phase transitions to the phase of intuitive thought around the age of 4 years. The phase of intuitive thought lasts until the age of 7 years.
  - Preschoolers make judgments based on visual appearances. Variations in thinking during this age include:
    - Magical thinking – Thoughts can cause events to occur.
    - Animism – Inanimate objects are alive.
    - Centration – Focus on one aspect instead of considering the whole.
  - Time – Preschoolers begin to understand the sequence of daily events. By the end of the preschool years, children have a better comprehension of time-oriented words and might comprehend days of the week.
  - Language Development
    - The vocabulary of preschoolers increases to more than 2,100 words by the end of the fifth year.
    - Preschoolers speak in sentences of three to four words at the ages of 3 and 4 years, and four to five words at the age of 4 to 5 years.
    - This age group enjoys talking, and language becomes their primary method of communication.

- Psychosocial Development
  - Erikson – initiative vs. guilt
    - Preschoolers become energetic learners, despite not having all of the physical abilities necessary to be successful at everything.
    - Guilt can occur when preschoolers believe they have misbehaved or when they are unable to accomplish a task.
    - Guiding preschoolers to attempt activities within their capabilities while setting limits is appropriate.
  - Moral Development
    - Early preschoolers continue in the good-bad orientation of the toddler years, and actions are taken based on whether it will result in a reward or punishment.
    - Older preschoolers primarily take actions based on satisfying personal needs, yet are beginning to understand the concepts of justice and fairness.
  - Self-Concept Development
    - Preschooler feels good about themselves with regard to mastering skills that allow independence (dressing, feeding). During stress, insecurity, or illness, preschoolers can regress to previous immature behaviors or develop habits (nose picking, bed-wetting, thumb sucking).
  - Body-Image Changes
    - Preschoolers begin to recognize differences in appearances, and identify what is considered acceptable and unacceptable.
    - By the age of 5 years, preschoolers begin comparing themselves with peers.
  - Social Development
    - Preschoolers generally do not exhibit stranger anxiety and have less separation anxiety.
    - Prolonged separation, such as during hospitalization, can provoke anxiety.
      - Favorite toys and appropriate play should be used to help ease preschoolers' fears.
    - Pretend play is healthy and allows preschoolers to determine the difference between reality and fantasy.
- Age-Appropriate Activities
  - Parallel play shifts to associative play during the preschool years. Play is not highly organized, but cooperation does exist between children. Appropriate activities include the following.
    - Playing ball
    - Putting puzzles together
    - Riding tricycles
    - Playing pretend and dress-up activities
    - Role playing
    - Painting
    - Simple sewing
    - Reading books
    - Wading pools
    - Skating
    - Computer programs
    - Electronic games

Health Promotion

- Immunizations
  - The Centers for Disease Control and Prevention (CDC) immunization recommendations for healthy preschoolers 3 to 6 years of age (www.cdc.gov) include:
    - 4 to 6 years – diphtheria and tetanus toxoids and pertussis (DTaP); measles, mumps, and rubella (MMR); varicella; and inactivated poliovirus (IPV).
    - 3 to 6 years – yearly seasonal influenza vaccine; two doses given at least 4 weeks apart are recommended for children through 8 years of age who are getting a flu vaccine for the first time.
- Nutrition
  - Preschoolers consume about half the amount of energy that adults do (1,800 kcal).
  - Picky eating can remain a behavior in preschoolers, but often by 5 years of age they become more willing to sample different foods.
  - Preschoolers need 13 to 19 g/day of protein in addition to adequate calcium, iron, folate, and vitamins A and C.
  - Parents should follow the United States Department of Agriculture's healthy diet recommendations (www.choosemyplate.gov).
- Sleep and Rest
  - On average, preschoolers need about 12 hr of sleep per day. Some still require a daytime nap.
  - Sleep disturbances frequently occur during early childhood, and problems range from difficulty going to bed to sleep terrors. Appropriate interventions vary, but can include the following.
    - Keep a consistent bedtime routine.
    - Use a night-light.
    - Reassure preschoolers who are frightened, but avoid allowing preschoolers to sleep with their parents.
- Dental health
  - Eruption of primary teeth is finalized by the beginning of the preschool years.
  - Parents need to assist and supervise brushing and flossing to ensure they are performed appropriately and to prevent dental caries.
  - Trauma to teeth is common in preschool-age children and should be assessed by a dentist immediately.
- Injury Prevention
  - Bodily harm
    - Firearms should be kept in locked cabinets or containers.
    - Preschoolers should be taught stranger safety.
    - Preschoolers should be taught to wear protective equipment (helmet, pads).
  - Burns
    - Thermostats should be turned down on hot water heaters.
    - Working smoke detectors should be kept in the home.
    - Preschoolers should have sunscreen applied when outside.

- Drowning
  - Preschoolers should not be left unattended in bathtubs.
  - Preschoolers should be closely supervised when near the pool or any other body of water.
  - Preschoolers should be taught to swim.
- Motor-vehicle injuries

  - Preschoolers should use a federally approved car restraint according to the manufacturer recommendations.
  - When the forward-facing car seat is outgrown, the preschooler transitions to a booster seat.
  - Children should use an approved car restraint system until they achieve a height of 145 cm (4 feet, 9 in).
  - The safest area for children is the backseat of the car.
  - Supervise preschool-age children when playing outside, and do not allow them to play near a curb or parked cars.
  - Teach pedestrian safety rules to preschool-age children.
    - Stand back from curb while waiting to cross the street.
    - Before crossing the street, look left, then right, then left again.
    - Walk on the left, facing traffic, when there are no sidewalks.
    - At night, wear light-colored clothing with fluorescent materials attached.

APPLICATION EXERCISES

1. A nurse is reinforcing teaching about methods to promote sleep to the parent of a preschool-age child. Which of the following statements by the parent indicates an understanding of the teaching?

    A. "I will sleep in the bed with my child if she wakes up during the night."

    B. "I will let my child stay up an additional 2 hours on weekend nights."

    C. "I will let my child watch television for 30 minutes just before bedtime each night."

    D. "I will keep a dim lamp on in my child's room during the night."

2. A nurse is assisting with a well-child visit with a child who is scheduled to receive the recommended immunizations for 4- to 6-year-olds. Which of the following immunizations should the nurse administer? (Select all that apply.)

    _____ A. Diphtheria, tetanus, pertussis (DTaP)

    _____ B. Inactivated poliovirus (IPV)

    _____ C. Measles, mumps, rubella (MMR)

    _____ D. Pneumococcal (PCV)

    _____ E. Haemophilus influenzae type b (Hib)

3. A nurse is assisting with preparation for an education program about nutrition for preschool-age children for a group of parents. Which of the following should the nurse include?

    A. Saturated fats should equal 20% of total caloric intake.

    B. Average daily intake should be 1,800 calories.

    C. Finicky eating habits develop around 5 years of age.

    D. Healthy diets include 8 g of protein each day.

4. A nurse is assisting with a developmental screening on a 3-year-old child. Which of the following skills should the child be able to perform?

    A. Ride a tricycle

    B. Hop on one foot

    C. Jump rope

    D. Throw a ball overhead

5. A nurse is caring for a preschool-age child who says she needs to leave the hospital because her doll is scared to be at home alone. Which of the following characteristics of preoperational thought is the child exhibiting?

    A. Egocentrism

    B. Centration

    C. Animism

    D. Magical thinking

6. A nurse is providing anticipatory guidance to the parents of a preschool-age child. Use the ATI Active Learning Template: Growth and Development to complete this item to include the following:

    A. Physical Development: Identify general expectations for height and weight during the preschool years.

    B. Cognitive Development: List two concepts related to language development in preschool-age children.

    C. Age-Appropriate Activities: List five activities appropriate for preschool-age children.

    D. Injury Prevention: Identify two pedestrian safety rules parents should teach children.

APPLICATION EXERCISES KEY

1. A. INCORRECT: The child should not be allowed to sleep in the same bed as the parent. This statement by the parent does not indicate an understanding of the teaching.

    B. INCORRECT: The parent should maintain a consistent bedtime routine and avoid allowing the child to stay up past a reasonable hour. This statement by the parent does not indicate an understanding of the teaching.

    C. INCORRECT: Watching television prior to bed can cause the child to resist and delay sleep. This statement by the parent does not indicate an understanding of the teaching.

    D. **CORRECT:** Leaving a light on in the child's room is an appropriate method to promote sleep for a preschool-age child. This statement by the parent indicates an understanding of the teaching.

    Ⓝ NCLEX® Connection: Basic Care and Comfort, Rest and Sleep

2. A. **CORRECT:** DTaP is a recommended immunization for 4- to 6-year-olds, and should be administered by the nurse.

    B. **CORRECT:** IPV is a recommended immunization for 4- to 6-year-olds, and should be administered by the nurse.

    C. **CORRECT:** MMR is a recommended immunization for 4- to 6-year-olds, and should be administered by the nurse.

    D. INCORRECT: PCV is given as a series of immunizations in the first 15 months of life, and is not recommended for 4- to 6-year-olds.

    E. INCORRECT: Hib is given as a series of immunizations in the first 15 months of life, and is not recommended for 4- to 6-year-olds.

    Ⓝ NCLEX® Connection: Health Promotion and Maintenance, Health Promotion/Disease Prevention

3. A. INCORRECT: Saturated fats should be less than 10% of total caloric intake.

    B. **CORRECT:** Preschool-age children should consume an average of 1,800 calories each day.

    C. INCORRECT: Finicky eating habits are more common during the toddler years, but children often become more willing to try new foods by the age of 5 years.

    D. INCORRECT: Healthy diets include 13 to 19 g of protein each day.

    Ⓝ NCLEX® Connection: Basic Care and Comfort, Nutrition and Oral Hydration

4. A. **CORRECT:** A 3-year-old child should be able to ride a tricycle.

    B. INCORRECT: A 4-year-old child should be able to hop on one foot.

    C. INCORRECT: A 5-year-old child should be able to jump rope.

    D. INCORRECT: A 4-year-old child should be able to throw a ball overhead.

    N NCLEX® Connection: Health Promotion and Maintenance, Developmental Stages and Transitions

5. A. INCORRECT: Egocentrism occurs when the child is unable to see another person's perspective.

    B. INCORRECT: Centration occurs when the child focuses on one aspect of something instead of considering the whole.

    C. **CORRECT:** Animism occurs when the child gives living qualities to inanimate objects, such as a doll feeling scared.

    D. INCORRECT: Magical thinking occurs when the child believes their thoughts cause an event to occur.

    N NCLEX® Connection: Health Promotion and Maintenance, Developmental Stages and Transitions

6. *Using the ATI Active Learning Template: Growth and Development*

    A. Physical Development
      - Height: Preschoolers should gain about 2 to 3 kg (4.4 to 6.6 lb) per year. *per yr*
      - Weight: Preschoolers should grow about 6.5 to 9 cm (2.6 to 3.5 in) per year.

    B. Cognitive Development
      - Vocabulary increases to more than 2,100 words by the end of the fifth year.
      - Speak in sentences of three to four words at the ages of 3 and 4 years.
      - Speak in sentences of four to five words at the age of 4 to 5 years.
      - Enjoy talking, and language becomes primary method of communication.

    C. Age-Appropriate Activities
      - Putting puzzles together
      - Playing pretend and dress-up activities
      - Painting
      - Simple sewing
      - Reading books
      - Wading pools
      - Skating
      - Electronic games

    D. Injury Prevention
      - Stand back from curb while waiting to cross the street.
      - Before crossing the street look left, then right, then left again.
      - Walk on the left, facing traffic, when there are no sidewalks.
      - At night, wear light-colored clothing with fluorescent materials attached.

    N NCLEX® Connection: Health Promotion and Maintenance, Aging Process

UNIT 1 **FOUNDATIONS OF NURSING CARE OF CHILDREN**
SECTION: PERSPECTIVES OF NURSING CARE OF CHILDREN

CHAPTER 6 **Health Promotion of School-Age Children (6 to 12 Years)**

Expected Growth and Development

- Physical Development
  - Weight – School-age children gain about 2 to 3 kg (4.4 to 6.6 lb) per year.
  - Height – School-age children grow about 5 cm (2 inches) per year.
  - Prepubescence
    - Preadolescence is typically when prepubescence occurs.
    - Onset of physiologic changes begins around the age of 9 years, particularly in girls.
    - Rapid growth in height and weight occurs.
    - Differences in the rate of growth and maturation between boys and girls becomes apparent.
    - Visible sexual maturation is minimal in boys during preadolescence.
    - Permanent teeth erupt.
    - Bladder capacity differs, but remains greater in girls than boys.
    - Immune system improves.
    - Bones continue to ossify.

- Cognitive Development
  - Piaget – Concrete operations
    - Transitions from perceptual to conceptual thinking
    - Masters the concept of conservation
    - Learns to tell time
    - Classifies more complex information
    - Able to see the perspective of others
    - Able to solve problems
  - Language
    - Defines many words and understands rules of grammar
    - Understands that a word can have multiple meanings

- Psychosocial Development
  - Erikson– industry vs. inferiority
    - A sense of industry is achieved through the development of skills.
    - A sense of accomplishment is gained through the ability to cooperate and compete with others.
    - Children should be taught that not everyone will master every skill.

- ○ Moral Development
  - Early school-age years
    - □ Do not understand the reasoning behind rules and expectations for behavior.
    - □ Believe what they think is wrong, and what others tell them is right.
    - □ Judgment is guided by rewards and punishment.
    - □ Sometimes interpret accidents as punishment.
  - Later school-age years
    - □ Able to judge the intentions of an act rather than just its consequences.
    - □ Understand different points of view instead of just whether or not an act is right or wrong.
    - □ Conceptualizes treating others as they like to be treated.
- ○ Self-Concept Development
  - School-age children develop an awareness of themselves in relation to others, as well as an understanding of personal values, abilities, and physical characteristics.
  - Confidence is gained through establishing a positive self-concept, which leads to feelings of worthiness and the ability to provide significant contributions.
  - Parents continue to influence the school-age child's self-ideals, but by middle childhood the opinions of peers and teachers become more valuable.
- ○ Body-Image Changes
  - Curiosity about sexuality should be addressed with education regarding sexual development and the reproductive process.
  - School-age children are more modest than preschoolers and place more emphasis on privacy issues.
- ○ Social Development
  - Peer groups play an important part in social development. Peer pressure begins to take effect.
  - Clubs and best friends are popular.
  - Bullying actions are intended to cause harm or to control someone, and are sometimes attributed to poor relationships with peers and difficulty identifying with a group.
  - Children prefer the company of same-gender companions, but begin developing an interest in the opposite sex toward the end of the school-age years.
  - Most relationships come from school associations.
  - Conformity becomes evident.

Q PCC

- • Age-Appropriate Activities
  - ○ Competitive and cooperative play is predominant.
  - ○ Children from 6 to 9 years of age:
    - Play simple board and number games.
    - Play hopscotch.
    - Jump rope.

- Collect rocks, stamps, cards, coins, or stuffed animals.
- Ride bicycles.
- Build simple models.
- Join organized sports (for skill building).
  ○ Children from 9 to 12 years of age:
    - Make crafts.
    - Build models.
    - Collect things/engage in hobbies.
    - Solve jigsaw puzzles.
    - Play board and card games.
    - Join organized competitive sports.

Health Promotion

- Immunizations
  ○ The Centers for Disease Control and Prevention (CDC) immunization recommendations for healthy school-age children 6 to 12 years of age (www.cdc.gov) include:
    - If not given between 4 and 5 years of age, children should receive the following vaccines by 6 years of age – diphtheria and tetanus toxoids and pertussis (DTaP); inactivated poliovirus (IPV); measles, mumps, and rubella (MMR); and varicella
    - Yearly seasonal influenza vaccine (two doses given at least 4 weeks apart are recommended for children aged 6 months through 8 years of age who are getting a flu vaccine for the first time) – trivalent inactivated influenza vaccine (TIV) or live, attenuated influenza vaccine (LAIV) by nasal spray.
    - 11 to 12 years – tetanus and diphtheria toxoids and pertussis vaccine (Tdap); human papillomavirus vaccine – HPV2 or HPV4 in three doses for females, HPV4 for males; and meningococcal (MCV4).
- Health Screenings
  ○ Scoliosis – School-age children should be screened for scoliosis by examining for a lateral curvature of the spine before and during growth spurts. Screening can take place at schools or at a health care facilities.

> **M**🎞 View Video: Scoliosis Screening

- Nutrition
  - By the end of the school-age years, children should eat adult portions of food. They need quality nutritious snacks.
  - Obesity is an increasing concern of this age group. Obesity predisposes children to low self-esteem, diabetes, heart disease, and high blood pressure. Advise parents to:
    - Avoid using food as a reward.
    - Emphasize physical activity.
    - Ensure that a balanced diet is consumed by following the U.S. Department of Agriculture's healthy diet recommendations (www.choosemyplate.gov).
    - Reinforce healthy food selections for meals and snacks.
    - Avoid eating fast-food frequently.
    - Avoid skipping meals.
    - Model healthy behaviors.
- Sleep and rest
  - Required sleep is highly variable in the school-age years, and is dependent on the following.
    - Age
    - Level of activity
    - Health status
  - Approximately 9 hr of sleep is needed each night at the age of 12 years.
  - Resistance to bedtime is sometimes experienced around the age of 8 and 9 years, and again around the age of 11 years, but is typically resolved by the age of 12 years.
- Dental health
  - Brush after meals and snacks, and at bedtime.
  - Floss daily.
  - Have regular checkups.
  - If necessary, have regular fluoride treatments.
- Injury Prevention
  - Bodily harm
    - Firearms should be kept in locked cabinets or boxes.
    - Safe play areas should be identified.
    - Stranger safety should be reinforced.
    - Children should be told to wear helmets and/or pads when roller skating, skateboarding, bicycling, riding scooters, skiing, and snowboarding.
  - Burns
    - Reinforce the importance of fire safety and potential burn hazards.
    - Working smoke detectors should be kept in the home.
    - Children should use sunscreen when outside.
    - Reinforce the importance of safety precautions while cooking.

- ○ Drowning
  - ▪ Children should be supervised when swimming or when near a body of water.
  - ▪ Children should be taught to swim.
  - ▪ Check depth of water before allowing child to dive.
  - ▪ Encourage breaks to prevent child from becoming over-tired.
- ○ Motor-vehicle injuries
  - ▪ Children should use an approved car restraint system until they achieve a height of 145 cm (4 feet, 9 inches).
  - ▪ Reinforce appropriate seat belt use when no longer using a car restraint system or booster seat.
  - ▪ The safest area for children is the backseat of the car.
  - ▪ Never let child ride in the bed of a pickup truck.
  - ▪ Reinforce safe pedestrian behaviors.
- ○ Poisoning/substance use
  - ▪ Cleaners and chemicals should be kept in locked cabinets or out of reach of younger children.
  - ▪ Children should be taught to say "no" to substance use.

APPLICATION EXERCISES

1. A nurse is discussing prepubescence and preadolescence with a group of parents of school-age children. Which of the following information should the nurse include in the discussion?

    A. Initial physiologic changes appear during early childhood.

    B. Changes in height and weight occur slowly during this period.

    C. Growth differences between boys and girls become evident.

    D. Signs of sexual maturation become highly visible in boys.

2. A nurse is conducting a well-child visit with a child who is scheduled to receive the recommended immunizations for 11- to 12-year-olds. Which of the following immunizations should the nurse administer? (Select all that apply.)

    _____ A. Trivalent inactivated influenza (TIV)

    _____ B. Pneumococcal (PCV)

    _____ C. Meningococcal (MCV4)

    _____ D. Tetanus and diphtheria toxoids and pertussis (Tdap)

    _____ E. Rotavirus (RV)

3. A nurse is reinforcing education about sleep and rest to a group of parents of school-age children. Which of the following statements by a parent indicates a need for further teaching?

    A. "My child's age influences the number of hours of sleep he needs."

    B. "My child's level of activity during the day influences the number of hours of sleep he needs."

    C. "My child's health status influences the number of hours of sleep he needs."

    D. "My child's family history of sleep apnea influences the number of hours of sleep he needs."

4. A nurse is reinforcing teaching about safety during the school-age years to a group of parents. Which of the following information should the nurse include? (Select all that apply.)

    _____ A. Gating stairs at the top and bottom

    _____ B. Wearing helmets when riding bicycles or skateboarding

    _____ C. Riding safely in beds of pickup trucks

    _____ D. Implementing firearm safety

    _____ E. Wearing seat belts

5. A nurse is providing anticipatory guidance to the parents of a school-age child. Use the ATI Active Learning Template: Growth and Development to complete this item to include the following:

    A. Developmental Stage: Identify the child's developmental stage according to Piaget and Erikson.

    B. Physical Development: Identify three facts relevant to the child's physical development.

    C. Nutrition: List three strategies the family can implement to reduce the risk of obesity.

APPLICATION EXERCISES KEY

1. A. INCORRECT: Initial physiologic changes appear toward the end of middle childhood, around the age of 9 years.

    B. INCORRECT: Changes in height and weight occur rapidly during this time period.

    C. **CORRECT:** The nurse should include in the discussion that growth differences between boys and girls become evident.

    D. INCORRECT: Visible signs of sexual maturation are minimal in boys.

     NCLEX® Connection: Health Promotion and Maintenance, Developmental Stages and Transitions

2. A. **CORRECT:** TIV is a recommended immunization for 11- to 12-year-olds, and should be administered by the nurse.

    B. INCORRECT: PCV is recommended as a series of immunizations in the first 15 months of life, and is not recommended for 11- to 12-year-olds.

    C. **CORRECT:** MCV4 is a recommended immunization for 11- to 12-year-olds, and should be administered by the nurse.

    D. **CORRECT:** Tdap is a recommended immunization for 11- to 12-year-olds, and should be administered by the nurse.

    E. INCORRECT: RV is recommended as a series of immunizations in the first 6 months of life, and is not recommended for 11- to 12-year-olds.

    NCLEX® Connection: Health Promotion and Maintenance, Health Promotion/Disease Prevention

3. A. INCORRECT: The child's age influences the number of hours of sleep he needs. This statement by a parent does not indicate a need for further teaching.

    B. INCORRECT: The child's level of activity during the day influences the number of hours of sleep he needs. This statement by a parent does not indicate a need for further teaching.

    C. INCORRECT: The child's health status influences the number of hours of sleep he needs. This statement by a parent does not indicate a need for further teaching.

    D. **CORRECT:** The child's family history of sleep apnea does not contribute to the number of hours of sleep he needs. This statement by the parent indicates a need for further teaching.

    NCLEX® Connection: Basic Care and Comfort, Rest and Sleep

4.   A. INCORRECT: Gating stairs at the top and bottom should not be included in the teaching. This is appropriate information to include when reinforcing teaching about safety during infant and toddler years.

   B. **CORRECT:** The nurse should include information about wearing helmets when riding bicycles or skateboarding when reinforcing teaching about safety in the school-age years.

   C. INCORRECT: Riding safely in beds of trucks should not be reinforced in the teaching. The nurse should teach that it is never safe to ride in the bed of a pickup truck.

   D. **CORRECT:** The nurse should include information about implementing firearm safety when reinforcing safety in the school-age years.

   E. **CORRECT:** The nurse should include information about wearing seat belts when teaching about safety in the school-age years.

   Ⓝ NCLEX® Connection: Safety and Infection Control, Accident/Error/Injury Prevention

5.   *Using the ATI Active Learning Template: Growth and Development*

   A. Developmental Stage
   • Piaget: concrete operations
   • Erikson: industry vs. inferiority

   B. Physical Development
   • Gain 2 to 3 kg (4.4 to 6.6 lb) per year.
   • Grow about 5 cm (2 in) per year.
   • Bladder capacity is variable with each child.
   • Immune system improves.
   • Bones continue to ossify.

   C. Nutrition
   • Avoid using food as a reward.
   • Emphasize physical activity.
   • Ensure a balanced diet is consumed.
   • Encourage children to select healthy foods and snacks.
   • Avoid eating fast foods frequently.
   • Avoid skipping meals.
   • Model healthy behaviors.

   Ⓝ NCLEX® Connection: Health Promotion and Maintenance, Aging Process

chapter 7

Expected Growth and Development

- Physical Development
  - The final 20% to 25% of height is achieved during puberty.
  - Acne can appear during adolescence.
  - Females stop growing at about 2 to 2.5 years after the onset of menarche. They grow 5 to 20 cm (2 to 8 in) and gain 7 to 25 kg (15.5 to 55 lb).
  - Males stop growing at around 18 to 20 years of age. They grow 10 to 30 cm (4 to 12 inches) and gain 7 to 30 kg (15.5 to 66 lb).
  - In females, sexual maturation occurs in the following order.
    - Breast development
    - Pubic hair growth (some females experience hair growth before breast development)
    - Axillary hair growth
    - Menstruation
  - In males, sexual maturation occurs in the following order.
    - Testicular enlargement
    - Pubic hair growth
    - Facial hair growth
    - Vocal changes
- Cognitive Development
  - Piaget – formal operations
    - Able to think through more than two categories of variables concurrently
    - Capable of evaluating the quality of their own thinking
    - Able to maintain attention for longer periods of time
    - Highly imaginative and idealistic
    - Increasingly capable of using formal logic to make decisions
    - Think beyond current circumstances
    - Able to understand how the actions of an individual influence others

Q
EBP

- Psychosocial Development
  - Erikson – identity vs. role confusion
    - Adolescents develop a sense of personal identity, and come to view themselves as unique individuals.
      - Group identity – Adolescents become part of a peer group that greatly influences behavior.
  - Sexual identity
    - Begins with close, same-sex friendships during early adolescence, which sometimes involve sexual experimentation driven by curiosity.
    - Self-exploration occurs through masturbation.
    - Transition from same-sex friendships to intimate relationships with the opposite sex during middle adolescence.
    - In late adolescence, sexual identity typically is formed through the integration of sexual experiences, feelings, and knowledge.
  - Health perceptions – Adolescents can view themselves as invincible to bad outcomes of risky behaviors.
  - Moral Development
    - Solve moral dilemma using internalized moral principles.
    - Question relevance of existing moral values to society and individuals.
  - Self-Concept Development
    - View themselves in relation to similarities with peers during younger adolescence.
    - View themselves according to their unique characteristics as the adolescent years progress.
  - Body-Image Changes
    - Base their own normality on comparisons with peers.
    - The image established during adolescence is retained throughout life.
  - Social Development
    - Peer relationships develop. These relationships act as a support system for adolescents.
    - Best-friend relationships are more stable and longer-lasting than they were in previous years.
    - Parent-child relationships change to allow a greater sense of independence.

Q
PCC

- Age-Appropriate Activities
  - Nonviolent video games
  - Nonviolent music
  - Sports
  - Caring for a pet
  - Career-training programs
  - Reading
  - Social events (going to movies, school dances)

Health Promotion

- Immunizations
  - The Centers for Disease Control and Prevention (CDC) recommendations for healthy adolescents 13 to 18 years of age (www.cdc.gov) include catch-up doses of any recommended immunizations not received at 11 to 12 years of age.
    - Yearly seasonal influenza vaccine – Trivalent inactivated influenza vaccine (TIV) or live, attenuated influenza vaccine (LAIV) by nasal spray.
    - 16 to 18 years – Meningococcal (MCV4) booster is recommended if first dose was received between the ages of 13 and 15 years. A booster dose is not needed if the first dose is received at age 16 or older.
- Health Screenings
  - Screenings for scoliosis should continue during the adolescent years. These screenings should include an examination for a lateral curvature of the spine before and during growth spurts. Screenings can take place at school or at a health care facility.
- Nutrition
  - Rapid growth and high metabolism require increases in quality nutrients, and make adolescents unable to tolerate caloric restrictions.
    - During times of rapid growth, additional calcium, iron, and zinc are needed.
    - Inadequate intake of folic acid, vitamin B_6, vitamin A, iron, calcium, and zinc is common.
  - Both overeating and undereating present special challenges during the adolescent years.
    - Yearly assessments of height, weight, and BMI for age are needed in order to identify nutritional issues and intervene early.
  - Advise parents to:
    - Avoid using food as a reward.
    - Emphasize physical activity.
    - Ensure that a balanced diet is consumed by following the U.S. Department of Agriculture's healthy diet recommendations (www.choosemyplate.gov).
    - Encourage adolescents to make healthy food selections for meals and snacks.
- Sleep and Rest
  - Sleep habits change with puberty due to increased metabolism and rapid growth.
  - Adolescents tend to stay up late, sleep in later in the morning, and sleep more than during the school-age years.
  - During periods of active growth, the need for sleep increases.
- Dental health
  - Corrective appliances are most common with this age group.
  - Brush after meals and snacks, and at bedtime.
  - Floss daily.
  - Have regular checkups.
  - If necessary, have regular fluoride treatments.

- Sexuality
  - Provide adolescents with accurate information and discuss what is heard from peers.
  - Emphasize abstinence and practicing safe sex.
  - Provide information about preventing sexually transmitted infections and pregnancy.
  - Promote an atmosphere where adolescents are comfortable asking questions.
  - Assist adolescents with problem-solving and decision-making skills.

- Injury Prevention
  - Bodily harm
    - Keep firearms unloaded and in a locked cabinet or box.
    - Reinforce proper use of sporting equipment prior to use.
    - Insist on helmet use and/or pads when roller skating, skateboarding, bicycling, riding scooters, skiing, and snowboarding.
    - Be aware of changes in mood. Monitor for self-harm in adolescents who are at risk. Watch for:
      - Poor school performance
      - Lack of interest in things that were of interest to the adolescent in the past
      - Social isolation
      - Disturbances in sleep or appetite
      - Expression of suicidal thoughts
  - Burns
    - Reinforce teaching about fire safety.
    - Instruct to apply sunscreen when outside.
    - Advise to avoid tanning beds.
  - Drowning
    - Instruct adolescents to swim.
    - Instruct adolescents not to swim alone.
  - Motor-vehicle injuries
    - Encourage attendance at drivers' education courses. Emphasize the need for adherence to seat belt use.
    - Insist on helmet use with bicycles, motorcycles, skateboards, roller skates, and snowboards.
    - Discourage use of cell phones while driving and enforce laws regarding use.
    - Reinforce the dangers of combining substance abuse with driving.
    - Role model desired behavior.
  - Substance abuse
    - Monitor for signs of substance use in adolescents who are at risk.
    - Instruct adolescents to say "no" to harmful substances and alcohol.
    - Present a no-tolerance attitude.

APPLICATION EXERCISES

1. A nurse is reinforcing teaching about expected changes during puberty to a group of parents of early adolescent females. Which of the following statements by one of the parents indicates an understanding of the teaching?

    A. "Females usually stop growing about 2 years after menarche."

    B. "Females are expected to gain about 65 pounds during puberty."

    C. "Females experience menstruation prior to breast development."

    D. "Females typically grow more than 10 inches during puberty."

2. A nurse is providing anticipatory guidance to the parent of a 13-year-old. The nurse should recommend which of the following screenings for the adolescent? (Select all that apply.)

    _____ A. Body mass index

    _____ B. Blood lead level

    _____ C. Height

    _____ D. Weight

    _____ E. Scoliosis

3. A nurse is caring for an adolescent whose mother expresses concerns about her son sleeping such long hours. The nurse should inform the mother that additional sleep is needed during adolescence due to which of the following?

    A. Sleep terrors

    B. Rapid growth

    C. Elevated zinc levels

    D. Slowed metabolism

4. A nurse is instructing a class about puberty in males. Which of the following should the nurse include as the first manifestation of sexual maturation?

    A. Pubic hair growth

    B. Vocal changes

    C. Testicular enlargement

    D. Facial hair growth

5. A nurse is preparing an educational program for a group of parents of adolescents. Use the ATI Active Learning Template: Growth and Development to complete this item to include the following:

    A. Developmental Stage: Identify adolescent developmental stages according to Piaget and Erikson.

    B. Cognitive Development: List five cognitive developmental tasks the adolescent should accomplish.

    C. Injury Prevention: Identify three injury prevention methods in each of the following categories:
        • Bodily harm
        • Motor vehicle injuries

APPLICATION EXERCISES KEY

1.   A. **CORRECT:** Females usually stop growing about 2 years after menarche. This statement by the parent indicates and understanding of the teaching.

   B. INCORRECT: Females are expected to gain 7 to 25 kg (15.5 to 55 lb) during puberty.

   C. INCORRECT: Breast development is usually the first manifestation of sexual maturity in females, and appears before menstruation.

   D. INCORRECT: Females typically grow 5 to 20 cm (2 to 8 in) during puberty.

    NCLEX® Connection: Health Promotion and Maintenance, Developmental Stages and Transitions

2.   A. **CORRECT:** The nurse should recommend that the adolescent have a body mass index screening annually.

   B. INCORRECT: Blood lead level screenings are recommended for children at the age of 1 and 2 years, and for children between the ages of 3 and 6 years who have not previously been screened.

   C. **CORRECT:** The nurse should recommend that the adolescent have a height screening annually.

   D. **CORRECT:** The nurse should recommend that the adolescent have a weight screening annually.

   E. **CORRECT:** The nurse should recommend that the adolescent have a scoliosis screening annually.

    NCLEX® Connection: Health Promotion and Maintenance, Health Promotion/Disease Prevention

3.   A. INCORRECT: Sleep terrors occur most often in preschool-age children, and do not contribute to the adolescent's need for additional sleep.

   B. **CORRECT:** Rapid growth during the adolescent years results in the need for additional sleep.

   C. INCORRECT: Zinc levels do not typically elevate during the adolescent years, and do not contribute to the adolescent's need for additional sleep. Zinc is often identified as a deficient due to inadequate dietary intake during adolescence.

   D. INCORRECT: An increased metabolism contributes to the adolescent's need for additional sleep.

    NCLEX® Connection: Health Promotion and Maintenance, Developmental Stages and Transitions

4.   A. INCORRECT: Pubic hair appears during early puberty, but is not the first manifestation of sexual maturation in males.

   B. INCORRECT: Vocal changes occur after the appearance of pubic hair, typically in early to midpuberty, and are not the first manifestation of sexual maturation in males.

   C. **CORRECT:** Testicular enlargement is the first manifestation of sexual maturation in males.

   D. INCORRECT: Facial hair growth typically appears about 2 years after pubic hair, and is not the first manifestation of sexual maturation in males.

   Ⓝ NCLEX® Connection: Health Promotion and Maintenance, Developmental Stages and Transitions

5.   *Using the ATI Active Learning Template: Growth and Development*

   A. Developmental Stage
   - Piaget: formal operations
   - Erikson: identity vs. role confusion

   B. Cognitive Development
   - Able to think through more than two categories of variables concurrently
   - Capable of evaluating the quality of own thinking
   - Able to maintain attention for longer periods of time
   - Highly imaginative and idealistic
   - Increasingly capable of using formal logic to make decisions
   - Think beyond current circumstances
   - Understand how the actions of an individual influence others

   C. Injury Prevention
   - Bodily injury
     ○ Keep firearms unloaded and in a locked cabinet or box.
     ○ Teach proper use of sporting equipment prior to use.
     ○ Insist on helmet use and/or pads when roller skating, skateboarding, bicycling, riding scooters, skiing, and snowboarding.
     ○ Be aware of changes in mood. Continuously monitor adolescents at risk for self-harm.
   - Motor vehicle injuries
     ○ Encourage attendance at drivers' education courses.
     ○ Emphasize the need for adherence to seat belt use.
     ○ Discourage use of cell phones while driving and enforce laws regarding use.
     ○ Teach the dangers of combining substance abuse with driving.
     ○ Role model desired behavior.

   Ⓝ NCLEX® Connection: Health Promotion and Maintenance, Aging Process

UNIT 1   Foundations of Nursing Care of Children

SECTION: SPECIAL CONSIDERATIONS OF NURSING CARE OF CHILDREN

› Safe Administration of Medication
› Pain Management
› Hospitalization, Illness, and Play
› Death and Dying

NCLEX® CONNECTIONS

When reviewing the chapters in this section, keep in mind the relevant sections of the NCLEX® outline, in particular:

Client Needs: Psychosocial Integrity

› Relevant topics/tasks include:
  » End-of-Life Care Concepts
    › Provide care or support for client/family at end-of-life

Client Needs: Basic Care and Comfort

› Relevant topics/tasks include:
  » Non-Pharmacological Comfort Interventions
    › Assist in planning comfort interventions for client with impaired comfort.
    › Monitor client non-verbal signs of pain/discomfort.
    › Evaluate pain using a rating scale.

Client Needs: Pharmacological Therapies

› Relevant topics/tasks include:
  » Expected Actions/Outcomes
    › Apply knowledge of pathophysiology when addressing client pharmacological agents.
  » Medication Administration
    › Administer medication by oral route.
    › Administer a subcutaneous, intradermal, or intramuscular medication.
    › Administer medication by ear, eye, nose, inhalation, rectum, vagina, or skin route.

Client Needs: Health Promotion and Maintenance

› Relevant topics/tasks include:
  » Aging Process
    › Provide care that meets the needs of the preschool, school age, and adolescent client ages 3 through 17 years.
  » Developmental Stages and Transitions
    › Identify occurrence of expected body image changes.
    › Compare client development to norms.
    › Modify approaches to care in accordance with client development stage.
  » Health Promotion/Disease Prevention
    › Provide assistance for screening examinations.

chapter 8

Overview

- Growth and organ system maturity affect the metabolism and excretion of medications in infants and children.
- Administration of medications to the pediatric population can be challenging, and requires that a nurse be patient and creative.
- Pediatric dosages are based on age, body weight, and body surface area (BSA).

Data Collection

- Medication and food allergies
- Appropriateness of medication dose for the child's age and weight
- Child's developmental age
- Tissue and skin integrity when administering IM, subcutaneous, and topical medications

Nursing Interventions

- Medication Administration
  - Calculate the safe dosage for medication.
  - Notify the provider if medication dosage is determined to be outside the safe dosage range, and for any questions about medication preparation or route.
  - Double-check high-risk and facility-regulated medications with a second nurse.
  - Perform the six rights of medication administration.
  - Use two client identifiers prior to administration: client name and date of birth. Use parent(s) for verification of infants or nonverbal children. However, two identifiers from the ID band must be confirmed: client name, date of birth, or hospital identification number.
  - Determine parental involvement with administration.
  - Allow the child to make appropriate choices regarding administration (choosing the left or right leg, whether the parent or nurse will administer the medication).
  - Prepare the child according to the developmental stage and age.

- Oral Medication
  - This route of medication administration is preferred for children.
  - Determine the child's ability to swallow pills.
  - Use the smallest measuring device for doses of liquid medication. Use an oral medication syringe for smaller amounts, and a medication cup for larger amounts.
  - Avoid measuring liquid medication in a teaspoon or tablespoon.
  - Avoid mixing medication with formula or putting it in a bottle of formula because the infant might not take the entire feeding, and the medication can alter the taste of the formula.
  - Hold the infant in a semi-reclining position similar to a feeding position.
  - Hold the small child in an upright position to prevent aspiration.
  - Administer the medication in the side of the mouth in small amounts. This allows the infant or child to swallow.
  - Only use the droppers that come with the medication for measurement.
  - Stroke the infant under the chin to promote swallowing while holding cheeks together.
  - Reinforce teaching for the child to swallow tablets that aren't available in liquid form and can't be crushed.
    - Explain in short sessions using verbal instruction, demonstration, and positive reinforcement.
  - Provide atraumatic care.
    - Mix the medication in a small amount of sweet fluid.
    - Offer juice, a soft drink, or snack after administration.
    - Have the child pinch her nose before, during, and shortly after administration.
    - Add flavoring to medications.
    - Use a nipple to allow the infant to suck the medication.
  - Administer medications via a feeding tube.
    - Confirm placement.
    - Use liquid formulation.
    - Do not add medication to the formula bag.
    - Flush with water to clear tubing of residual medication.
- Optic Medication
  - Place the child in a supine or sitting position.
  - Extend the child's head and ask the child to look up.
  - Pull the lower eye lid downward, and apply medication in the pocket.
  - Administer ointments before nap or bedtime.
  - Provide atraumatic care.
    - If infants clench their eyes closed, place the drops in the nasal corner. When the infant opens his eyes, the medication will enter the eye.
    - Apply light pressure to the lacrimal punctum for 1 min to prevent unpleasant taste.
    - Play games with younger children.

- Otic Medication
  - Place the child in a prone or supine position with the affected ear upward.
  - Children younger than 3 years: pull the pinna downward and straight back.
  - Children older than 3 years: pull the pinna upward and back.
  - Provide atraumatic care.
    - Allow refrigerated medications to warm to room temperature prior to administration.
    - Massage the outer area for a few minutes following administration.
    - Play games with younger children.
- Nasal Medication
  - Position the child with the head extended.
  - Use a football hold for infants.
  - Provide atraumatic care.
    - Insert the tip into the naris vertically, then angle it prior to administration.
    - Play games with younger children.
- Aerosol Medication
  - Use a mask for younger children.
  - Provide atraumatic care.
    - Allow parents to hold during treatment.
    - Use distraction.
- Rectal Medication
  - Insert beyond both rectal sphincters.
  - Hold the buttocks gently together for 5 to 10 minutes.
  - Halve the medication lengthwise, if necessary.
  - Provide atraumatic care.
    - Perform the procedure quickly.
    - Use distraction.
- Injection Medications
  - Change needle if it pierced a rubber stopper on a vial.
  - Secure the infant or child prior to injections.
  - Determine the need for assistance.
  - Avoid tracking of medication.
  - When selecting sites, consider:
    - Medication amount, viscosity, and type.
    - Muscle mass, condition, access of site, and potential for contamination.
    - Treatment course and number of injections.
    - Age and size of child.

- Intradermal
  - Administer on the inside surface of the forearm.
  - Use a TB syringe with a 26- to 30-gauge needle with an intradermal bevel.
  - Insert needle at a 15° angle.
  - Do not aspirate.
- Subcutaneous
  - Give anywhere there is subcutaneous tissue. Common sites are the lateral aspect of the upper arm, abdomen, and anterior thigh.
  - Inject volumes of less than 0.5 mL.
  - Use a 1 mL syringe with a 26- to 30-gauge needle.
  - Insert at a 90° angle. Use a 45° angle for children who are thin.
  - Check policy for aspiration practices.
- Intramuscular (IM)
  - Use a 22- to 25-gauge, ½- to 1-inch needle.
  - Vastus lateralis is the recommended site in infants and small children.
    - Position the child supine, side lying, or sitting.
    - Inject up to 0.5 mL for infants.
    - Inject up to 2 mL in children.
  - Ventrogluteal
    - Position the child supine, side-lying, or prone.
    - Inject up to 0.5 mL for infants.
    - Inject up to 2 mL in children.
  - Deltoid
    - Position the child sitting or standing.
    - Inject up to 1 mL.
  - Provide atraumatic care
    - Apply eutectic mixture of lidocaine and prilocaine (EMLA) to the site for 60 min prior to injection.
    - Change needle after puncturing a rubber stopper.
    - Use the smallest gauge of needle possible.
    - Secure the child firmly to decrease movement of the needle while injecting.
    - Use distraction.
    - Use play therapy.
    - Offer sucrose pacifiers to infants.

 View Video: Pediatric IM Injections

- Intravenous (IV) Medications
  - Peripheral venous access devices
    - Use a 24- to 20-gauge catheter.
    - Use for continuous and intermittent IV medication administration.
    - A child who requires short-term IV therapy can complete it at home with the assistance of a home health nurse.
  - Central venous access devices
    - Short term: nontunneled catheter or peripherally inserted central catheters (PICC)
    - Long term: tunneled catheter or implanted infusion ports
  - Provide atraumatic care
    - Decide to insert a PICC before multiple peripheral attempts.
    - Use a transilluminator to assist in vein location.
    - Avoid terminology such as a "bee sting" or "stick."
    - Attach an extension tubing to decrease movement of the catheter.
    - Use play therapy.
    - Apply EMLA to the site for 60 min prior to attempt.
    - Keep equipment out of site until procedure begins.

    - Perform procedure in a treatment room.
    - Use nonpharmacologic therapies.
    - Allow parents to stay if they prefer.
    - Use therapeutic holding.
    - Avoid using the dominant or sucking hand.
    - Cover site with a colorful wrap.
    - Swaddle infants.
    - Offer nonnutritive sucking to infants before, during, and after the procedure.

APPLICATION EXERCISES

1. A nurse is planning to administer the influenza vaccination to a toddler. Which of the following is an appropriate action for the nurse to take?

    A. Administer subcutaneously in the abdomen.

    B. Use a 20-gauge needle.

    C. Divide the medication into two injections.

    D. Place the child in the supine position.

2. A nurse is preparing to administer an intramuscular (IM) injection to a child. Which of the following muscle groups is contraindicated?

    A. Deltoid

    B. Ventrogluteal

    C. Vastus lateralis

    D. Dorsal gluteal

3. A nurse is reinforcing teaching with a parent of an infant about administration of oral medications. Which of the following should the nurse include in the teaching? (Select all that apply.)

    _____ A. Use a universal dropper for medication administration.

    _____ B. Ask the pharmacy to add flavoring to the medication.

    _____ C. Add the medication to the formula bottle before feeding.

    _____ D. Use the nipple of the bottle to administer the medication.

    _____ E. Hold the infant in an semi-reclining position.

4. A nurse is preparing to administer medication to a toddler. Which of the following are appropriate actions for the nurse to take? (Select all that apply.)

    _____ A. Identify the toddler by asking the parent.

    _____ B. Tell the parent to administer the medication.

    _____ C. Calculate the safe dosage.

    _____ D. Ask the toddler what toy he wants to hold during administration.

    _____ E. Offer juice after the medication.

5. A nurse is caring for an infant who needs otic medication. Which of the following is an appropriate action for the nurse to take?

      A. Hold the infant in an upright position.

      B. Pull the pinna downward and straight back.

      C. Hyperextend the infant's neck.

      D. Ensure that the medication is cool.

6. A nurse is planning to initiate IV access for a toddler. What actions should the nurse plan to take? Use the ATI Active Learning Template: Basic Concepts to complete this item to include Nursing Interventions: Describe 10 atraumatic care interventions.

APPLICATION EXERCISES KEY

1. A. INCORRECT: The influenza vaccination is administered IM.

   B. INCORRECT: A 22- to 25-gauge needle is recommended for IM injections.

   C. INCORRECT: The total volume of the influenza vaccination is 0.5 mL, which can be administered in the vastus lateralis.

   D. **CORRECT:** The vastus lateralis is recommended for administering IM medications. Therefore, placing the toddler in a supine position is the appropriate action for the nurse to take.

   Ⓝ NCLEX® Connection: Pharmacological Therapies, Medication Administration

2. A. INCORRECT: Once the deltoid muscle has developed, it can be used in children for IM injections of medication containing up to 1 mL of fluid.

   B. INCORRECT: The ventrogluteal muscle can be used for IM injections in children for medication containing up to 2 mL of fluid.

   C. INCORRECT: The vastus lateralis muscle can be used for intramuscular injections in children for medication containing up to 2 mL of fluid.

   D. **CORRECT:** The dorsal gluteal site has major nerves and blood vessels and is not a recommended site for IM injections for children.

   Ⓝ NCLEX® Connection: Pharmacological Therapies, Medication Administration

3. A. INCORRECT: Medication has different viscosities, and droppers do not have a standard opening. Therefore, a universal dropper is not an accurate way to measure medications.

   B. **CORRECT:** Multiple flavorings are available to add to medications and can assist in masking the taste.

   C. INCORRECT: Because an infant might not finish an entire bottle of formula, it is not recommended to add medication to the bottle.

   D. **CORRECT:** Administering medications through an empty nipple can assist with successful administration of the medication.

   E. **CORRECT:** For successful medication administration, the infant should be held in a semi-reclining position, similar to feeding.

   Ⓝ NCLEX® Connection: Pharmacological Therapies, Medication Administration

4.   A. INCORRECT: For safe medication administration, confirm two identifiers by looking at the identification band or having the toddler state his name and date of birth.

      B. INCORRECT: The nurse should determine the preferred level of involvement of the parents prior to medication administration.

      C. **CORRECT:** For safe medication administration, the nurse should calculate safe dosage prior to administering medication.

      D. **CORRECT:** Offering choices to the toddler is an example of atraumatic care.

      E. **CORRECT:** Offering juice after the medication is an example of atraumatic care.

       NCLEX® Connection: Health Promotion and Maintenance, Developmental Stages and Transitions

5.   A. INCORRECT: Position the infant supine or prone for administration of otic medication.

      B. **CORRECT:** Pulling the pinna downward and straight back will straighten the ear canal to allow medication to flow into the ear.

      C. INCORRECT: Hyperextending the infant's neck could occlude the airway and should not be performed during otic medication administration.

      D. INCORRECT: Allowing the otic medication to warm up to room temperature is recommended to provide atraumatic care.

       NCLEX® Connection: Pharmacological Therapies, Medication Administration

6.   *Using the ATI Active Learning Template: Basic Concepts*

    • Nursing Interventions

      ◦ Decide to insert a peripherally inserted catheter before multiple peripheral attempts.

      ◦ Use a transilluminator to assist in vein location.

      ◦ Avoid terminology such as a "bee sting" or "stick."

      ◦ Attach extension tubing to decrease movement of the catheter.

      ◦ Use play therapy.

      ◦ Apply eutectic mixture of lidocaine and prilocaine (EMLA) to the site for 60 minutes prior to attempts.

      ◦ Keep equipment out of sight until procedure begins.

      ◦ Perform the procedure in a treatment room.

      ◦ Use nonpharmacologic therapies.

      ◦ Allow parents to stay if they prefer.

      ◦ Use therapeutic holding.

      ◦ Avoid using the dominant or sucking hand.

      ◦ Cover site with a colorful wrap.

      ◦ Swaddle infants.

      ◦ Offer nonnutritive sucking to infants before, during, and after the procedure.

     NCLEX® Connection: Health Promotion and Maintenance, Developmental Stages and Transitions

chapter 9

Overview

- Determination of pain depends on the child's cognitive, emotional, and physical development.
- Atraumatic care is the use of interventions that minimize or eliminate physical and psychological distress.
- Pain is managed by atraumatic, nonpharmacological, and pharmacological interventions.

Influential Factors

- Influential factors that can have a positive or negative effect on pain perception
  - Age
  - Development stage
  - Chronic or acute disease
  - Prior experiences with pain
  - Personality
  - Family dynamics
  - Culture
  - Socioeconomic status

Data Collection

 View Video: Pain Evaluation in Children

- Subjective and Objective Data
  - Developmental Characteristics
    - Young infant
      - Loud cry
      - Rigid body or thrashing
      - Local reflex withdrawal from pain stimulus
      - Expressions of pain (eyes tightly closed, mouth open in a squarish shape, eyebrows lowered and drawn together)
      - Lack of association between stimulus and pain

- Older infant
  - Loud cry
  - Deliberate withdrawal from pain
  - Facial expression of pain
- Toddler
  - Loud cry or screaming
  - Verbal expressions of pain
  - Thrashing of extremities
  - Attempt to push away or avoid stimulus
  - Noncooperation
  - Clinging to significant person
  - Behaviors occur in anticipation of painful stimulus
- School-age child
  - Stalling behavior
  - Muscular rigidity
  - Any behaviors of the toddler, but less intense in the anticipatory phase and more intense with painful stimulus
- Adolescent
  - More verbal expressions of pain with less protest
  - Muscle tension with body control
- Pain Intensity
  - Data collection includes behavioral measures, physiologic measures, and self-report.
  - Self-report is used for children older than 4 years of age. Children under 4 are unable to accurately report their pain.
  - Multiple tools have been developed and researched as reliable.
  - A nurse should choose an appropriate pain tool that will adequately determine the infant's or child's pain.
  - Include the parent or caregiver in rating the infant's or child's pain.
  - Determine the location, quality, and severity of pain.

PAIN ASSESSMENT TOOL FOR EVALUATION BY AGE

FLACC (2 months to 7 years)

› Pain rated on a scale of 0 to 10.

› Observe behaviors of the child.

› Face (F)

0 – Smile or no expression	1 – Occasional frown or grimace, withdrawn	2 – Frequent or constant frown, clenched jaw, quivering chin

› Legs (L)

0 – Relaxed or normal position	1 – Uneasy, restless, tense	2 – Kicking or legs drawn up

› Activity (A)

0 – Lying quietly, moves easily, normal position	1 – Squirming, shifting, tense	2 – Arched, ridged, or jerking

› Cry (C)

0 – No cry	1 – Moans or whimpers, occasional complaints	2 – Crying, screaming, sobbing, frequent complaints

› Consolability (C)

0 – Content or relaxed	1 – Reassured by occasional touching, or hugging; able to distract	2 – Difficult to console or comfort

FACES (3 years and older)

› Pain rated on a scale of 0 to 5 using a diagram of six faces.

› Substitute 0, 2, 4, 6, 8, 10 for 0 to 5 to convert to the 0 to 10 scale.

› Explain each face to the child; ask the child to choose a face that best describes how they are feeling.

0 – No hurt	2 – Hurts a little more	4 – Hurts a whole lot
1 – Hurts a bit	3 – Hurts even more	5 – Hurts worst

Oucher (3 to 13 years)

› Pain rated on a scale of 0 to 5 using six photographs.

› Substitute 0, 2, 4, 6, 8, 10 for 0 to 5 to convert to the 0 to 10 scale.

› Have the child organize the photographs in order of no pain to the worst pain. Ask the child to choose a picture that best describes how they are feeling.

0 – No hurt	2 – Hurts a little more	4 – Hurts a whole lot
1 – Hurts a bit	3 – Hurts even more	5 – Hurts worst

PAIN ASSESSMENT TOOL FOR EVALUATION BY AGE
Numeric scale (5 years and older)
› Pain rated on a scale of 0 to 10.
› Explain to the child that 0 means "no pain" and 10 means "worst pain."
› Have the child verbally report a number or point to their level of pain on a visual scale.
Non-communicating children's pain checklist (3 to 18 years)
› Behaviors are observed for 10 min.
› Six subcategories are scored on a scale 0 to 3.
› Subcategories are vocal, social, facial, activity, body and limbs, and physiological, each with observable behaviors to be scored. 0 – Not at all   1 – Just a little   2 – Fairly often   3 – Very often
› Cutoff scores 11 or higher indicates moderate to severe pain.   6 to 10 indicates mild pain.

Nursing Interventions

- Determine the child's pain level frequently.
- Use nonpharmacological, pharmacological, or both approaches to manage pain.
- Ask parent or caregiver to reassess the child's pain level.
- Ask the parent or caregiver about their satisfaction of the pain management.
- Observe child for adverse reactions to pain medications.
- Review laboratory reports.
- Observe the child's physical functioning following pain management intervention.
- Monitor for negative affect or distress the child might be experiencing related to the pain, such as anxiety, withdrawal, fear, depression, or unhappiness.
- Atraumatic measures
  - Use a treatment room for painful procedures.
  - Avoid procedures in "safe places," such as the play room and the child's bed.
  - Use developmentally appropriate terminology when explaining procedures.
  - Offer choices to the child.
  - Allow parents to stay with the child during painful procedures.
  - Use play therapy to explain procedures, allowing the child to perform the procedure on a doll or toy.

- Pharmacological measures
  - Optimal dosage of medications will control pain without causing severe adverse effects.
  - Select the least traumatic route for medication administration.
  - Give medications routinely, vs. PRN (as needed), to manage pain that is expected to last for an extended period of time.
  - Combine adjuvant medications (steroids, antidepressants, sedatives, antianxiety medications, muscle relaxants, anticonvulsants) with other analgesics.
  - Use nonopioid and opioid medications.
    - Acetaminophen (Tylenol) and NSAIDs are acceptable for mild to moderate pain.
    - Opioids are acceptable for moderate to severe pain. Medications used include morphine sulfate, oxycodone (OxyContin), and fentanyl (Duragesic).
    - Combining a nonopioid and an opioid medication treats pain peripherally and centrally. This offers greater analgesia with fewer adverse effects (respiratory depression, constipation, nausea).
  - IM injections are not recommended for pain control in children.
  - Intranasal medications are not recommended for children younger than 18 years.
  - Rectal medications have variable absorption rates, and children dislike them.
  - Intradermal medications are used for skin anesthesia prior to procedures.
- Appropriate Routes

ROUTE	NURSING IMPLICATIONS
Oral	› Route is preferred due to convenience, cost, and ability to maintain steady blood levels. › Take 1 to 2 hr to reach peak analgesic effects. Oral medications are not suited for children experiencing pain that requires rapid relief or pain that is fluctuating in nature.
Topical/ transdermal	› Eutectic mixture of local anesthetics (EMLA) contains equal quantities of lidocaine and prilocaine in the form of a cream or disk. » Used for any procedure in which the skin will be punctured (IV insertion, biopsy) 60 min prior to a superficial puncture and 2.5 hr prior to a deep puncture. » Place an occlusive dressing over the cream after application. » Prior to procedure, remove the dressing or disk and clean the skin. Indication of an adequate response is reddened or blanched skin. » Demonstrate to the child that the skin is not sensitive by tapping or scratching lightly. » Instruct parents to apply EMLA at home prior to coming to a health care facility for the procedure. › Fentanyl » Use for children older than 12 years of age. » Use to provide continuous pain control. Onset of 12 to 24 hr and a duration of 72 hr. » Use an immediate-release opioid for breakthrough pain. » Treat respiratory depression with naloxone (Narcan).

Q
PCC

- Nonpharmacological Measures
  - Strategies
    - Distraction
      - Use play, radio, computer game, movie.
      - Tell jokes or a story to the child.
    - Relaxation
      - Hold or rock the infant or young child.
      - Assist older children into a comfortable position.
      - Assist with breathing techniques.
    - Guided imagery
      - Assist the child in an imaginary experience.
      - Have the child describe the details.
    - Positive self-talk
      - Have the child say positive things during a procedure or through a painful episode.
    - Behavioral contracting
      - Use stickers or tokens as rewards.
      - Give time limits for the child to cooperate.
      - Reinforce cooperation with a reward.
    - Containment
      - Swaddle the infant.
      - Place rolled blankets around the child.
      - Maintain proper positioning.
    - Nonnutritive sucking
      - Offer pacifier with sucrose before, during, and after painful procedures.
      - Offer nonnutritive sucking during episodes of pain.
    - Kangaroo care – skin-to-skin contact between infants and parents

APPLICATION EXERCISES

1. A nurse is determining the level of pain an infant is experiencing. Which of the following pain scales should the nurse use?

    A. FACES

    B. FLACC

    C. Oucher

    D. Non-communicating children's pain checklist

2. A nurse is planning care for a child following a surgical procedure. Which of the following interventions should be included in the plan of care?

    A. Administer NSAIDs for pain rated greater than 7 on a 0 to 10 scale.

    B. Administer intranasal analgesics PRN.

    C. Administer IM analgesics for pain.

    D. Administer IV analgesics on a schedule.

3. A nurse is checking an infant. Which of the following are clinical manifestations of pain in an infant? (Select all that apply.)

    _____ A. Pursed lips

    _____ B. Loud cry

    _____ C. Lowered eyebrows

    _____ D. Rigid body

    _____ E. Pushes away stimulus

4. A nurse is caring for a hospitalized toddler. Which of the following methods should the nurse use when checking the toddler for pain?

    A. Ask the toddler about the pain.

    B. Observe the toddler for restlessness.

    C. Show the toddler a numeric pain scale.

    D. Look for changes in the toddler's temperature.

5. A nurse is planning care for an infant who is experiencing pain. Which of the following should be included in the plan of care? (Select all that apply.)

   _____ A. Offer a pacifier.

   _____ B. Use guided imagery.

   _____ C. Use swaddling.

   _____ D. Initiate a behavioral contract.

   _____ E. Encourage kangaroo care.

6. A nurse educator is reviewing pain determination tools with a group of pediatric nurses. What should be included in this discussion? Use the ATI Active Learning Template: Nursing Skill to describe four different pain tools used with pediatric clients.

APPLICATION EXERCISES KEY

1. A. INCORRECT: The FACES pain assessment scale is recommended for children 3 years or older.

    B. **CORRECT:** The FLACC pain assessment scale is recommended for infants and children between 2 months and 7 years of age.

    C. INCORRECT: The Oucher pain assessment scale is recommended for children between the ages of 3 and 13 years.

    D. INCORRECT: The non-communicating children's pain checklist is recommended for non-communicating children between the ages of 3 and 18 years.

    Ⓝ NCLEX® Connection: Basic Care and Comfort, Non-Pharmacological Comfort Interventions

2. A. INCORRECT: NSAIDs are used for mild to moderate pain.

    B. INCORRECT: Intranasal analgesics are used for clients older than 18 years.

    C. INCORRECT: IM analgesics are not recommended for pain management in children.

    D. **CORRECT:** IV analgesics should be administered on a schedule to achieve optimal pain management.

    Ⓝ NCLEX® Connection: Pharmacological Therapies, Expected Actions/Outcomes

3. A. INCORRECT: Infant who experience pain will have their mouth open in a squarish shape.

    B. **CORRECT:** Infants who experience pain will exhibit a loud cry.

    C. **CORRECT:** Infants who experience pain will lower and draw together their eyebrows.

    D. **CORRECT:** Infants who experience pain will exhibit a rigid body.

    E. INCORRECT: Infants who experience pain will exhibit a local reflex to withdraw from the stimulus.

    Ⓝ NCLEX® Connection: Basic Care and Comfort, Non-Pharmacological Comfort Interventions

4. A. INCORRECT: The nurse should not ask the toddler about the pain because a toddler is unable to understand or describe the level of her pain due to a lack of verbal and cognitive skills at this age.

    B. **CORRECT:** The nurse should observe the toddler for restlessness because toddlers express pain through behaviors such as restlessness, facial grimacing, irritability and crying.

    C. INCORRECT: The nurse should not show the toddler a numeric pain scale because pain scales are appropriate methods of determining pain in children who are school-age or older.

    D. INCORRECT: The nurse should not look for changes in the toddler's temperature. Changes in behavior would be noticed first, before changes in vital signs.

     NCLEX® Connection: Basic Care and Comfort, Non-Pharmacological Comfort Interventions

5. A. **CORRECT:** Nonnutritive sucking is a therapeutic nonpharmacological strategy for pain management with infants.

    B. INCORRECT: Guided imagery is a nonpharmacological strategy used with children.

    C. **CORRECT:** Swaddling the infant is a therapeutic nonpharmacological strategy for pain management.

    D. INCORRECT: Behavioral contracts are a nonpharmacological strategy used with children.

    E. **CORRECT:** Skin-to-skin touch is a relaxation technique and should be encouraged for infants who have pain.

    NCLEX® Connection: Basic Care and Comfort, Non-Pharmacological Comfort Interventions

6. *Using the ATI Active Learning Template: Nursing Skill*
   - FLACC (2 months to 7 years)
     - Pain rated on a scale of 0 to 10.
     - Determine behaviors of the child.
     - Face (F)
       - 0 – Smile or no expression
       - 1 – Occasional frown or grimace, withdrawn
       - 2 – Frequent or constant frown, clenched jaw, quivering chin
     - Legs (L)
       - 0 – Relaxed or normal position
       - 1 – Uneasy, restless, tense
       - 2 – Kicking or legs drawn up
     - Activity (A)
       - 0 – Lying quietly, moves easily, normal position
       - 1 – Squirming, shifting, tense
       - 2 – Arched, ridged, or jerking
     - Cry (C)
       - 0 – No cry
       - 1 – Moans or whimpers, occasional complaints
       - 2 – Crying, screaming, sobbing, frequent complaints
     - Consolability (C)
       - 0 – Content or relaxed
       - 1 – Reassured by occasional touching, or hugging. Able to distract
       - 2 – Difficult to console or comfort
   - FACES (3 years and older)
     - Pain rated on a scale of 0 to 5 using a diagram of six faces.
     - Substitute 0, 2, 4, 6, 8, 10 for 0 to 5 to convert to the 0 to 10 scale.
     - Explain each face to the child.
       - 0 – No hurt
       - 1 – Hurts a bit
       - 2 – Hurts a little more
       - 3 – Hurts even more
       - 4 – Hurts a whole lot
       - 5 – Hurts worst
     - Ask the child to choose a face that best describes how they are feeling
   - Oucher (3 to 13 years)
     - Pain rated on a scale of 0 to 5 using six photographs.
     - Substitute 0, 2, 4, 6, 8, 10 for 0 to 5 to convert to the 0 to 10 scale.
     - Have the child organize the photographs in order of no pain to the worst pain.
       - 0 – No hurt
       - 1 – Hurts a bit
       - 2 – Hurts a little more
       - 3 – Hurts even more
       - 4 – Hurts a whole lot
       - 5 – Hurts worst
     - Ask the child to choose a picture that best describes how they are feeling.
   - Numeric scale (5 years and older)
     - Pain rated on a scale of 0 to 10.
     - Explain to the child that 0 means "no pain" and 10 means "worst pain."
     - Have the child verbally report a number or point on a visual scale their pain level.
   - Non-communicating children's pain checklist (3 to 18 years)
     - Behaviors are observed for 10 min.
     - Six subcategories are scored on a scale 0 to 3.
     - Subcategories are vocal, social, facial, activity, body and limbs, and physiological, each with observable behaviors to be scored.
       - 0 – Not at all
       - 1 – Just a little
       - 2 – Fairly often
       - 3 – Very often
     - Cutoff scores:
       - 11 or more indicates moderate to severe pain.
       - 6 to 10 indicates mild pain.

Ⓝ NCLEX® Connection: Basic Care and Comfort, Non-Pharmacological Comfort Interventions

chapter 10

Overview

- A nurse is likely to encounter children who are ill and hospitalized. When caring for these children, it is important to know what play activities are considered appropriate.

HOSPITALIZATION AND ILLNESS

Overview

- Families and children can experience major stress related to hospitalization. The nurse should be alert to evidence of stress and intervene as appropriate.
- Families should be considered clients when children are ill.
- Separation anxiety during hospitalization manifests in three behavioral responses.
  - Protest (screaming, clinging to parents, verbal and physical aggression toward strangers)
  - Despair (withdrawal from others, depression, decreased communication, developmental regression)
  - Detachment (interacts with strangers, forms new relationships, appears happy)
- Each child's understanding of illnesses and hospitalization is dependent on the child's stage of development and cognitive ability.

Impact Based on Development

INFANT	
Level of Understanding	› Inability to describe illness and follow directions › Lack of understanding the need for therapeutic procedures
Impact of Hospitalization	› Experiences stranger anxiety between 6 to 18 months of age › Displays physical behaviors as expressions of discomfort due to inability to verbalize › Can experience sleep deprivation due to strange noises, monitoring devices, and procedures
TODDLER	
Level of Understanding	› Limited ability to describe illness › Poorly developed sense of body image and boundaries › Limited understanding of the need for therapeutic procedures › Limited ability to follow directions
Impact of Hospitalization	› Experiences separation anxiety › Can exhibit an intense reaction to any type of procedure due to the intrusion of boundaries › Behavior can regress

PRESCHOOLER	
Level of Understanding	› Limited understanding of the cause of illness but knows what illness feels like › Limited ability to describe clinical manifestations › Fears related to magical thinking › Ability to understand cause and effect inhibited by concrete thinking
Impact of Hospitalization	› Can experience separation anxiety › Can harbor fears of bodily harm › Can believe illness and hospitalization are a punishment
SCHOOL-AGE CHILD	
Level of Understanding	› Beginning awareness of body functioning › Ability to describe pain › Increasing ability to understand cause and effect
Impact of Hospitalization	› Fears loss of control › Seeks information as a way to maintain a sense of control › Can sense when not being told the truth › Can experience stress related to separation from peers and regular routine
ADOLESCENT	
Level of Understanding	› Increasing ability to understand cause and effect › Perceptions of illness severity based on the degree of body image changes
Impact of Hospitalization	› Develops body image disturbance › Attempts to maintain composure but is embarrassed about losing control › Experiences feelings of isolation from peers › Worries about outcome and impact on school/activities › Might not adhere to treatments/medication regimen due to peer influence

Family Responses

- Fear and guilt regarding not bringing the child in for care earlier.
- Frustration due to the perceived inability to care for the child.
- Altered family roles.
- Worry regarding finances if work is missed.
- Worry regarding care of other children within the household.
- Fear related to lack of knowledge regarding illness or treatments.
- Siblings experience loneliness, jealousy, guilt, fear, or anger.

Data Collection

- Child's and family's understanding of the illness or the reason for hospitalization
- Stressors unique to the child and family (needs of other children in the family, socioeconomic situation, health of other extended family members)
- Past experiences with hospitalization and illness
- Developmental level and needs of child/family
- Parenting role and the family's perception of role changes
- Support available to the child/family

Nursing Interventions

- Inform the child and family what to expect during hospitalization.
- Encourage parents or family members to stay with the child during the hospital experience to reduce the stress.
- Attempt to maintain routine as much as possible.

AGE	INTERVENTIONS
Infant	› Place infants whose parents are not in attendance close to nurses' stations so that their needs can be quickly met. › Provide consistency in assigning caregivers.
Toddler	› Encourage parents to provide routine care for the child, such as changing diapers and feeding. › Encourage the child's autonomy by offering appropriate choices. › Provide consistency in assigning caregivers.
Preschooler	› Explain procedures using simple, clear language. Avoid medical jargon and terms that can be misinterpreted. › Encourage independence by letting the child provide self-care. › Encourage the child to express feelings. › Validate the child's fears and concerns. › Provide toys that allow for emotional expression, such as a pounding board to release feelings of protest. › Provide consistency in assigning caregivers. › Give choices when possible, such as, "Do you want your medicine in a cup or a spoon?" › Allow younger children to handle equipment if it is safe.

AGE	INTERVENTIONS
School-age	› Provide factual information. › Encourage expression of feelings. › Try to maintain a normal routine for long hospitalizations, including time for school work. › Encourage contact with peer group.
Adolescent	› Provide factual information. › Include the adolescent in the planning of care to relieve feelings of powerlessness and lack of control. › Encourage contact with peer group.

M View Video: Interventions for Hospitalization

PLAY

Overview

- Play allows children to express feelings and fears.
- Play facilitates mastery of developmental stages and assists in the development of problem-solving abilities.
- Play allows children to learn socially acceptable behaviors.
- Play activities should be specific to each child's stage of development.
- Play can be used to teach children.
- Play is a means of protection from everyday stressors.

Content of Play

- Social affective – taking pleasure in relationships
- Sense-pleasure – objects in the environment catching the child's attention
- Skill – demonstrating new abilities
- Unoccupied behavior – focusing attention on something of interest
- Dramatic – pretending and fantasizing
- Games – imitative, formal, or competitive

Social Character of Play

- Onlooker – the child observing others
- Solitary – the child playing alone
- Parallel – children playing independently but among other children, which is characteristic of toddlers
- Associative – children playing together without organization, which is characteristic of preschoolers
- Cooperative play – organized playing in groups, which is characteristic of school-age children

Functions of Play

- Play helps in the development of the following types of skills.
  - Intellectual
  - Sensorimotor
  - Social
  - Self-awareness
  - Creativity
  - Therapeutic and moral values

Play Activities Related to Age

- Infants
  - Birth to 3 months – colorful moving mobiles, music/sound boxes
  - 3 to 6 months – noise-making objects and soft toys
  - 6 to 9 months – teething toys and social interaction
  - 9 to 12 months – large blocks, toys that pop apart, and push-and-pull toys
- Toddlers
  - Cloth books, puzzles with large pieces
  - Large crayons and paper
  - Push-and-pull toys, balls
  - Tricycles
  - Educational television
  - Videos for children
- Preschoolers
  - Imitative and imaginative play
  - Drawing, painting, riding a tricycle, swimming, jumping, and running
  - Educational television and videos

- School-age children
  - Games that can be played alone or with another person
  - Team sports
  - Musical instruments
  - Arts and crafts
  - Collections
- Adolescents
  - Team sports
  - School activities
  - Reading and listening to music
  - Peer interactions

Therapeutic Play

- Makes use of dolls and/or stuffed animals
- Encourages the acting out of feelings of fear, anger, hostility, and sadness
- Enables the child to learn coping strategies in a safe environment
- Assists in gaining cooperation for medical treatment

Data Collection

- Developmental level of the child
- Motor skills
- Level of activity tolerance
- Child's preferences

Nursing Interventions

- Select toys that are safe for the child.
- Consider isolation precautions and the child's illness in relation to toy selection.
- Select activities that enhance development.
- Observe the child's play for clues to the child's fears or anxieties.
- Encourage parents to bring one favorite toy from home.
- Use dolls or stuffed animals to demonstrate a procedure before it is done.
- Provide play opportunities that meet the child's level of activity tolerance.
- Allow the child to go to the play room if able.
- Encourage the adolescent's peers to visit.
- Involve a child life specialist in planning activities.

APPLICATION EXERCISES

1. A nurse is caring for a preschooler. Which of the following is an expected behavior of a preschool-age child?

    A. Describing manifestations of illness

    B. Relating fears to magical thinking

    C. Understanding cause of illness

    D. Awareness of body functioning

2. A nurse on a pediatric unit is caring for a toddler. Which of the following behaviors is an effect of hospitalization? (Select all that apply.)

_____ A. Believes the experience is a punishment

_____ B. Experiences separation anxiety

_____ C. Displays intense emotions

_____ D. Exhibits regressive behaviors

_____ E. Manifests disturbance in body image

3. A nurse is reinforcing teaching to a parent about parallel play in children. Which of the following statements by the nurse is appropriate?

    A. "Children sit and observe others playing."

    B. "Children exhibit organized play when in a group."

    C. "The child plays alone."

    D. "The child plays independently when in a group."

4. A nurse is reinforcing teaching to a group of parents about separation anxiety. Which of the following should be included in the teaching?

    A. It is often observed in the school-age child.

    B. Detachment is the stage exhibited in the hospital.

    C. It results in prolonged issues of adaptability.

    D. Kicking a stranger is an example.

5. A nurse on a pediatric unit is caring for a group of children of different ages and planning play activities. What activities should the nurse include in the plan of care? Use the ATI Active Learning Template: Basic Concept to complete this item to identify appropriate toys and activities for children in three age groups.

APPLICATION EXERCISES KEY

1. A. INCORRECT: Preschool-age children have limited ability to describe manifestations of illness.

    B. **CORRECT:** Preschool-age children are egocentric and relate fears to magical thinking.

    C. INCORRECT: Preschool-age children have limited understanding of cause-and-effect relationship, but understand what illness feels like.

    D. INCORRECT: Awareness of body functioning is a behavior of an adolescent.

    Ⓝ NCLEX® Connection: Health Promotion and Maintenance, Developmental Stages and Transitions

2. A. INCORRECT: Preschool children believe hospitalization is a punishment.

    B. **CORRECT:** Separation anxiety is a potential effect of hospitalization in a toddler.

    C. **CORRECT:** Intense emotions are a potential impact of hospitalization in a toddler.

    D. **CORRECT:** Behavior regression is a potential impact of hospitalization in a toddler.

    E. INCORRECT: Body image disturbances can be seen in adolescents who are hospitalized.

    Ⓝ NCLEX® Connection: Health Promotion and Maintenance, Developmental Stages and Transitions

3. A. INCORRECT: Onlooker play is when a child sits and observes others playing.

    B. INCORRECT: Cooperative play is when a child exhibits organized play in a group.

    C. INCORRECT: Solitary play is when a child plays alone.

    D. **CORRECT:** Parallel play is when the toddler plays independently but is among other children in a group.

    Ⓝ NCLEX® Connection: Health Promotion and Maintenance, Developmental Stages and Transitions

4. A. INCORRECT: Separation anxiety is commonly observed in the toddler.

    B. INCORRECT: The detachment stage is rarely seen in the hospital setting.

    C. INCORRECT: Children are adaptable, and permanent issues are rare.

    D. **CORRECT:** Physical aggression toward strangers is a behavior seen in the protest stage of separation anxiety.

    Ⓝ NCLEX® Connection: Health Promotion and Maintenance, Developmental Stages and Transitions

5. *Using the ATI Active Learning Template: Basic Concept*
   - Appropriate Toys and Activities for Children by Age
     - Infants
       - Birth to 3 months – colorful moving mobiles, music/sound boxes
       - 3 to 6 months – noise-making objects and soft toys
       - 6 to 9 months – teething toys and social interaction
       - 9 to 12 months – large blocks, toys that pop apart, and push-and-pull toys
     - Toddlers
       - Cloth books
       - Large crayons and paper
       - Push-and-pull toys
       - Tricycles
       - Balls
       - Puzzles with large pieces
       - Educational television
       - Videos for children
     - Preschoolers
       - Imitative and imaginative play
       - Drawing, painting, riding a tricycle, swimming, jumping, and running
       - Educational television and videos
     - School-age children
       - Games that can be played alone or with another person
       - Team sports
       - Musical instruments
       - Arts and crafts
       - Collections
     - Adolescents
       - Team sports
       - School activities
       - Reading and listening to music
       - Peer interactions

   Ⓝ NCLEX® Connection: Health Promotion and Maintenance, Developmental Stages and Transitions

chapter 11

Overview

- A nurse is tasked with meeting the physical, psychological, spiritual, and emotional needs of a client and the family during illness and at the time of death.
- Palliative care is a multidisciplinary approach that focuses on the process of dying rather than prolonging life in cases in which cures are no longer possible.
  - Focus on control of managing manifestations and offering supportive care.
- Hospice care specializes in the care of a client who is dying.
  - Family members are the primary caregivers.
  - Nursing focus is on pain control and comfort.
  - Family and client needs are equal.
  - Provide support for the family grieving process, which can continue after the client's death.
- End-of-life decisions require honest information regarding prognosis, disease progression, treatment options, and the effect of treatments. These decisions are made during a highly stressful time. It is important that all health care personnel are aware of the child and family's decisions.
- Nurses may experience personal grief when caring for children with whom they have developed rapport and intimacy.

Factors Influencing Loss, Grief, and Coping Ability

- Interpersonal relationships and social support networks
- Type and significance of loss
- Culture and ethnicity
- Spiritual and religious beliefs and practices
- Prior experience with loss
- Socioeconomic status
- Grief and mourning
  - Anticipatory grief: when death is expected or a possible outcome
  - Complicated grief: extends for more than 1 year following the loss
    - Intense thoughts
    - Distressing yearning
    - Feelings of loneliness
    - Distressing emotions and feelings
    - Disturbances in personal activities, such as sleep
    - May require referral to an expert in grief counseling

- ○ Parental grief
  - ▪ Intense, long-lasting, and complex
  - ▪ Secondary losses related to the death of the child, such as absence of hope and dreams, disruption of the family unit, and loss of identity as a parent
  - ▪ Differences between maternal and paternal grief
- ○ Sibling grief
  - ▪ Differs from adult/parental grief
  - ▪ Reactions depend on age and developmental stage
- Current stage of development

AGE	RELEVANT FACTORS
Infants/toddlers (birth to 3 years)	› Have little to no concept of death › Egocentric thinking prevents their understanding death (toddlers) › Mirror parental emotions (sadness, anger, depression, anxiety) › React in response to the changes brought about by being in the hospital (change of routine, painful procedures, immobilization, less independence, separation from family) › May regress to an earlier stage of behavior
Preschool children (3 to 6 years)	› Egocentric thinking › Magical thinking allows for the belief that thoughts can cause an event such as death (as a result, child may feel guilt and shame) › Interpret separation from parents as punishment for bad behavior › View dying as temporary because of the lack of a concept of time and because the dead person can still have attributes of the living (sleeping, eating, breathing)
School-age children (6 to 12 years)	› Start to respond to logical or factual explanations › Begin to have an adult concept of death (inevitable, irreversible, universal), which generally applies to older school-age children (9 to 12 years) › Experience fear of the disease process, the death process, the unknown, and loss of control » Fear often displayed through uncooperative behavior › May be curious about funeral services and what happens to the body after death
Adolescents (12 to 20 years)	› May have an adultlike concept of death › May have difficulty accepting death because they are discovering who they are, establishing an identity, and dealing with issues of puberty › Rely more on peers than the influence of parents, which can result in the reality of a serious illness causing adolescents to feel isolated › May be unable to relate to peers and communicate with parents › May become increasingly stressed by changes in physical appearance due to medications or illness than the prospect of death › May experience guilt and shame

- Factors that can increase the family's potential for dysfunctional grieving following the death of a child
  - Lack of a support system
  - Presence of inadequate coping skills
  - Association of violence or suicide with the death of a child
  - Sudden and unexpected death of a child
  - Lack of hope or presence of pre-existing mental health issues

Data Collection

- Physical manifestations of impending death
  - Sensation of heat when the body feels cool
  - Decreased sensation and movement in the lower extremities
  - Loss of senses (hearing is the last to be lost)
  - Confusion or loss of consciousness
  - Decreased appetite and thirst
  - Swallowing difficulties
  - Loss of bowel and bladder control
  - Bradycardia, hypotension
  - Cheyne-Stokes respirations
- Knowledge regarding diagnosis, prognosis, and care
- Perceptions and desires regarding diagnosis, prognosis, and care
- Nutritional status, as well as growth and development patterns
- Activity and energy level of the child and siblings
- Parents' wishes regarding the child's end-of-life care
- Presence of a do-not-resuscitate (DNR) order
- Family coping and available support
- The stage of grief the child and family are experiencing

Nursing Interventions

- Allow an opportunity for anticipatory grieving, which affects the way a family will cope with the death of a child.
- Provide consistency among nursing personnel who are caring for the client and family.
- Encourage parents to remain with the client.
- Attempt to maintain a normal environment.
- Communicate with the client honestly and respectfully.
- Encourage independence.

- Stay with the client as much as possible.
- Administer analgesics to control pain.
- Provide privacy.
- Soften lights.
- Offer soft music if desired.
- Assist with arranging religious or cultural rituals desired by the client and family.
- Assist the client with unfinished tasks.
- Provide support for the family and client.
- Palliative care
  - Consider the client, siblings, and parents as the units of care.
  - Provide an environment that is as close to being like home as possible.
  - Consult with the client and family for desired measures.
  - Respect the family's cultural and religious preferences and rituals.
  - Provide and clarify information and explanations.
  - Encourage physical contact; address feelings; and show concern, empathy, and support.
  - Provide comfort measures (warmth, quiet, noise control, dry linens).
  - Provide adequate nutrition and hydration.
  - Control pain.
    - Give medications on a regular schedule.
    - Treat breakthrough pain.
    - Increase doses as necessary to control pain.
    - Encourage use of relaxation, imagery, and distraction to help manage pain.
- Care for grieving families during the dying process.
  - Provide information to the client and family about the disease, medications, procedures, and expected events.
  - Encourage and support parents to participate in caring for the client.
  - Encourage parents to remain near the child as much as possible.
  - Encourage the client's independence and control as developmentally and physically appropriate.
  - Allow for visitation of family and friends as desired.
  - Emphasize open, honest communication among the client, family, and health care team.
  - Provide support to the client and family with decision-making.
  - Provide opportunities for the client and family to ask questions.
  - Assist parents to cope with their feelings, and help them to understand the client's behaviors.
  - Use books, movies, art, music, and play therapy to stimulate discussions and provide an outlet for emotions.
  - Provide and encourage professional support and guidance from a trusted member of the health care team.

- Remain neutral and accepting.
- Give reassurance that the client is not in pain and that all efforts are being made to maintain comfort and support of the client's life.
- Recognize and support the individual differences of grieving. Advise families that each member may react differently on any given day.
- Give families privacy, unlimited time, and opportunities for any cultural or religious rituals. Respect the family's decisions regarding care of the client.
- Encourage discussion of special memories and people, reading of favorite books, providing favorite toys or objects, physical contact, sibling visits, and continued verbal communication, even if the client seems unconscious.

- After death
  - Allow family to stay with the body as long as they desire.
  - Allow family to rock the infant/toddler, if desired.
  - Assist with the removal of tubes and equipment.
  - Offer family the option to assist with the preparation of the body.
  - Assist with preparations involving the death ritual.
  - Encourage parents to prepare siblings for the funeral and related death rituals.
  - Remain with the family and offer support.
  - Allow family to share stories about the client's life.
  - Refer to the client by name.
  - Allow all family members to communicate feelings.
- Nurses caring for a client who is dying should:
  - Express personal feelings of loss to someone who can offer support.
  - Maintain good general health.
  - Develop the ability for empathy.
  - Take time off from work as needed.
  - Develop well-rounded interests.
  - Develop professional and social support systems.
  - Focus on the positive aspects of caring for children who are dying.
  - Attend funeral services if desired.
  - Maintain contact with the family.

APPLICATION EXERCISES

1. A nurse is caring for a child who has a terminal illness. Which of the following are physical manifestations of impending death? (Select all that apply.)

_____ A. Heightened sense of hearing

_____ B. Tachycardia

_____ C. Difficulty swallowing

_____ D. Sensation of being cold

_____ E. Cheyne-Stokes respirations

2. A nurse is reinforcing teaching with a parent about complicated grief. Which of the following statements by the nurse is appropriate?

A. "It is considered complicated grief if you are still grieving 6 months after your loss."

B. "Personal activities are affected when experiencing complicated grief."

C. "Parents will experience complicated grief together."

D. "Complicated grief self-resolves in 12 months."

3. A nurse is reinforcing teaching with a parent of a preschool child about factors that affect the child's perception of death. Which of the following should be included in the information session?

A. Preschool children have no concept of death.

B. Preschool children perceive death as temporary.

C. Preschool children often regress to an earlier stage of behavior.

D. Preschool children experience fear related to the disease process.

4. A nurse is caring for a child who is dying. Which of the following are appropriate actions for the nurse to take during and after the death of a child? (Select all that apply.)

_____ A. Remain in contact with the family after their loss.

_____ B. Develop a professional support system.

_____ C. Take time off from work.

_____ D. Suggest that a hospital representative attend the funeral.

_____ E. Demonstrate feelings of sympathy toward the family.

5. A nurse is caring for a child who has a terminal illness and reviews palliative care with an assistive personnel (AP). Which of the following statements by the AP indicates understanding of this review?

    A. "I'm sure the family is hopeful that the new medication will stop the illness."

    B. "I'll miss working with this client now that only nurses will be caring for him."

    C. "I will get all the client's personal objects out of his room."

    D. "I will listen and respond as the family talks about their child's life."

6. A nurse is planning care for a client who is nearing the end of life. What interventions should the nurse include in the plan of care? Use the ATI Active Learning Template: Basic Concept to complete this item to describe at least eight nursing interventions to be used.

APPLICATION EXERCISES KEY

1. A. INCORRECT: A decrease in the senses of smell, sight, and hearing are physical manifestations of approaching death.

    B. INCORRECT: Bradycardia is a physical manifestation of approaching death.

    C. **CORRECT:** Difficulty swallowing is a physical finding of approaching death.

    D. INCORRECT: A client's sensation of heat when the body feels cool is a physical manifestation of approaching death.

    E. **CORRECT:** Cheyne-Stokes respirations are an abnormal breathing pattern with periods of apnea that is a physical finding of impending death.

     NCLEX® Connection: Psychosocial Integrity, End of Life Concepts

2. A. INCORRECT: A parent who is still experiencing intense grieving after 1 year is evaluated for complicated grief.

    B. **CORRECT:** A parent who is experiencing complicated grief experiences intense emotions that affect personal activities.

    C. INCORRECT: Parents grieve differently, and not all parents experience complicated grief.

    D. INCORRECT: A nurse should refer the parent to an expert in grief counseling if complicated grief is identified.

     NCLEX® Connection: Psychosocial Integrity, End of Life Concepts

3. A. INCORRECT: Toddlers have no concept of death.

    B. **CORRECT:** Preschool children perceive death as temporary because they have no concept of time.

    C. INCORRECT: Toddlers often regress to an earlier stage of behavior.

    D. INCORRECT: School-age children experience fear related to the disease process.

     NCLEX® Connection: Psychosocial Integrity, End of Life Concepts

4.   A. **CORRECT:** Maintaining contact with the family after their loss is an act of support for the family.

   B. **CORRECT:** Developing professional support systems is a strategy the nurse can use to maintain effectiveness when working with the client who is dying and their family.

   C. **CORRECT:** Taking time off from work is a strategy the nurse can use to maintain effectiveness when working with the client who is dying and their family.

   D. INCORRECT: Nurses should be encouraged to participate in funeral rituals as an act of support for the family.

   E. INCORRECT: A nurse should develop the ability for empathy when dealing with clients who are dying.

    NCLEX® Connection: Psychosocial Integrity, End of Life Concepts

5.   A. INCORRECT: Palliative care is provided when there is no longer hope for a disease cure.

   B. INCORRECT: Palliative care focuses on providing consistency among the multidisciplinary team and nursing personnel to offer supportive care and a normal environment.

   C. INCORRECT: Palliative care focuses on offering support and a normal environment as the dying process occurs.

   D. **CORRECT:** Palliative care focuses on the process of dying and grieving, which includes using therapeutic communication.

    NCLEX® Connection: Psychosocial Integrity, End of Life Concepts

6.   *Using the ATI Active Learning Template: Basic Concept*
   • Nursing Interventions
      ○ Allow an opportunity for anticipatory grieving, which affects the way a family will cope with the death of a child.
      ○ Provide consistency among nursing staff caring for the client and family.
      ○ Encourage parents to remain with the client.
      ○ Attempt to maintain a normal environment.
      ○ Communicate with the client honestly and respectfully.
      ○ Encourage independence.
      ○ Stay with the client as much as possible.
      ○ Administer analgesics to control pain.
      ○ Provide privacy.
      ○ Soften lights.
      ○ Offer soft music if desired.
      ○ Assist with arranging religious or cultural rituals desired by the client and family.
      ○ Assist the client with unfinished tasks.
      ○ Provide support for the family and client.

    NCLEX® Connection: Psychosocial Integrity, End of Life Concepts

UNIT 2 Nursing Care of Children with System Disorders

SECTION: NEUROSENSORY DISORDERS

› Acute Neurological Disorders
› Seizures

NCLEX® CONNECTIONS

When reviewing the chapters in this section, keep in mind the relevant sections of the NCLEX® outline, in particular:

Client Needs: Reduction of Risk Potential	Client Needs: Physiological Adaptations

› Relevant topics/tasks include:
» Laboratory Values
  › Monitor diagnostic or laboratory test results.
» Potential for Alterations in Body Systems
  › Compare current client clinical data to baseline information.
  › Perform neurological checks.
  › Reinforce client teaching on methods to prevent complications associated with activity level/ diagnosed illness/disease.
» Therapeutic Procedures
  › Reinforce client teaching on treatments and procedures.
	› Relevant topics/tasks include:
	» Alterations in Body Systems
	  › Provide care to client who has experienced a seizure.
	» Medical Emergencies
	  › Respond /intervene to a client life-threatening situation.

chapter 12

Overview

- Meningitis is an inflammation of the cerebrospinal fluid (CSF) and meninges, which are the membranes that protect the brain and spinal cord.

- Reye syndrome is a life-threatening disease that involves acute encephalopathy and fatty changes of the liver.

- Meningitis and Reye syndrome have similar manifestations, and both sometimes are preceded by viral infections. Testing is necessary to differentiate between the two.

- Head injuries can be classified as open (skull integrity is compromised – penetrating trauma) or closed (skull integrity is maintained – blunt trauma). Head injuries also are classified as mild, moderate, or severe, depending upon Glasgow Coma Scale (GCS) ratings and length of loss of consciousness.

MENINGITIS

Overview

- Viral, or aseptic, meningitis usually requires only supportive care for recovery.

- Bacterial, or septic, meningitis is a contagious infection. The prognosis depends on how quickly care is initiated.

Data Collection

- Risk Factors

  - Viral Meningitis

    - Viral illnesses, such as cytomegalovirus, mumps, herpes simplex virus, and arbovirus

  - Bacterial Meningitis

    - Infections caused by bacterial agents (Neisseria meningitidis [meningococcal], Streptococcus pneumoniae [pneumococcal], Haemophilus influenzae type B [HIB], Escherichia coli)

    - Immunosuppression

    - Injuries that provide direct access to cerebrospinal fluid (skull fracture, penetrating head wound)

    - Crowded living conditions

- Subjective Data

  - Children may report photophobia, nausea, irritability, or headache.

  - Parents may report that children are irritable, have vomited, and are drowsy.

- Objective Data
  - Physical Findings
    - Newborns
      - No illness is present at birth, but it progresses within a few days.
      - Clinical manifestations can be vague and difficult to diagnose.
        - ▸ Poor muscle tone, weak cry, poor suck, vomiting, or diarrhea
        - ▸ Fever or hypothermia
      - Nuchal rigidity is not usually present.
      - Bulging fontanels are a late sign.
    - 2 months to 2 years
      - Seizures with a high-pitched cry
      - Fever and irritability
      - Bulging fontanels
      - Possible nuchal rigidity
      - Poor feeding
      - Vomiting
      - Brudzinski's sign (flexion of extremities occurring with deliberate flexion of the child's neck) and Kernig's sign (resistance to extension of the child's leg from a flexed position) do not assist with the diagnosis.
    - 2 years through adolescence
      - Seizures (often initial sign)
      - Nuchal rigidity
      - Positive Brudzinski's sign
      - Positive Kernig's sign
      - Fever and chills
      - Headache
      - Vomiting
      - Photophobia
      - Irritability and restlessness that can progress to drowsiness, delirium, stupor, and coma
      - Petechia or purpuric-type rash (seen with meningococcal infection)
      - Involvement of joints (seen with meningococcal and Haemophilus influenza)
      - Chronic draining ear (seen with pneumococcal infection)
  - Laboratory Tests
    - Blood cultures are sometimes positive when the CSF culture is negative
    - Complete blood counts

- Cerebrospinal fluid
  - Results indicative of meningitis
    - Bacterial
      - Cloudy color
      - Elevated WBC count
      - Elevated protein content
      - Decreased glucose content
      - Positive Gram stain
    - Viral
      - Clear color
      - Slightly elevated WBC count
      - Normal or slightly elevated protein content
      - Normal glucose content
      - Negative Gram stain
- Diagnostic Procedures
  - CSF analysis
    - This is the best diagnostic test for meningitis.
    - The collection of CSF with a lumbar puncture (performed by a health care provider)
    - Nursing Actions
      - Have children empty the bladder if appropriate.
      - Place children in the fetal position, and assist in maintaining the position. Older children may be placed in the sitting position.
      - Administer sedatives as prescribed.
      - Apply a eutectic mixture of local anesthetics (EMLA), which contains equal quantities of lidocaine and prilocaine, over the area between L3 and L5 45 to 60 min prior to the procedure.
      - Appropriately label the three test tubes of CSF and deliver them to the laboratory.
      - Monitor the site for hematoma and infection.
    - Client Education
      - Children should be encouraged to remain in bed for 4 to 8 hr in a flat position to prevent leakage and a resulting spinal headache. This might not be possible for infants, toddlers, or preschoolers.
  - CT or MRI scans
    - These may be performed to identify increased intracranial pressure (ICP) or an abscess.
    - Nursing Actions
      - Assist with positioning.
      - Administer sedatives.

Patient-Centered Care

- Nursing Care

  - The presence of petechia or a purpuric-type rash requires immediate medical attention.

  - Isolate children as soon as meningitis is suspected, and maintain droplet precautions per facility protocol.

  - Maintain isolation precautions (droplet precautions) per facility protocol. This requires a private room, the wearing of a surgical mask within 3 feet of children, appropriate hand hygiene, and the use of designated equipment, such as blood pressure cuff and thermometer. Continue for 24 hr after the first antibiotic has been administered.

  - Monitor for manifestations of increased intracranial pressure (severe headache, deteriorating level of consciousness, restlessness, irritability, agitation).

  - Continue frequent monitoring of vital signs, urine output, fluid status, pain level, neurologic status, and head circumference (for infants).

  - Monitor I&O hourly for children receiving IV fluids.

  - Maintain NPO status if the child has a decreased level of consciousness. As the child's condition improves, advance to clear liquids and then to a diet that the child can tolerate and is suitable for the child's age.

  - Decrease environmental stimuli.

    - Provide a quiet environment.

    - Minimize the child's exposure to bright light (natural and electric).

  - Provide comfort.

    - Keep the child's room cool.

    - Position children without a pillow and slightly elevate the head of the bed. Children may prefer a side-lying position to take pressure off the neck.

    - Maintain safety (keep the bed in a low position, implement seizure precautions).

    - Keep the family informed of the child's condition.

- Medications

  - Antibiotics – usually a cephalosporin

    - Ordered by provider for bacterial infections via an IV route. Length of therapy is determined by the child's condition and CSF results (normal blood glucose levels, negative culture). Therapy may last as long as 10 days.

    - Nursing Considerations

      - Check for allergies.

      - Monitor children receiving IV infusions for signs of irritation or swelling. Report changes in site immediately.

    - Client Education

      - Provide support for children and families.

      - Reinforce teaching to the family about the need to complete the entire course of medication.

- ○ Corticosteroids – dexamethasone
  - ▪ Prescribed by provider to prevent neurologic complications for children with bacterial meningitis.
  - ▪ Nursing Considerations
    - ▫ Check for effectiveness of medication.
  - ▪ Client Education
    - ▫ Provide support for children and their families.
    - ▫ Reinforce teaching on the administration of the medication and side effects that can occur.
- ○ Antiepileptics
  - ▪ Prophylaxis for seizures
  - ▪ Nursing Considerations
    - ▫ Watch for effectiveness of the medication.
    - ▫ Monitor therapeutic medication levels.
  - ▪ Client Education
    - ▫ Reinforce teaching to children and their families about the need to administer the medication on schedule.
- ○ Analgesics
  - ▪ Nonopioids should be used to avoid masking changes in the level of consciousness.
  - ▪ Nursing Considerations
    - ▫ Monitor respiratory status.
    - ▫ Monitor level of consciousness.
  - ▪ Client Education
    - ▫ Provide support for children and their families.
- • Care After Discharge
  - ○ Client Education
    - ▪ Recommend early and complete treatment for upper respiratory infections.
    - ▪ Encourage parents to maintain appropriate immunizations for children. Children should receive the Hib vaccine; pneumococcal conjugate vaccine (PCV) at 2, 4, and 6 months of age and then again between 12 and 15 months of age; and meningococcal vaccine (MCV4) between 11 and 12 years of age.

REYE SYNDROME

Overview

- Reye syndrome primarily affects the liver and brain, causing:
  - Liver dysfunction
    - Bleeding and poor blood clotting
  - Cerebral edema (with increased intracranial pressure).
    - Lethargy progressing to coma
    - Potential for cerebral herniation
- Reye syndrome has been mistaken for a variety of other disorders, including encephalitis, meningitis, poisoning, sudden infant death syndrome (SIDS), diabetes mellitus, and psychiatric illness.
- The prognosis for Reye syndrome is best with early recognition and aggressive treatment.

Data Collection

- Risk Factors
  - The cause of Reye syndrome is unknown. However, research has revealed an association between using aspirin (salicylate) products for treating viral infections and the development of Reye syndrome.
  - Manifestations most often appear at the end of a viral illness (viral upper respiratory infection, typically influenza or varicella).
- Subjective Data
  - History of recent viral illness or recent use of aspirin
- Objective Data
  - Physical Findings
    - Reye syndrome presents in clinical stages based on the severity of liver and neurologic findings.
      - Lethargy
      - Irritability
      - Combativeness
      - Confusion
      - Delirium
      - Profuse vomiting
      - Convulsions
      - Loss of consciousness
  - Laboratory Tests
    - Liver enzymes (alanine aminotransferase [ALT], aspartate aminotransferase [AST]) – elevated
    - Serum ammonia level – elevated
    - Serum electrolytes – altered due to cerebral edema and liver changes
    - Coagulation times can be extended.

- Diagnostic Procedures

  - Nursing Actions

    - Liver biopsy – A piece of liver tissue is taken using a large-bore needle and sent to the pathology department (performed by the provider).

      - Maintain NPO status prior to the procedure.

      - Monitor for hemorrhage postprocedure.

      - Monitor vital signs frequently postprocedure.

    - Client Education

      - Encourage the parents to limit the child's postprocedure activities to decrease the risk of hemorrhage.

  - CSF analysis

    - A lumbar puncture should be performed to collect CSF and rule out meningitis as a cause of manifestations (performed by a provider, usually a physician).

Patient-Centered Care

- Nursing Care

  - Maintain hydration.

    - Monitor IV site for signs of irritation or swelling. Report changes to site immediately.

    - Maintain accurate I&O.

    - Insert indwelling urinary catheter as ordered.

  - Position children to avoid extreme flexion, extension, or rotation.

    - Maintain the head in a midline neutral position.

    - Keep the head of the bed elevated 30°.

  - Monitor appropriateness of coagulation.

    - Note unexplained or prolonged bleeding.

    - Apply pressure after procedures.

    - Vitamin K may be ordered.

  - Monitor pain status and response to painful stimuli. Administer pain medications when appropriate.

  - Monitor the child's nasogastric tube.

  - Implement seizure precautions.

  - Keep the family informed of the child's status.

  - Provide private time for the family to be with the child if death is imminent.

  - Contact support for families.

- Medications
  - Osmotic diuretic – mannitol (Osmitrol)
    - To decrease cerebral swelling
    - Nursing Considerations
      - Monitor the child for increased intracranial pressure.
- Teamwork and Collaboration
  - Occupational and physical therapy may be needed to help the client adapt to neurologic deficits.
  - Dietitian may be involved if indicated.
- Care After Discharge
  - Client Education
    - Reinforce teaching to parents to avoid giving salicylates for pain or fever in children.
    - Recommend to parents to read labels of over-the-counter medications to check for the presence of salicylates.

HEAD INJURY

Overview

- Concussion is a injury to the brain that alters the way the brain functions.
- Contusion is bruising of the cerebral tissue.
- Laceration is tearing of the cerebral tissue.
- Fractures can be linear, depressed, comminuted, basilar, open, or growing.

Data Collection

- Risk Factors
  - Lack of supervision
  - Poor/absent safety practices
  - Improper use of safety devices (helmets, seat belts)
- Subjective Data
  - History of events leading up to the injury, including any reports of dizziness, headache, diplopia, and/or vomiting
  - Amnesia (loss of memory) before or after injury
  - Alcohol or drug ingestion

- Objective Data
  - Physical Findings
    - Loss of consciousness – The length of time the client is unconscious is significant.
    - Minor Injury
      - Possible loss of consciousness
      - Confusion
      - Vomiting
      - Pallor
      - Irritability
      - Drowsiness
    - Progression of Injury
      - Changes in vital signs
      - Altered mental status
    - Severe Injury
      - Increased ICP
        - ▸ Infants: bulging fontanel, separation of cranial sutures, irritability, increased sleeping, high-pitched cry, poor feeding, setting-sun sign
        - ▸ Children: nausea, headache, vomiting, blurred vision, increased sleeping, inability to follow simple commands, seizures
        - ▸ Late Signs: alterations in pupillary response, posturing (decorticate and decerebrate), bradycardia, decreased motor response, decreased sensory response, Cheyne-Stokes respirations, coma
        - ▸ Decorticate (dysfunction of the cerebral cortex) – Demonstrates the arms, wrists, and fingers flexed and bent inward onto the chest and the legs extended and adducted
        - ▸ Decerebrate (dysfunction at the midbrain) – Demonstrates a backward arching of the head and arms with legs rigidly extended and toes pointing downward

View Images
  › Decorticate Posturing   › Decerebrate Posturing

        - ▸ Flaccidity – Demonstrates no muscle tone
      - It is considered a medical emergency when a child is comatose and has asymmetric pupils or one pupil that is dilated and nonreactive.
    - CSF leakage from the nose and ears.
      - A sample of fluid that tests positive for glucose indicates CSF leakage.
    - Glasgow Coma Scale (GCS)
      - GCS score of 3, indicates deep coma.
      - GCS score of 8 or below generally defined as coma.
      - GCS score of 15 is defined as an unaltered LOC.

- Laboratory Tests
  - Arterial blood gases (ABGs)
  - Alcohol level and drug screen
  - CBC with differential
- Diagnostic Procedures
  - Cervical spine films
    - Rule out cervical spine injury.
  - CT and/or MRI scans of head and/or neck
    - Perform with and without contrast if indicated.
  - Measurement of ICP
    - The expected reference range is 10 to 15 mm Hg.
    - Client Education
      - Provide support to the children and their families.

Patient Centered Care

- Nursing Care
  - Ensure the child's spine is stabilized until spinal cord injury is ruled out.
  - Monitor vital signs, level of consciousness, pupils, ICP, motor activity, sensory perception, and verbal responses at frequent intervals. Use the Glasgow Coma Scale as indicated.
  - Maintain a patent airway. Monitor children receiving mechanical ventilation.
  - Administer oxygen as indicated to maintain an O_2 saturation level greater than 95%.
  - Maintain cervical spine stability if indicated.
  - Implement actions that will decrease ICP.
    - Keep the head of the bed elevated to 30°, which also promotes venous drainage.
    - Avoid extreme flexion, extension, or rotation of the head, and maintain in midline neutral position.
    - Keep the child's body in alignment, avoiding hip flexion/extension.
    - Minimize endotracheal or oral suctioning.
    - Instruct the child to avoid coughing and blowing her nose, because these activities increase ICP.
  - Restrain extremities as indicated to prevent pulling on tubes.
  - Implement measures to prevent complications of immobility (turn every 2 hr, maintain foot alignment and splints). Use specialty beds if indicated.
  - Maintain and monitor an indwelling urinary catheter.
  - Administer stool softener to prevent straining (Valsalva maneuver).

- Report to the provider the presence of CSF from nose or ears.
- Provide a calm, restful environment (limit visitors, minimize noise).
- Use energy conservation measures. Alternate activities with rest periods.
- Implement seizure precautions.
- Monitor fluid and electrolyte values and osmolarity to detect changes in sodium regulation, the onset of diabetes insipidus, or severe hypovolemia.
- Provide adequate fluids to maintain cerebral perfusion. When a large amount of IV fluids is ordered, monitor the child carefully for excess fluid volume, which can increase ICP.
- Maintain the child's safety (side rails up, padded side rails, call light within reach).
- Provide nutritional support (enteral nutrition).
- Maintain ongoing communication with the child.
- Reinforce teaching to the family on effective ways to communicate with the child (touching, talking, assisting with care as appropriate).

- Medications
  - Corticosteroids – dexamethasone and methylprednisolone (Solu-Medrol)
    - Decrease cerebral edema
  - Mannitol (Osmitrol)
    - Osmotic diuretic used to treat cerebral edema
    - Nursing Considerations
      - Monitor the child receiving IV infusion to treat acute cerebral edema.
      - Maintain indwelling urinary catheter to monitor fluid status and renal function.
  - Antiepileptics
    - Used to prevent or treat seizures that can occur
    - Nursing Considerations
      - Monitor therapeutic medication levels.
      - Check for medication interactions.
  - Analgesics – acetaminophen (Tylenol)
    - Used for headache/pain management
- Teamwork and Collaboration
  - Care for the child who has a head injury should include professionals from other disciplines as indicated. These may include physical, occupational, recreational and/or speech therapists.
  - Social services should be involved to provide links to social service agencies and schools.
  - Rehabilitation services may be needed.
- Surgical Interventions
  - Craniotomy – removal of part of the skull. The bone is replaced once the edema has resolved.

Complications

- Epidural Hemorrhage – bleeding between the dura and the skull
  - Clinical manifestations: short period of unconsciousness followed by a normal period leading to herniation, coma, and death
- Subdural Hemorrhage – bleeding between the dura and the arachnoid membrane
  - Can be a result of birth injury, falls or violent shaking
  - Clinical manifestations: irritability, vomiting, seizures
- Cerebral Edema – can develop within 24 to 72 hr posttrauma
  - Clinical manifestations: increased ICP
- Brain Herniation – downward shift of brain tissue
  - Clinical manifestations: loss of blinking, loss of gag reflex, pupils fail to react to light, coma, respiratory arrest

APPLICATION EXERCISES

1. A nurse is caring for a child with photophobia. Which of the following should the nurse do to reduce sensitivity?

    A. Avoid using the television.

    B. Lower the volume of the child's portable CD player.

    C. Lower the room temperature.

    D. Keep the door to the closet open at night.

2. A nurse is caring for an adolescent who has sustained a closed head injury. Which of the following are clinical manifestations of increased intracranial pressure (ICP)? (Select all that apply.)

    _____ A. Report of headache

    _____ B. Alteration in pupillary response

    _____ C. Increased motor response

    _____ D. Increased sleeping

    _____ E. Increased sensory response

3. A nurse is reviewing cerebrospinal fluid (CSF) analysis for a client who has suspected meningitis. Which of the following results indicate viral meningitis? (Select all that apply.)

    _____ A. Negative Gram stain

    _____ B. Normal glucose content

    _____ C. Cloudy color

    _____ D. Decreased WBC count

    _____ E. Normal protein content

4. A nurse in a clinic is monitoring a child who has suspected Reye syndrome. Which of the following questions should be asked of the parents when collecting data to assist in confirming the diagnosis? (Select all that apply.)

    _____ A. "Have you given your child aspirin?"

    _____ B. "Has your child had chickenpox recently?"

    _____ C. "Did your child receive ibuprofen in the last few days?"

    _____ D. "Does your child have a history of any recent upper respiratory infections?"

    _____ E. "Does your child drink adequate fluids?"

5. A nurse is caring for a toddler who has meningitis. Which of the following is the skin change that can be seen in bacterial meningitis?

    A. Discrete rose-pink macules or papules first appearing on the trunk, and then spreading outward

    B. Red pinhead-sized lesions mostly in the skin folds that scab over and slough in 5 to 7 days

    C. Reddish-purple, non-raised, bruise-like areas that appear under the skin; can be pinpoint at first and then spread rapidly

    D. Begins as a macule, becomes a papule, and finally a vesicle that is highly pruritic and then crusts over

6. A nurse is assisting with admitting a client who has Reye Syndrome. Use the ATI Active Learning Template: Systems Disorder complete this item to include the following:

    A. Description of Disorder/Disease Process

    B. Objective and Subjective Data: Identify five.

    C. Laboratory Tests: List two results indicative of Reye syndrome.

APPLICATION EXERCISES KEY

1. A. **CORRECT:** Photophobia is an abnormal sensitivity to light. Keeping the television off, closing window curtains, and using minimal lighting will decrease light exposure.

   B. INCORRECT: Regulating the volume of sounds will not affect light sensitivity.

   C. INCORRECT: Lowering the room temperature will not affect light sensitivity.

   D. INCORRECT: Keeping the closet door open at night will not affect light sensitivity.

   Ⓝ NCLEX® Connection: Reduction of Risk Potential, Potential for Alterations in Body Systems

2. A. **CORRECT:** A headache is a clinical manifestation of ICP.

   B. **CORRECT:** Alterations in pupillary response are a clinical manifestation of ICP.

   C. INCORRECT: Decreased motor response is a clinical manifestation of ICP.

   D. **CORRECT:** Increased sleeping is a clinical manifestation of ICP.

   E. INCORRECT: Decreased sensory response is a clinical manifestation of ICP.

   Ⓝ NCLEX® Connection: Reduction of Risk Potential, Potential for Alterations in Body Systems

3. A. **CORRECT:** A negative Gram stain indicates viral meningitis.

   B. **CORRECT:** Normal glucose content indicates viral meningitis.

   C. INCORRECT: A clear color indicates viral meningitis.

   D. INCORRECT: A slightly elevated WBC count indicates viral meningitis.

   E. **CORRECT:** Normal protein content indicates viral meningitis.

   Ⓝ NCLEX® Connection: Reduction of Risk Potential, Laboratory Values

4. A. INCORRECT: The cause of Reye syndrome is unknown, but there is an association with having taken aspirin for treatment of a viral infection.

   B. **CORRECT:** Manifestations of Reye syndrome most often appear at the end of a viral illness (varicella).

   C. **CORRECT:** There is no known association with ingesting ibuprofen and Reye syndrome.

   D. **CORRECT:** Manifestations most often appear at the end of a viral illness (upper respiratory infection) and Reye syndrome.

   E. INCORRECT: There is no known association with an inadequate fluid intake and Reye syndrome.

   Ⓝ NCLEX® Connection: Reduction of Risk Potential, Potential for Alterations in Body Systems

5. A. INCORRECT: Roseola rash is characterized by rose-pink macules that spread.

   B. INCORRECT: The rash of scarlet fever appears as pinhead-sized lesions mostly in skin folds that then slough.

   C. **CORRECT:** Purpura and petechia are seen with meningococcal meningitis. This skin change is characterized as a reddish-purple, non-raised, bruise-like area that appears under the skin. It can begin as pinpoint areas that then spread rapidly.

   D. INCORRECT: Chickenpox rash begins as macules, then papules, and finally progresses to vesicles.

   (N) NCLEX® Connection: Reduction of Risk Potential, Potential for Alterations in Body Systems

6. *Using the ATI Active Learning Template: Systems Disorder*

   A. Description of Disorder/Disease Process
   - Reye syndrome is a life-threatening disorder involving acute encephalopathy and fatty changes of the liver.

   B. Objective and Subjective Data
   - Recent viral illness
   - Recent use of aspirin (Bayer Children's)
   - Lethargy
   - Irritability
   - Combativeness
   - Confusion
   - Delirium
   - Profuse vomiting
   - Convulsions
   - Loss of consciousness

   C. Laboratory Tests
   - Altered serum electrolytes due to cerebral edema and liver changes
   - Possible extended coagulation times
   - Elevated liver enzymes
   - Elevated serum ammonia levels

   (N) NCLEX® Connection: Reduction of Risk Potential, Potential for Alterations in Body Systems

chapter 13

Overview

- Seizures are abnormal, excessive electrical discharges of neurons within the brain caused by a disease process.

- Seizures are classified according to their type and etiology.

- Epilepsy is chronic, recurring, and diagnosed after all other possible etiologies for the seizures have been ruled out.

Data Collection

- Risk Factors for Seizures

    ○ Some seizures have no known etiology

    ○ Febrile episode

    ○ Cerebral edema

    ○ Intracranial infection or hemorrhage

    ○ Brain tumors or cysts

    ○ Anoxia

    ○ Toxins or drugs

    ○ Lead poisoning

    ○ Tetanus, *Shigella*, or *Salmonella*

    ○ Hypoglycemia, hypocalcemia, alkalosis, hyponatremia, hypernatremia, or hypomagnesemia

- Risk Factors for Epilepsy

    ○ Trauma

    ○ Hemorrhage

    ○ Congenital defects

    ○ Anoxia

    ○ Infection

    ○ Toxins

    ○ Hypoglycemic injury

    ○ Uremia

    ○ Migraine

    ○ Cardiovascular dysfunction

- Subjective and Objective Data
  - Generalized
    - Tonic-clonic seizure (previously referred to as grand mal)
      - Onset without warning
      - Tonic phase (10 to 20 seconds)
        - Eyes roll upward
        - Loss of consciousness
        - Tonic contraction of entire body, with arms flexed and legs, head, and neck extended
        - Possible piercing cry
        - Increased salivation
        - Loss of swallowing reflex
        - Apnea leading to cyanosis
      - Clonic phase (time varies)
        - Violent jerking movements of the body
        - Can having foaming in the mouth
        - Can be incontinent
        - Gradual slowing of movements until cessation
      - Postictal state
        - Arouses with difficulty
        - Confused for several hours
        - Impairment of fine motor movements
        - Lack of coordination
        - Possible vomiting, headache, visual or speech difficulties
        - Sleeps for several hours
        - No recollection of the seizure
    - Absence seizure (previously referred to petit mal)
      - Onset between age 4 to 12 years and ceases by puberty
      - Loss of consciousness lasting 5 to 10 seconds
      - Minimal or no change in behavior
      - Resembles daydreaming or inattentiveness
      - Can drop items being held
      - Lip smacking, twitching of eyelids or face, or slight hand movements
      - Unable to recall episodes

- ○ Partial (focal/local)
  - Simple partial seizures with motor signs
    - □ Aversive seizure: eyes and head turn away from the side of focus, with or without loss of consciousness
    - □ Rolandic seizure: tonic-clonic movements involving the face and most common during sleep
  - Complex partial seizures
    - □ Altered behavior
    - □ Inability to respond to the environment
    - □ Impaired consciousness
    - □ Confusion and unable to recall event
    - □ Complex sensory aura: strange feeling in stomach that rises to the throat, auditory or visual hallucinations, feelings of fear, distorted sense of time and self
- ○ Laboratory tests depend on age, history, and physical condition.
  - Lead level
  - WBC
  - Blood glucose
  - Serum electrolytes
  - Metabolic panel
  - Chromosomal analysis
  - Toxicology screen
- ○ Diagnostic Procedures
  - Electroencephalogram (EEG) records electrical activity and can identify the origin of seizure activity.
    - □ Client Education
      - ▸ Abstain from caffeine for several hours prior to the procedure.
      - ▸ Wash hair (no oils or sprays) before and after the procedure to remove electrode gel.
      - ▸ Inform the client that he may be asked to take deep breaths or be exposed to flashes of light during the procedure.
      - ▸ If prescribed, instruct a parent to withhold sleep from the child prior to test.
        - ▹ Inform the client that he may be allowed to sleep during the test. Sleep might be withheld prior to test and might be induced during the test.
      - ▸ Inform the client that the test will not be painful.
  - Magnetic resonance imaging (MRI) is used to detect malformations, cortical dysplasia, or tumors.
  - Lumbar puncture (LP) detects infection.
  - Computed tomography (CT) scan detects hemorrhage, infarction or malformations.

Patient-Centered Care

- Nursing Care
  - Initiate seizure precautions for any child at risk.
    - Pad side rails of bed, crib, and wheelchair.
    - Keep bed free of objects that could cause injury.
    - Have suction and oxygen equipment available.
  - During a seizure
    - Protect from injury (move furniture away, hold head in lap if on the floor).
    - Maintain a position to provide a patent airway.
    - Be prepared to suction oral secretions.
    - Turn the client to the side (decreases risk of aspiration).
    - Loosen restrictive clothing.
    - Do not attempt to restrain the child.
    - Do not attempt to open the jaw or insert an airway during seizure activity (this can damage teeth, lips, or tongue). Do not use padded tongue blades.
    - Remove glasses.
    - Administer oxygen.
    - Remain with the child.
    - Note onset, time, and characteristics of seizure.
    - Allow the seizure to end spontaneously.
  - Postseizure
    - Maintain in a side-lying position to prevent aspiration and to facilitate drainage of oral secretions.
    - Check vital signs.
    - Check for injuries, including the mouth (tongue, teeth).
    - Allow for rest if necessary.
    - Reorient and calm the client (due to agitation or confusion).
    - Maintain seizure precautions, including placing the bed in the lowest position and padding the side rails to prevent future injury.
    - Note the time of the postictal period.
    - Remain with the client.
    - Do not offer food or liquids until completely awake and swallow reflex is present.
    - Encourage the client to describe the period before, during, and after the seizure activity.
    - Determine if the client experienced an aura, which can indicate the origin of seizure in the brain.
    - Try to determine the possible trigger, such as fatigue or stress.
    - Document the onset and duration of seizure and client findings/observations prior to, during, and following the seizure (level of consciousness, apnea, cyanosis, motor activity, incontinence).

- Medications
  - Antiepileptic drugs (AEDs) – diazepam (Valium), phenytoin (Dilantin), carbamazepine (Tegretol), valproic acid (Depakene), and fosphenytoin sodium (Cerebyx)
    - Medication selection is based on the client's age, type of seizure, and other medical factors.
    - A single medication is initiated at low dosage and gradually increased until seizures are controlled.
    - A second medication can be added to achieve seizure control.
    - Nursing Considerations
      - Monitor for seizure control.
      - Monitor for adverse affects.
      - Monitor therapeutic serum medication levels.
    - Client Education
      - Medications should be taken at the same time every day to enhance effectiveness.
      - Be aware of medication and food interactions that are specific to each medication.
      - Instruct the child and family about adverse affects of the medications.
- Teamwork and Collaboration
  - The school nurse should be involved in providing for the child's safety in the school setting. This can include implementation of an individualized education plan or another specialized program.
  - Referral to nutrition services if a ketogenic diet (high-fat, low-carbohydrate, and adequate protein) is prescribed.
- Surgical Interventions
  - Removal of a tumor, lesion, or hematoma
  - Focal resection of an area of the brain to remove epileptogenic zone
  - Hemispherectomy: removal of one hemisphere of the brain
  - Corpus callosotomy: separation of the two hemispheres in the brain
- Vagal nerve stimulator
  - Under general anesthesia, the stimulator is implanted into the left chest wall and connected to an electrode that is placed at the left vagus nerve. The device is then programmed to administer intermittent vagal nerve stimulation at a rate specific to the client's needs.
  - In addition to routine stimulation, the client can initiate vagal nerve stimulation by holding a magnet over the implantable device at the onset of seizure activity. This will either abort the seizure or lessen its severity.
- Client Education
  - Educate the client and family about the importance of periodic laboratory testing to monitor AED levels.
  - Encourage medication adherence.
  - Encourage the child to wear a medical alert bracelet or necklace at all times.
  - Encourage the child to wear safety devices, such as helmets, with activities.

Complications

- Status epilepticus is prolonged seizure activity that lasts longer than 30 min or continuous seizure activity in which the client does not enter a postictal phase. This acute condition requires immediate treatment to prevent loss of brain function, which can become permanent.
  - Nursing Actions
    - Maintain airway, administer oxygen, monitor IV access, assist with ECG monitoring, and monitor pulse oximetry and ABG results.
  - Client Education – Provide support for the client/family.

APPLICATION EXERCISES

1. A nurse is caring for a child who has absence seizures. Which of the following findings can the nurse expect? (Select all that apply.)

_____ A. Loss of consciousness

_____ B. Appearance of daydreaming

_____ C. Dropping held objects

_____ D. Falling to the floor

_____ E. Having a piercing cry

2. A nurse is caring for a child who just experienced a generalized seizure. Which of the following is the priority action for the nurse to take?

A. Maintain in a side-lying position.

B. Monitor vital signs.

C. Reorient the child to the environment.

D. Check for injuries.

3. A nurse is reinforcing teaching to the parent of a child who is to have an electroencephalogram (EEG). Which of the following statements by the nurse should be included in the teaching?

A. "Decaffeinated beverages should be offered on the morning of the procedure."

B. "Do not wash your child's hair the night before the procedure."

C. "Withhold all foods the morning of the procedure."

D. "Give your child an analgesic the night before the procedure."

4. A nurse is reinforcing teaching to a group of parents about the risk factors for seizures. Which of the following should be included in the teaching? (Select all that apply.)

_____ A. Febrile episodes

_____ B. Hypoglycemia

_____ C. Sodium imbalances

_____ D. Low serum lead levels

_____ E. Presence of diphtheria

5. A nurse is reviewing treatment options with the parent of a child who has worsening seizures. Which of the following should be included in the discussion? (Select all that apply.)

_____ A. Vagal nerve stimulator

_____ B. Additional antiepileptic medications

_____ C. Corpus callosotomy

_____ D. Focal resection

_____ E. Radiation therapy

6. A nurse is planning care for a child who has tonic-clonic seizures. What nursing actions should be included in the plan of care? Use the ATI Active Learning Template: Systems Disorder to complete this item to include Nursing Care: Describe nursing actions during and after a seizure.

APPLICATION EXERCISES KEY

1. A. **CORRECT:** Loss of consciousness for 5 to 10 seconds is a clinical manifestation of an absence seizure.

    B. **CORRECT:** Behavior that resembles daydreaming is a clinical manifestation of an absence seizure.

    C. **CORRECT:** A child who is having absence seizures can drop a held object.

    D. INCORRECT: Falling to the floor is a clinical manifestation of a tonic-clonic seizure.

    E. INCORRECT: The presence of a piercing cry is a clinical manifestation of a tonic-clonic seizure.

    Ⓝ NCLEX® Connection: Reduction of Risk Potential, Potential for Alterations in Body Systems

2. A. **CORRECT:** Using the airway, breathing, and circulation priority-setting framework, the first action is to place the child in a side-lying position to maintain a patent airway and prevent aspiration of secretions.

    B. INCORRECT: Monitoring the child's vital signs is an appropriate action. However, it is not the priority action.

    C. INCORRECT: Reorienting the child to the environment following a generalized seizure is an appropriate action. However, it is not the priority action.

    D. INCORRECT: Checking for injuries is an appropriate action. However, it is not the priority action.

    Ⓝ NCLEX® Connection: Physiological Adaptations, Medical Emergencies

3. A. **CORRECT:** Caffeine can alter the results of an EEG and should be avoided prior to the test.

    B. INCORRECT: The child's hair should be washed to remove oils that permit adherence of the EEG electrodes.

    C. INCORRECT: Foods are not withheld prior to an EEG.

    D. INCORRECT: Analgesics can alter the results of an EEG and should be avoided prior to the test.

    Ⓝ NCLEX® Connection: Reduction of Risk Potential, Therapeutic Procedures

4. A. **CORRECT:** Febrile episodes can cause general tonic-clonic seizures in infants and young children.

    B. **CORRECT:** Seizure activity is a late manifestation of hypoglycemia.

    C. **CORRECT:** Seizure activity is a manifestation of hyponatremia and hypernatremia.

    D. INCORRECT: High serum lead levels is a risk factor for seizure activity.

    E. INCORRECT: Diphtheria is a respiratory illness causing difficulty breathing and is not a risk factor for seizures.

    Ⓝ NCLEX® Connection: Reduction of Risk Potential, Potential for Alterations in Body Systems

5. A. **CORRECT:** The implantation of a vagal nerve stimulator is an option to provide seizure control.

B. **CORRECT:** Additional antiepileptic medication can be added to the current medication regime to control seizures.

C. **CORRECT:** A corpus callosotomy can be performed for uncontrolled seizures.

D. **CORRECT:** A focal resection can be performed for uncontrolled seizures.

E. INCORRECT: Radiation therapy is used in cancer treatment and is not used to control seizures.

 NCLEX® Connection: Reduction of Risk Potential, Potential for Alterations in Body Systems

6. *Using the ATI Active Learning Template: Systems Disorder*

- During a seizure
  - Protect the child from injury. (Move furniture away. Hold head in lap if on the floor.)
  - Position the child to maintain a patent airway.
  - Be prepared to suction oral secretions.
  - Turn the child to the side (decreases risk of aspiration).
  - Loosen restrictive clothing.
  - Do not attempt to restrain the child.
  - Do not attempt to open the jaw or insert an airway during seizure activity. (This can damage teeth, lips, or tongue.) Do not use padded tongue blades.
  - Remove glasses.
  - Administer oxygen.
  - Remain with the child.
  - Note the onset, time, and characteristics of the seizure.
  - Allow the seizure to end spontaneously.

- Postseizure
  - Maintain the child in a side-lying position to prevent aspiration and to facilitate drainage of oral secretions.
  - Check vital signs.
  - Check for injuries, including the mouth.
  - Perform neurologic checks.
  - Allow the child to rest if necessary.
  - Reorient and calm the child (she can be agitated or confused).
  - Maintain seizure precautions, including placing the bed in the lowest position and padding the side rails to prevent future injury.
  - Note the time of the postictal period.
  - Remain with the child.
  - Do not offer food or liquids until completely awake and has a swallow reflex.
  - Encourage the child to describe the period before, during, and after the seizure activity.
  - Determine if the child experienced an aura, which can indicate the origin of seizure in the brain.
  - Try to determine the possible trigger, such as fatigue or stress.
  - Document the onset and duration of seizure and client findings/observations prior to, during, and following the seizure (level of consciousness, apnea, cyanosis, motor activity, incontinence).

 NCLEX® Connection: Physiological Adaptations, Alterations in Body Systems

UNIT 2   Nursing Care of Children with System Disorders

SECTION: RESPIRATORY DISORDERS

› Oxygen and Inhalation Therapy
› Acute and Infectious Respiratory Illnesses
› Asthma
› Cystic Fibrosis

NCLEX® CONNECTIONS

When reviewing the chapters in this section, keep in mind the relevant sections of the NCLEX® outline, in particular:

Client Needs: Pharmacological Therapies	Client Needs: Reduction of Risk Potential	Client Needs: Physiological Adaptations
› Relevant topics/tasks include: » Expected Actions/Outcomes › Apply knowledge of pathophysiology when addressing client pharmacological agents. › Reinforce education to client regarding medications.	› Relevant topics/tasks include: » Diagnostic Tests › Perform diagnostic testing. » Potential for Complications from Surgical Procedures and Health Alterations › Identify client response to surgery or health alterations. » Therapeutic Procedures › Reinforce client teaching on treatments and procedures.	› Relevant topics/tasks include: » Alterations in Body Systems › Intervene to improve client respiratory status. › Reinforce education to client regarding care and condition. » Basic Pathophysiology › Identify pathophysiology related to an acute or chronic condition. › Consider general principles of client disease process when providing care. › Apply knowledge of pathophysiology to monitoring client for alterations in body systems. » Medical Emergencies › Respond/intervene to a client life-threatening situation.

chapter 14

Overview

- Oxygen is used to maintain adequate cellular oxygenation. It is used in the treatment of many acute and chronic respiratory problems (hypoxemia, cystic fibrosis, asthma). Supplemental oxygen can be delivered using a variety of methods, depending on individual circumstances.

- Pulse oximetry is used to monitor the effectiveness of inhalation therapies.

- Common treatment methods for children with respiratory issues (acute or chronic)
  - Nebulized aerosol therapy
  - Metered-dose inhaler (MDI) or dry powder inhaler (DPI)
  - Chest physiotherapy (CPT)
  - Oxygen therapy
  - Suctioning
  - Artificial airway

Pulse Oximetry

- A noninvasive measurement of the oxygen saturation (SaO_2) of arterial blood.

- A pulse oximeter is a device that is operated by battery or electricity and has a sensor probe that is attached securely to the child's fingertip, toe, earlobe, or around the foot with a clip or band.

- Indications – Pulse oximetry is used for a variety of situations in which quick assessments of a child's respiratory status are needed.

- Interpretation of Findings
  - The expected reference range for SaO_2 is 95% to 100%. Acceptable levels can range from 91% to 100%. Some illnesses can allow for an SaO_2 of 85% to 89%.
  - Results less than 91% require nursing intervention to assist the child to regain acceptable SaO_2 levels. An SaO_2 of less than 86% is a life-threatening emergency. The lower the SaO_2 level, the less accurate the value.

- Preprocedure
  - Nursing Actions
    - Find an appropriate probe site. The probe site must be dry and have adequate circulation. Remove polish from nails or remove earring if using the earlobe.
    - Be sure the child is in a comfortable position and that the arm is supported if a finger is used as a probe site.

- Intraprocedure
  - Nursing Actions
    - Note the pulse reading and compare it with the child's radial pulse. Any discrepancy warrants further investigation.
    - If continuous monitoring is required, make sure the alarms are set for a low and a high limit, the alarms are functioning, and the sound is audible. Move the probe every 4 hr or per facility policy.
- Postprocedure
  - Nursing Actions – Report unexpected findings to the provider.
    - If a child's SaO_2 is less than prescribed range (usually 90 to 92%)
      - Confirm that the sensor probe is properly placed.
      - Confirm that the oxygen delivery system is functioning and that the child is receiving the prescribed oxygen flow rate. Increase oxygen rate as needed.
      - Place the child in a semi-Fowler's or Fowler's position to maximize ventilation.
      - Encourage deep breathing.
      - Report significant findings to the provider.
      - Remain with the child, and provide emotional support to decrease anxiety.

Nebulized Aerosol Therapy

- The process of nebulization breaks up medications into minute particles that are then dispersed throughout the respiratory tract. These droplets are much finer than those created by inhalers.
- Indications – Respiratory conditions that necessitate bronchodilators, corticosteroids, mucolytics, or antibiotics.
- Nursing Actions
  - Preparation of the Client
    - Instruct the child and family that the treatment can take 10 to 15 min.
    - Determine if the child should use a mouthpiece, mask, or blow-by.
    - Obtain vital signs and oxygen saturation.
    - Pour the medication into the small container and attach the device to an air or oxygen source.
  - Ongoing Care
    - Encourage the child to take slow, deep breaths by mouth.
    - Monitor the child during the treatment.
    - Check vital signs, oxygen saturation, and lung sounds at the completion of treatment.
    - Assist the family with obtaining a nebulizer for home use if needed.
    - Enforce recommendations for aerosolized medications.
    - Monitor for adverse reactions to medications.
- Client Education
  - Inform the family how to operate a home nebulizer.
  - Inform the family about adverse affects of the prescribed medications.

Metered-Dose Inhaler (MDI) or Dry Powder Inhaler (DPI)

- These are handheld devices that allow children to self-administer medications on an intermittent basis.
- Indications – respiratory conditions that necessitate bronchodilators or corticosteroids
- Nursing Actions
  - Provide instructions to the child and parents for use of an MDI.

> **M**▷   View Animation: Metered-Dose Inhaler

  - Remove the cap from the inhaler.
  - Shake the inhaler five to six times.
  - Attach the spacer. (A spacer should be encouraged for children to facilitate proper inhalation of the medication.)
  - Hold the inhaler with the mouthpiece at the bottom.
  - Hold the inhaler with the thumb near the mouthpiece, and the index and middle fingers at the top.
  - Instruct the child on an MDI placement technique.
    - Open-mouth method: Hold the inhaler approximately 2 to 4 cm (0.8 to 1.6 in) away from the front of the mouth.
    - Closed-mouth method: Place the inhaler between the lips, and instruct the child to form a seal around the MDI.
  - Take a deep breath and then exhale.
  - Tilt the head back slightly, and press the inhaler. While pressing the inhaler, begin a slow, deep breath that lasts for 3 to 5 seconds to facilitate delivery to the air passages.
  - Hold the breath for approximately 10 seconds to allow the medication to deposit in the airways.
  - Take the inhaler out of the mouth and slowly exhale through the nose.
  - Resume normal breathing.
  - Provide instructions to the child and parents for the use of a DPI.
    - Do not shake the device.
    - Take the cover off the mouthpiece.
    - Follow the directions of the manufacturer, such as turning the wheel of the inhaler, for preparing the medication.
    - Exhale completely.
    - Place the mouthpiece between the lips, and take a deep breath through the mouth.
    - Hold breath for 5 to 10 seconds.
    - Take the inhaler out of the mouth, and slowly exhale through pursed lips.
    - Resume normal breathing.
  - If more than one puff is prescribed, instruct the child to wait the length of time directed before administering the second puff.
  - Instruct the child to remove the canister and rinse the inhaler, cap, and spacer once a day with warm running water. Instruct the child to dry the inhaler before reuse.

- Complications
  - Fungal infections
    - Fungal infections of the oral cavity can occur with corticosteroid use.
    - Nursing Actions
      - Check the mouth for signs of infection.
      - Assist the child with rinsing his mouth after administration.
    - Client Education – Instruct the child and parents to clean the MDI and spacer after each use and to have the child rinse his mouth and expectorate.

Chest Physiotherapy (CPT)

- Chest physiotherapy is a set of techniques that include percussion, vibration, and postural drainage. Gravity and positioning loosen respiratory secretions and move them into the central airways, where they can be eliminated by coughing or suctioning to rid excessive secretions from specific areas of the lungs.
- Indications
  - Client Presentation
    - Thick secretions with an inability to clear the airway
    - Contraindications – decreased cardiac reserves, pulmonary embolism, or increased intracranial pressure
- Preprocedure
  - Nursing Actions
    - Schedule treatments 1 hr before or 2 hr after meals and at bedtime to decrease the likelihood of vomiting or aspirating.
    - Administer a bronchodilator medication or nebulizer treatment prior to postural drainage if prescribed.
    - Offer an emesis basin and facial tissues.
- Intraprocedure
  - Nursing Actions
    - Perform hand hygiene, provide privacy, and explain the procedure to the child and parents.
    - Ensure proper positioning to promote drainage of specific areas of the lungs.
      - Apical sections of the upper lobes – Fowler's position
      - Posterior sections of the upper lobes – side-lying position
      - Right lobe – on the left side with a pillow under the chest wall
      - Left lobe – Trendelenburg position
    - Apply manual percussion by using cupped hand or a special device to clap rhythmically on the chest wall to break up secretions.
    - Electronic percussion is applied by a vest device worn by the child.
    - Have the child remain in each postural drainage position for 10 to 15 min to allow time for percussion, vibration, and postural drainage.
    - Discontinue the procedure if the child reports faintness or dizziness.

- Postprocedure
  - Nursing Actions
    - Perform lung auscultation and check the amount, color, and character of the expectorated secretions.
    - Document interventions and repeat the procedure as prescribed (typically two to four times per day).
- Complications
  - Hypoxia (decrease in SaO_2)
    - Nursing Actions
      - Monitor respiratory status during the procedure.
      - Discontinue the procedure if dyspnea occurs.

Oxygen Therapy

- Oxygen therapy increases the oxygen concentration of the air that is being breathed.
- Oxygen can be delivered via nasal cannula, face mask, hood, or ventilator.
  - Humidification of oxygen moistens the airways, which promotes loosening and mobilization of pulmonary secretions and prevents drying and injury of respiratory structures.
- Indication – Diagnosis of Hypoxemia
  - Hypoxemia develops when there is an inadequate level of oxygen in the blood. Hypovolemia, hypoventilation, and interruption of arterial flow can lead to hypoxemia.

EARLY SIGNS	LATE SIGNS
› Tachypnea	› Confusion and stupor
› Tachycardia	› Cyanosis of skin and mucous membranes
› Restlessness	› Bradypnea
› Pallor of the skin and mucous membranes	› Bradycardia
› Evidence of respiratory distress (use of accessory muscles, nasal flaring, tracheal tugging, adventitious lung sounds)	› Hypotension or hypertension

- Nursing Actions
  - Preparation of the Client
    - Warm oxygen to prevent hypothermia.
    - Use a calm, nonthreatening approach.
    - Explain all procedures to the child and parents.
    - Place the client in a semi-Fowler's or Fowler's position to facilitate breathing and to promote chest expansion.
    - Ensure that equipment is working properly.

- ○ Ongoing Care
  - Provide oxygen therapy at the lowest flow rate that corrects hypoxemia.
  - Monitor lung sounds and respiratory rate, rhythm, and effort to determine the need for supplemental oxygen.
  - Do not allow oxygen to blow directly onto the faces of infants.
  - Change linens and clothing frequently.
  - Monitor temperature for hypothermia.
  - Monitor oxygenation status with pulse oximetry and ABGs.
  - Apply the oxygen delivery device prescribed.
  - Provide oral hygiene as needed.
  - Promote turning, coughing, deep breathing, and use of incentive spirometry and suctioning.
  - Promote rest and decrease environmental stimuli.
  - Provide emotional support for children who appear anxious.
  - Monitor nutritional status and provide supplements as prescribed.
  - Monitor skin integrity. Provide moisture and pressure-relief devices as indicated.
  - Monitor and document response to oxygen therapy.
  - Titrate oxygen to maintain the prescribed oxygen saturation.
  - Discontinue oxygen gradually.

DELIVERY SYSTEM	NURSING IMPLICATIONS
› Oxygen hood – small plastic hood that fits over the infant's head	› Use a minimum flow rate of 4 to 5 L/min to prevent carbon dioxide buildup. › Ensure that neck, chin, or shoulders do not rub against the hood. › Secure a pulse oximeter for continuous SaO_2 monitoring.
› Nasal cannula – disposable plastic tube with two prongs for insertion into the nostrils that delivers an oxygen concentrations of 24% to 40% FiO_2 at a flow rate of 1 to 6 L/min	› Nasal cannulas are safe, easy to apply, and well tolerated. › The child is able to eat, talk, and ambulate while wearing a cannula. › Cannulas can be used by infants and older children who are cooperative. › Check the patency of the nares. › Ensure that the prongs fit in the nares properly. › A nasal cannula can cause skin breakdown and dry mucous membranes. › Supply the child with a water-soluble gel if the nares are dry. › Provide humidification for flow rates greater than 4 L/min. › Prongs can become dislodged easily. Monitor the child frequently.
› Pediatric face mask – pediatric-size mask that covers the nose and mouth	› Face masks require a snug fit and may not be tolerated. › Used for supplying high oxygen flow rate or for children who are mouth breathers.

- • Complications
  - ○ Combustion – Oxygen is combustible.
    - Nursing Actions
      - □ Place "No Smoking" or "Oxygen in Use" signs to alert others of the combustion hazard.
      - □ Know where the closest fire extinguisher is located.
      - □ Have the child wear a cotton gown, because synthetics or wools can create sparks of static electricity.

□ Ensure that all electric machinery (monitors, suction machines) are grounded.

□ Avoid toys that can induce a spark.

□ Do not use volatile, flammable materials (alcohol, acetone) near children who are receiving oxygen.

■ Client Education – Educate the child and others about the fire hazards of smoking with oxygen use.

○ Oxygen toxicity

■ Oxygen toxicity can result from high concentrations of oxygen, long duration of oxygen therapy, and the child's degree of lung disease.

□ Hypoventilation and increased $PaCO_2$ levels allow for rapid progression into unconscious state.

■ Nursing Actions

□ Use the lowest level of oxygen necessary to maintain an adequate SaO_2.

□ Monitor ABGs, and notify the provider if $PaCO_2$ levels rise outside of the expected reference range.

□ Use of an oxygen mask with continuous positive airway pressure (CPAP), bilevel positive airway pressure (BiPAP), or positive end-expiratory pressure (PEEP) while a child is on a mechanical ventilator can decrease the amount of oxygen needed.

□ Decrease the oxygen flow rate gradually.

Suctioning

• Suctioning can be accomplished orally, nasally, endotracheally, or through a tracheostomy tube.

• Indications – to remove mucus plugs and excessive secretions

○ Client Presentation

■ Early signs of hypoxemia (restlessness, tachypnea, tachycardia, decreased SaO_2 levels, adventitious breath sounds, visualization of secretions, cyanosis, absence of spontaneous cough)

• Nasal suctioning

○ Use clean technique.

○ Use a mushroom tip catheter.

• Oral suctioning

○ Use clean technique.

○ Use a hard catheter tip.

○ Insert in sides of mouth.

• Endotracheal and tracheal suctioning

○ Preprocedure

■ Nursing Actions

□ Perform hand hygiene, provide privacy, and explain the procedure to the child.

□ Don the required personal protective equipment. Assist the child to a high-Fowler's or Fowler's position for suctioning if possible.

   ▫ Perform through a tracheostomy or an endotracheal tube. Obtain a suction catheter with an outer diameter of no more than 1 cm (0.4 in) of the internal diameter of the tube.

   ▫ Ask for assistance if necessary.

   ▫ Hyperoxygenate the child using a bag-valve-mask (BVM) resuscitator or specialized ventilator function with an FiO_2 of 100%.

   ▫ Obtain baseline breath sounds and vital signs, including oxygen saturation (SaO_2) by pulse oximeter. Oxygen saturation can be monitored continually during the procedure.

   ○ Intraprocedure

      ▪ Nursing Actions

         ▫ Use correct surgical aseptic technique as identified in appropriate resources.

         ▫ Monitor oxygen status while performing the procedure.

   ○ Postprocedure

      ▪ Nursing Actions – Document the child's response.

- Complications

   ○ Hypoxia

      ▪ Nursing Actions

         ▫ Stop the procedure.

         ▫ Hyperoxygenate the child.

Artificial Airways

- A tracheotomy is a sterile surgical incision into the trachea through the skin and muscles for the purpose of establishing an airway.

- A tracheotomy can be performed as an emergency procedure or as a scheduled surgical procedure.

- A tracheostomy is the stoma/opening that results from a tracheotomy to provide and secure a patent airway. A tracheostomy can be permanent or temporary.

- Artificial airways can be placed orotracheally, nasotracheally, or through a tracheostomy to assist with respiration.

   ○ Pediatric tracheostomy tubes made of plastic have a more acute angle than adult tubes. Pediatric tracheostomy tubes soften with body temperature to shape to the contour of the child's trachea. No inner cannula is necessary, because this material resists the accumulation of dried secretions.

- Indications

   ○ Client Presentation – obstruction of the upper airway requiring the use of artificial ventilation

- Nursing Actions

   ○ Monitor:

      ▪ Oxygenation, ventilation (respiratory rate, effort, SaO_2), and vital signs hourly.

      ▪ Thickness, quantity, odor, and color of mucous secretions.

      ▪ The stoma and the skin surrounding the stoma for signs of inflammation or infection (redness, swelling, or drainage).

- ○ Provide adequate humidification and hydration to thin secretions and decrease the risk of mucus plugging.

- ○ Do not suction routinely. This can cause mucosal damage, bleeding, and bronchospasm.

- ○ Monitor the need for suctioning. Suction on a PRN basis when assessment findings indicate the need to do so (audible/noisy secretions, crackles, restlessness, tachypnea, tachycardia, and mucus in the airway).

- ○ Maintain surgical aseptic technique when suctioning to prevent infection.

- ○ Provide emotional support to the child and parents.

- ○ Provide oral hygiene, usually every 2 hr.

- ○ For cuffed tubes, keep the pressure below 20 mm Hg to reduce the risk of tracheal necrosis due to prolonged compression of tracheal capillaries.

- ○ Provide tracheostomy care every 8 hr.

- ○ Change nondisposable tracheostomy tubes every 6 to 8 weeks or per protocol.

- ○ Reposition the client every 2 hr to prevent atelectasis and pneumonia.

- ○ Keep an emergency tracheostomy tube (one size smaller) at the bedside.

- ○ Client Education

  - ▪ Provide discharge instructions regarding the following.

    - ▫ Tracheostomy care

    - ▫ Findings that the family should immediately report to the provider (signs of infection or copious secretions)

    - ▫ Ways to promote improved nutrition

- • Complications

  - ○ Accidental decannulation

    - ▪ Accidental decannulation in the first 72 hr after surgery is an emergency because the tracheostomy tract has not matured and replacement can be difficult.

    - ▪ Nursing Actions – Always have an additional staff member present when moving the tube or during any situation in which decannulation can occur.

    - ▪ Client Education

      - ▫ When caring for the tube at home, have a second tube available in the event of dislodgement.

      - ▫ Have scissors available to cut the old strings in an emergency.

  - ○ Occlusion

    - ▪ Occlusion is a situation in which the tube is clogged with secretions and prevents adequate air exchange.

    - ▪ Nursing Actions – Maintain a patent airway with suctioning.

    - ▪ Client Education – Instruct the parents about the need to suction to prevent occlusion.

APPLICATION EXERCISES

1. A nurse is reinforcing teaching to an adolescent on how to self-administer a corticosteroid medication per dry powder inhaler (DPI). Which of the following should be included in the teaching? (Select all that apply.)

_____ A. Shake the device prior to use.

_____ B. Rinse and expectorate after administration.

_____ C. Inhale with medication administration.

_____ D. Exhale quickly after medication administered.

_____ E. Attach a spacer to the device prior to use.

2. A nurse is caring for a child who is receiving oxygen therapy and is on a continuous oxygen saturation monitor that is reading 89%. Which of the following is the priority action for the nurse to take?

A. Increase the oxygen flow rate.

B. Encourage the child to take deep breaths.

C. Ensure proper placement of the sensor probe.

D. Place the child in the Fowler's position.

3. A nurse is checking a child. Which of the following is an early indication of hypoxemia?

A. Nonproductive cough

B. Hypoventilation

C. Nasal flaring

D. Nasal stuffiness

4. A nurse is caring for a child who is receiving oxygen. Which of the following is a clinical manifestations of oxygen toxicity?

A. Increased blood pressure

B. Hyperventilation

C. Decreased $PaCO_2$

D. Unconsciousness

5. A nurse is caring for a child who is receiving a bronchodilator medication by nebulized aerosol therapy. Which of the following are appropriate actions for the nurse to take? (Select all that apply.)

_____ A. Instruct the child that the treatment will last 30 min.

_____ B. Obtain vital signs prior to the procedure.

_____ C. Tell the child to take slow deep breaths.

_____ D. Determine if the child should use a mask.

_____ E. Attach the device to an air source.

6. A nurse is reinforcing teaching a child how to use a metered-dose inhaler. What information should be included in the teaching? Use the ATI Active Learning Template: Nursing Skill to complete this item.

APPLICATION EXERCISES KEY

1. A. INCORRECT: A DPI is a powder medication and should not be shaken prior to administration.

    B. **CORRECT:** Corticosteroids can cause an oral fungal infection. The client should rinse and expectorate following medication administration.

    C. **CORRECT:** The client should take a quick, deep inhalation from the device to administer the medication into the lungs.

    D. INCORRECT: After inhalation of the medication, the client should hold his breath for 5 to 10 seconds.

    E. INCORRECT: A spacer is not used with a DPI device.

    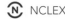 NCLEX® Connection: Pharmacological Therapies, Medication Administration

2. A. INCORRECT: Increasing the oxygen flow rate for a child who has an oxygen saturation of 89% is important, but this is not the priority action.

    B. INCORRECT: Encouraging the child to take deep breaths to increase oxygenation is important, but this is not the priority action.

    C. **CORRECT:** The first action the nurse should take using the nursing process approach is to assess. Ensuring the sensor probe is properly placed is the priority action.

    D. INCORRECT: Placing the child in Fowler's position to increase oxygenation is important, but this is not the priority action.

    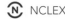 NCLEX® Connection: Physiological Adaptations, Alterations in Body Systems

3. A. INCORRECT: Nonproductive cough is a clinical manifestation of a respiratory infection.

    B. INCORRECT: Hypoventilation is a clinical manifestation of oxygen toxicity.

    C. **CORRECT:** Early signs of hypoxemia include indications of respiratory distress, such as nasal flaring.

    D. INCORRECT: Nasal stuffiness is a clinical manifestation of a respiratory infection.

    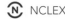 NCLEX® Connection: Physiological Adaptations, Basic Pathophysiology

4. A. INCORRECT: Increased blood pressure is not a clinical manifestation of oxygen toxicity.

    B. INCORRECT: Hypoventilation is a clinical manifestation of oxygen toxicity.

    C. INCORRECT: An increased $PaCO_2$ is a clinical manifestation of oxygen toxicity.

    D. **CORRECT:** Children who exhibit oxygen toxicity progress into an unconscious state rapidly.

    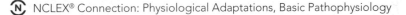 NCLEX® Connection: Physiological Adaptations, Basic Pathophysiology

5. A. INCORRECT: Nebulized medications take approximately 10 to 15 min to deliver.

    B. **CORRECT:** Baseline vital signs should be obtain prior to a nebulized medication for purposes of comparison with how the client tolerates the medication.

    C. **CORRECT:** The client should take slow, deep breaths to inhale the medication deeply into the respiratory tract.

    D. **CORRECT:** Nebulized medications can be delivered by mask, mouthpiece, or blow-by. The nurse should determine the best method of delivery.

    E. **CORRECT:** Nebulized medications need to have an air source to break the medication into small particles for inhalation.

    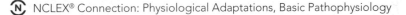 NCLEX® Connection: Pharmacological Therapies, Expected Actions/Outcomes

6. *Using the ATI Active Learning Template: Nursing Skill*
    - How To Use a Metered-Dose Inhaler
      ○ Remove the cap from the inhaler
      ○ Shake the inhaler five or six times.
      ○ Attach the spacer. (A spacer should be encouraged for children to facilitate proper inhalation of the medication.)
      ○ Hold the inhaler with the mouthpiece at the bottom.
      ○ Hold the inhaler with the thumb near the mouthpiece and the index and middle fingers at the top.
        - Open-mouth technique: Hold the inhaler approximately 2 to 4 cm (0.8 to 1.6 in) away from the front of the mouth.
        - Closed-mouth method: Place the inhaler between the lips and instruct the child to form a seal around the inhaler.
      ○ Take a deep breath, and then exhale.
      ○ Tilt the head back slightly, and press the inhaler. While pressing the inhaler, begin a slow, deep breath that lasts for 3 to 5 seconds to facilitate delivery to the air passages.
      ○ Hold the breath for approximately 10 seconds to allow the medication to deposit in the airways.
      ○ Take the inhaler out of the mouth and slowly exhale through the nose.
      ○ Resume normal breathing.

     NCLEX® Connection: Pharmacological Therapies, Medication Administration

chapter 15

Overview

- Acute and infectious respiratory illnesses prevalent in children include tonsillitis, nasopharyngitis, pharyngitis, croup syndromes, bacterial tracheitis, bronchitis, bronchiolitis, allergic rhinitis, and pneumonia.

TONSILLITIS AND TONSILLECTOMY

Overview

- Tonsils are masses of lymph-type tissue found in the pharyngeal area. They filter pathogenic organisms (viral and bacterial), which helps to protect the respiratory and gastrointestinal tracts. In addition, they contribute to antibody formation.

- Palatine tonsils are located on both sides of the oropharynx. These are the tonsils removed during a tonsillectomy.

- Other tonsils are the pharyngeal tonsils, also known as the adenoids. These are removed during an adenoidectomy.

- Tonsils are highly vascular, which helps them to protect against infection because foreign materials, such as viral or bacterial organisms, enter the body through the mouth.

- In some instances, enlarged tonsils can block the nose and throat. This can interfere with breathing, nasal and sinus drainage, sleeping, swallowing, and speaking.

- Enlarged tonsils also can disrupt the function of the eustachian tube, which can impede hearing.

- Acute tonsillitis occurs when the tonsils become inflamed and reddened. Small patches of yellowish pus also can become visible. Acute tonsillitis can become chronic.

Data Collection

- Risk Factors
  - Exposure to a viral or bacterial agent
  - Immature immune systems (younger children)
- Subjective Data
  - Report of sore throat with difficulty swallowing
  - History of otitis media and hearing difficulties

- Objective Data
  - Physical Assessment Findings
    - Mouth odor
    - Mouth breathing
    - Snoring
    - Nasal qualities in the voice
    - Fever
    - Tonsil inflammation with redness and edema
  - Laboratory Tests
    - Throat culture for group A β-hemolytic Streptococci (GABHS)

Patient-Centered Care

- Nursing Care
  - Tonsillitis
    - Provide symptomatic treatment for viral tonsillitis (rest, cool fluids, warm salt-water gargles).
    - Administer antibiotic therapy for bacterial tonsillitis.
- Medications
  - Antipyretics – acetaminophen (Tylenol) or ibuprofen (Advil)
    - Antipyretics decrease fever and manage pain.
    - Nursing Considerations – Be aware of allergies.
    - Client Education – Advise parents of the appropriate dosing for acetaminophen and ibuprofen.
  - Antibiotics – IM penicillin G, erythromycin, azithromycin, cephalosporins, amoxicillin
    - Nursing Considerations – Be aware of allergies.
    - Client Education – Tell parents to administer antibiotics for the full course of treatment.
- Therapeutic Procedures
  - Tonsillectomy
    - Nursing Actions
      - Preoperative – Maintain NPO status.
      - Postoperative

NURSING CONSIDERATION	NURSING ACTIONS
Positioning	› Place in side-lying position or on abdomen to facilitate drainage. › Elevate head of bed when child is fully awake.
Data Collection	› Observe for evidence of bleeding (frequent swallowing, clearing the throat, restlessness, bright red emesis, tachycardia, pallor). › Monitor the airway and vital signs. › Monitor for difficulty breathing related to oral secretions, edema, or bleeding.

NURSING CONSIDERATION	NURSING ACTIONS
Comfort measures	› Administer analgesics (acetaminophen and codeine). › Provide an ice collar. › Offer ice chips or sips of water to keep throat moist. › Administer pain medication on a regular schedule.
Diet	› Encourage clear liquids and fluids after a return of the gag reflex, initially avoiding red-colored liquids, citrus juice, and milk-based foods. › Advance the diet with soft, bland foods.
Instruction	› Discourage coughing, throat clearing, and nose blowing in order to protect the surgical site. › Refrain from placing pointed objects in the back of the mouth. › Alert parents that there can be clots or blood-tinged mucus in vomitus.

- Client Education
    - Instruct the family to notify the provider if bright-red bleeding occurs.
    - Encourage the child to rest.
- Care After Discharge
    - Client Education
        - Instruct the parents to contact the provider if the child experiences difficulty breathing, lack of oral intake, increase in pain, or indications of infection.
        - Tell the parents to ensure that the child does not put anything sharp (popsicle stick, straw, pointed object) in the mouth.
        - Tell the parents to administer pain medications for discomfort.
        - Encourage fluid intake and diet advancement to a soft diet with no spicy foods or hard, sharp foods like corn chips until full recovery.
        - Instruct the child and family to limit strenuous activity and physical play with no swimming for 2 weeks as prescribed.
        - Instruct the child and family that full recovery usually occurs in approximately 14 days.
        - Inform the family of clinical manifestations of hemorrhage, dehydration, and infection, and when to notify the provider.

Complications

- Hemorrhage
    - Nursing Actions
        - Use a good light source and possibly a tongue depressor to directly observe the throat.
        - Monitor for findings of bleeding (tachycardia, repeated swallowing and clearing of throat, hemoptysis). Hypotension is a late sign of shock.
        - Contact the provider immediately if there is any indication of bleeding.
    - Client Education
        - Instruct the family to report indications of bleeding (frequent swallowing, clearing the throat, restlessness, bright red emesis, tachycardia, pallor).

- Dehydration
  - Nursing Actions
    - Encourage oral fluids.
    - Monitor I&O.
  - Client Education
    - Instruct the family to encourage oral fluids.
    - Inform the family about clinical manifestations of dehydration.
- Chronic infection
  - Chronically infected tonsils with group A β-hemolytic streptococci can pose a potential threat to other parts of the body. Some children who frequently have tonsillitis can develop other diseases, such as rheumatic fever and kidney infection.
  - Client Education – Instruct the family to seek medical attention when the child presents with manifestations of tonsillitis.

COMMON RESPIRATORY ILLNESSES

Overview

- Disorders can affect both the upper (nasopharynx, pharynx, larynx, and upper part of the trachea) and lower (lower trachea, mainstem bronchi, segmental bronchi, subsegmental bronchioles, terminal bronchioles, and alveoli) respiratory tracts.
- Infections of the respiratory tract can affect more than one area.

Data Collection

- Risk Factors
  - Age
    - Infants between 3 and 6 months of age are at an increased risk due to the decrease of maternal antibodies acquired at birth and the lack of antibody protection.
    - Viral infections are more common in toddlers and preschoolers. The incidence of these infections decreases by age 5.
    - Certain viral agents can cause serious illness during infancy, but only cause a mild illness in older children.
  - Anatomy
    - A short, narrow airway can become easily obstructed with mucus or edema.
    - A short respiratory tract allows infections to travel quickly to the lower airways.
    - Infants and young children have small surface areas for gas exchange.
    - Infectious agents have easy access to the middle ear through the short and open eustachian tubes of infants and young children.

- ○ Decreased resistance
  - ▪ Compromised immune system
  - ▪ Anemia
  - ▪ Nutritional deficiencies
  - ▪ Allergies
  - ▪ Chronic medical conditions (asthma, cystic fibrosis, congenital heart disease)
  - ▪ Exposure to second-hand smoke
- ○ Seasonal variables
  - ▪ Children with asthma have a greater incidence of respiratory infections during cold weather.
  - ▪ Respiratory syncytial virus (RSV) and other common respiratory infections are more common during the winter and spring.
  - ▪ Infections caused by *Mycoplasma pneumoniae* are more frequent during autumn and early winter.
- Subjective Data
  - ○ Nursing history that includes recent infections, medications taken, immunization status, and family coping
  - ○ Reports of sore throat, decreased activity level, chest pain, fatigue, difficulty breathing, shortness of breath, cough, and decreased appetite
- Objective Data
  - ○ Physical Assessment Findings

RESPIRATORY ILLNESS	CLINICAL MANIFESTATIONS
› Nasopharyngitis (common cold) » Self-limiting virus that persists for 7 to 10 days	› Nasal inflammation, rhinorrhea, cough, dry throat, sneezing, and nasal qualities in voice › Fever, decreased appetite, and irritability
› Bacterial tracheitis » Infection of the lining of the trachea	› Thick, purulent drainage from the trachea that can obstruct the airway and cause respiratory distress › Fever, croupy cough, stridor
› Bronchitis (tracheobronchitis) » Associated with an upper respiratory infection (URI) and inflammation of large airways » Self-limiting and requires symptomatic relief	› Persistent cough as a result of inflammation › Resolves in 5 to 10 days
› Bronchiolitis » Mostly caused by RSV » Primarily affects the bronchi and bronchioles » Occurs at the bronchiolar level	› Rhinorrhea – intermittent fever, cough, and wheezing › Coughing that progresses toward wheezing, increased respiratory rate, nasal flaring, retractions, and cyanosis › Possible posttussive vomiting due to coughing

RESPIRATORY ILLNESS	CLINICAL MANIFESTATIONS
› Allergic rhinitis » Caused by seasonal reaction to allergens most often in the autumn or spring	› Watery rhinorrhea › Nasal congestion › Itchiness of the nose, eyes, and pharynx › Itchy, watery eyes › Nasal quality of the voice › Dry, scratchy throat › Snoring › Poor sleep leading to poor performance in school › Fatigue
› Pneumonia (RSV, *Streptococcus pneumoniae, Haemophilus influenzae, Mycoplasma pneumoniae*)	› High fever › Cough that can be unproductive or productive of white sputum › Retractions and nasal flaring › Rapid, shallow respirations › Report of chest pain › Adventitious breath sounds (rhonchi, crackles) › Pale color that progresses to cyanosis › Irritability, anxiety, agitation, and fatigue › Abdominal pain, diarrhea, lack of appetite, and vomiting › Sudden onset, usually following a viral infection (bacterial pneumonia)
Croup Syndromes	
› Bacterial epiglottitis (acute supraglottitis) » Medical emergency » Caused by *Haemophilus influenzae*	› Predictive signs – absence of cough, drooling, and agitation › Sitting with chin pointing out, mouth opened, and tongue protruding › Dysphonia (hoarseness or difficulty speaking) › Dysphagia (difficulty swallowing) › Inspiratory stridor (noisy inspirations) › Sore throat, high fever, and restlessness
› Acute laryngotracheobronchitis » Causative agents include RSV, influenza A and B, and *Mycoplasma pneumoniae*	› Low-grade fever › Restlessness › Hoarseness › Barky cough › Dyspnea › Inspiratory stridor › Retractions

RESPIRATORY ILLNESS	CLINICAL MANIFESTATIONS
Croup Syndromes	
› Acute spasmodic laryngitis » Self-limiting illness that can result from allergens	› Barky cough › Restlessness › Difficulty breathing › Hoarseness › Nighttime episodes of laryngeal obstruction
› Influenza A and B » Mild, moderate, or severe	› Sudden onset of fever and chills › Dry throat and nasal mucosa › Dry cough › Flushed face › Photophobia › Myalgia › Fatigue

- ○ Laboratory Tests
  - ▪ Blood samples
    - ▫ Elevated serum antistreptolysin O (ASO) titer
    - ▫ Elevated C-reactive protein (CRP) or sedimentation rate in response to an inflammatory reaction
    - ▫ CBC to check for anemia and infection
  - ▪ Sputum culture and sensitivity to detect infection
- ○ Diagnostic Procedures
  - ▪ Collection of direct aspiration of nasal secretions
    - ▫ The secretions are collected for immunofluorescence analysis to detect RSV. Instill 1 to 3 mL of 0.9% sodium chloride into one of the child's nostrils. The fluid is then aspirated for evaluation.
    - ▫ Nursing Actions
      - ▸ Place the child in a supine position.
      - ▸ Use a sterile syringe without a needle.
    - ▫ Client Education – Caregivers should be educated about the potential need for isolation, dependent on the results of laboratory tests.
  - ▪ Chest x-ray
    - ▫ Identifies infiltration in pneumonia
    - ▫ Nursing Actions – Ensure the child is positioned correctly to avoid the need for a repeat x-ray.
    - ▫ Client Education – Inform adolescents of childbearing age of the need for confirmation of nonpregnant status.

Patient-Centered Care

- Nursing Care
  - Closely monitor progression of illness and ensuing respiratory distress. Observe for increased heart and respiratory rate, retractions, nasal flaring, and restlessness.
  - Make emergency equipment for intubation readily accessible.
  - Position the child to have optimal ventilation without increasing distress that would contribute to increasing respiratory distress.
  - Implement isolation precautions if indicated.
- Nasopharyngitis – Instruct parents about home management.
  - Administer antipyretic for fever.
  - Encourage rest.
  - Provide vaporized air (cool mist).
  - Administer decongestants for children older than 1 year.
  - Administer cough suppressants with caution (avoid oversedation).
  - Antihistamines are not recommended.
  - Antibiotics are not indicated.
- Bacterial tracheitis
  - Administer oxygen.
  - Monitor continuous oximetry.
  - Administer antipyretics for fever.
  - Administer IV antibiotics.
- Bronchitis – Instruct parents about home management.
  - Administer antipyretics for fever.
  - Administer a cough suppressant.
  - Provide increased humidity (cool mist vaporizer).
- Bronchiolitis
  - Provide humidified oxygen.
  - Monitor continuous oximetry.
  - Encourage fluid intake if tolerated.
  - Administer IV fluids if oral intake not tolerated.
  - Suction nasopharynx as needed.
  - Administer nebulized bronchodilator.
  - Corticosteroids and antihistamines are not recommended.
  - Antibiotics are not recommended for RSV.
  - Chest percussion and postural drainage is not recommended.
  - Ribavirin administration is controversial.

- Allergic rhinitis – Instruct parents about home management.
  - Avoid allergens.
  - Administer antihistamines.
  - Administer nasal corticosteroids.
- Pneumonia
  - Viral (symptom management)
    - Administer oxygen with cool mist.
    - Monitor continuous oximetry.
    - Administer antipyretics for fever.
    - Monitor I&O.
  - Bacterial
    - Encourage rest.
    - Promote increased oral intake.
    - Monitor I&O.
    - Administer antipyretics for fever.
    - Chest percussion and postural drainage are controversial.
    - Administer IV fluids.
    - Administer oxygen.
    - Monitor continuous oximetry.
    - Administer IV antibiotics.
- Bacterial epiglottitis
  - Protect airway.
    - Avoid throat culture or using a tongue blade.
  - Prepare for intubation.
  - Provide humidified oxygen.
  - Monitor continuous oximetry.
  - Administer racemic epinephrine, corticosteroids, and IV fluids.
  - Administer antibiotic therapy (ceftriaxone sodium or cephalosporin), starting with IV, then transition to oral to complete a 10-day course.
- Acute laryngotracheobronchitis and acute spasmodic laryngitis
  - Provide humidity with cool mist.
  - Administer oxygen if needed.
  - Monitor continuous oximetry.
  - Administer nebulized racemic epinephrine.
  - Administer corticosteroids: oral (prednisone), IM (dexamethasone), or nebulized (budesonide).
  - Encourage oral intake if tolerated.
  - Administer IV fluids.

- Influenza – Instruct parents about home management.
  - Promote increased fluid intake.
  - Suggest rest.
  - Administer medications.
    - Amantadine (Symmetrel) – for type A
      - Shortens the length of the illness.
      - Administer within 24 to 48 hr of onset of symptoms.
    - Rimantadine (Flumadine) – for type A
      - Treats manifestations.
      - Administer orally two times per day for 7 days for children older than 1 year.
    - Zanamivir (Relenza) – for type A and B
      - Treatment of influenza for children 7 and older or for prophylaxis for children 5 and older.
      - Start within 48 hr of manifestations.
      - Inhaled two times per day for 5 days.
    - Oseltamivir (Tamiflu) – for type A and B
      - Decreases manifestations.
      - Give orally for 5 days for children older than 1 year.
      - Start within 48 hr of manifestations.
    - Influenza vaccine – prevention
      - Recommended for children 6 months and older.
      - Live vaccination should not be used in clients who are immunocompromised, have respiratory conditions, are pregnant, or have a history of Guillain-Barre syndrome.
    - Antipyretic (pain or fever)
- Care After Discharge
  - Use a cool-air vaporizer to provide humidity.
  - Recommend rest during febrile illness.
  - Maintain adequate fluid intake. Infants can be given commercially prepared oral rehydration solutions, and older children can be given sports drinks.
  - Apply ice or warm pack to the neck to decrease pain from enlarged cervical nodes.
  - Administer medications using accurate dosages and appropriate time intervals.
  - Recommend strategies to decrease the spread of infection: performing good hand hygiene; covering the nose and mouth with tissues when sneezing and coughing; properly disposing of tissues; not sharing cups, eating utensils, or towels; and keeping infected children from contact with children who are well.
  - Seek further medical attention for the child if manifestations worsen or respiratory distress occurs.

Complications

- Pneumothorax – accumulation of air in the pleural space
  - ○ Clinical manifestations – dyspnea, chest pain, back pain, labored respirations, decreased oxygen saturations, and tachycardia
  - ○ Nursing Interventions
    - ▪ Prepare client for an emergent needle aspiration with insertion of chest tube to closed drainage.
    - ▪ Provide for chest tube management.
    - ▪ Monitor respiratory status.
    - ▪ Administer oxygen.
- Pleural effusion – accumulation of fluid in the pleural space
  - ○ Clinical manifestations – dyspnea, chest pain, back pain, labored respirations, decreased oxygen saturations, and tachycardia
  - ○ Nursing Interventions
    - ▪ Prepare the client for an emergent needle aspiration with insertion of chest tube to closed drainage.
    - ▪ Provide for chest tube management.
    - ▪ Monitor respiratory status.
    - ▪ Administer oxygen.

APPLICATION EXERCISES

1. A nurse is caring for a child who has bronchiolitis. Which of the following are appropriate actions for the nurse to take? (Select all that apply.)

_____ A. Administer oral prednisone.

_____ B. Initiate chest percussion and postural drainage.

_____ C. Administer humidified oxygen.

_____ D. Suction the nasopharynx as needed.

_____ E. Administer oral penicillin.

2. A nurse is reinforcing teaching to a group of parents about influenza. Which of the following should be included in the teaching?

A. "Amantadine will prevent the illness."

B. "Rimantadine is administered intramuscularly."

C. "Zanamivir can be given to children 1 year and older."

D. "Oseltamivir should be given within 48 hours of onset of symptoms."

3. A nurse is caring for a child who is in the postoperative period following a tonsillectomy. Which of the following is a clinical finding of postoperative bleeding?

A. Hgb 11.6 and Hct 37%

B. Inflamed and reddened throat

C. Frequent swallowing and clearing of the throat

D. Blood-tinged mucus

4. A nurse is caring for a child in the postoperative period following a tonsillectomy. Which of the following is an appropriate action for the nurse to take?

A. Encourage the child to blow her nose gently.

B. Administer analgesics on a schedule.

C. Offer orange juice.

D. Position the child supine.

5. A nurse is checking a child. Which of the following are clinical manifestations of epiglottitis? (Select all that apply.)

_____ A. Hoarseness and difficulty speaking

_____ B. Difficulty swallowing

_____ C. Low-grade fever

_____ D. Drooling

_____ E. Dry, barky cough

_____ F. Stridor

6. A nurse is reinforcing teaching to the parent of a child who has an infectious respiratory illness. What should be included in the teaching? Use the ATI Active Learning Template: Basic Concept to complete this item to include Related Content: Identify at least three strategies to decrease the spread of infection.

APPLICATION EXERCISES KEY

1. A. INCORRECT: Corticosteroids are not indicated for a client who has bronchiolitis.

    B. INCORRECT: Chest percussion and postural drainage are not indicated for a client who has bronchiolitis.

    C. **CORRECT:** Administering humidified oxygen provides moisture to the airway and is an appropriate action for the nurse to take.

    D. **CORRECT:** Suctioning the nasopharynx will assist the client to clear secretions and is an appropriate action for the nurse to take.

    E. INCORRECT: Antibiotics are not indicated for a client who has bronchiolitis.

    Ⓝ NCLEX® Connection: Physiological Adaptations, Alterations in Body Systems

2. A. INCORRECT: Amantadine can shorten the length of the illness.

    B. INCORRECT: Rimantadine is administered orally two times per day for 7 days.

    C. INCORRECT: Zanamivir is approved for children over the age of 5 years.

    D. **CORRECT:** Oseltamivir decrease flu manifestations in clients who have findings for less than 48 hr.

    Ⓝ NCLEX® Connection: Pharmacological Therapies, Expected Actions/Outcomes

3. A. INCORRECT: Hgb 11.6 and Hct 37% are within the expected reference range.

    B. INCORRECT: An inflamed and reddened throat is an expected finding following a tonsillectomy.

    C. **CORRECT:** Frequent swallowing and clearing of the throat indicates that there is an increased amount of fluid in the back of the throat, which is a clinical finding in the client who is experiencing postoperative bleeding.

    D. INCORRECT: Blood-tinged mucus is an expected finding following a tonsillectomy.

    Ⓝ NCLEX® Connection: Reduction of Risk Potential, Potential for Complications from Surgical Procedures and Health Alterations

4. A. INCORRECT: Blowing the nose causes pressure and could increase the risk of bleeding.

   B. **CORRECT:** Analgesics should be administered on a scheduled basis to provide pain relief.

   C. INCORRECT: Citrus juices, such as orange juice, can cause discomfort and should be avoided postoperatively.

   D. INCORRECT: The client should be positioned on the abdomen or side-lying following a tonsillectomy.

   (N) NCLEX® Connection: Pharmacological Therapies, Expected Actions/Outcomes

5. A. **CORRECT:** Hoarseness and difficulty speaking are clinical manifestations of epiglottitis.

   B. **CORRECT:** Difficulty swallowing is a clinical manifestation of epiglottitis.

   C. INCORRECT: A high fever is a clinical manifestation of epiglottitis.

   D. **CORRECT:** Drooling is a clinical manifestation of epiglottitis.

   E. INCORRECT: Dry, barky cough is a clinical manifestation of croup.

   F. **CORRECT:** Stridor is a clinical manifestation of epiglottitis.

   (N) NCLEX® Connection: Physiological Adaptations, Medical Emergencies

6. *Using the ATI Active Learning Template: Basic Concept*
   - Related Content
     - Perform appropriate hand hygiene.
     - Cover the nose and mouth with tissues when sneezing and coughing.
     - Dispose of tissues properly.
     - Do not share cups, eating utensils, or towels.
     - Keep infected children from contact with children who are well.

   (N) NCLEX® Connection: Physiological Adaptations, Alterations in Body Systems

UNIT 2   NURSING CARE OF CHILDREN WITH SYSTEM DISORDERS
         SECTION: RESPIRATORY DISORDERS

CHAPTER 16   Asthma

Overview

- Asthma is a chronic inflammatory disorder of the airways that results in intermittent and reversible airflow obstruction of the bronchioles.

- The obstruction occurs either by inflammation or airway hyper-responsiveness.

 View Video: Asthma

- Asthma diagnoses are based on symptoms and classified into four categories.

  - Intermittent – Symptoms occur two or fewer times per week. Nighttime symptoms two or fewer per month. No interference with normal activity. Uses short-acting β-agonist less than two times per week.

  - Mild persistent – Symptoms occur more than twice a week, but not daily. Nighttime symptoms one to two times per month for 0- to 4-year-old and three to four times per month for 5- to 11-year-old. Minor limitations with activity. Uses short-acting β-agonist more than 2 days per week but not daily.

  - Moderate persistent – Daily symptoms. Nighttime symptoms three to four times a month for 0- to 4-year-old and more than one time per week, but not daily for 5- to 11-year-old. Some limitation in activity. Uses short-acting β-agonist daily.

  - Severe persistent – Symptoms occur continually. Nighttime symptoms more than one time per week for 0- to 4-year-old and nightly for 5- to 11-year-old. Limited activity. Uses short-acting β-agonist several times per day.

Data Collection

- Risk Factors

  - Family history of asthma

  - Family history of allergies

  - Allergies

- Triggers to asthma

  - Allergens

    - Indoor: mold, cockroach, house dust mites

    - Outdoor: grass, pollen, trees, shrubs, molds, spores, air pollution

  - Exercise/activity

  - Cold air or changes in weather

- ○ Tobacco smoke
- ○ Infections/colds
- ○ Animal hair or dander
- ○ Medications
- ○ Strong odors
- ○ Emotions
- ○ Gastroesophageal reflux
- ○ Food allergies or additives
- Subjective Data
  - ○ Chest tightness
  - ○ History regarding current and previous asthma exacerbations
    - Onset and duration
    - Precipitating factors
    - Changes in medication regimen
    - Medications that relieve symptoms
    - Other medications
    - Self-care methods used to relieve symptoms
- Objective Data
  - ○ Physical Findings
    - Dyspnea
    - Cough
    - Audible wheezing
    - Coarse lung sounds, wheezing throughout possible crackles
    - Mucus production
    - Restlessness
    - Anxiety
    - Red ears, dark red lips
    - Sweating
    - Use of accessory muscles
    - Decreased oxygen saturation (low SaO_2)
  - ○ Laboratory Tests – CBC

○ Diagnostic Procedures

▪ Pulmonary function tests (PFTs) are the most accurate tests for diagnosing asthma and its severity.

□ Baseline test at time of diagnosis

□ After treatment is initiated and child is stabilized

□ Yearly testing

▪ Peak expiratory flow rates

□ Measures the amount of air that can be forcefully exhaled in 1 second

□ Each child needs to establish personal best

▪ Bronchoprovocation testing

□ Exposure to methacholine, cold air, or histamine

□ Exercise challenge

▪ Skin prick testing (SPT)

□ Identify allergens that trigger asthma

▪ Chest x-ray showing hyperexpansion and infiltrates

Patient-Centered Care

• Nursing Care

○ Monitor airway patency, respiratory rate, symmetry, effort, and use of accessory muscles.

○ Check breath sounds in all lung fields.

○ Monitor for shortness of breath, dyspnea, and audible wheezing. An absence of wheezing can indicate severe constriction of the alveoli.

○ Monitor vital signs and oxygen saturation.

○ Check CBC, chest x-ray results, and possible ABGs.

○ Position the child to maximize ventilation.

○ Administer oxygen therapy as prescribed.

○ Initiate and maintain IV access as prescribed.

○ Maintain a calm and reassuring demeanor.

○ Encourage appropriate vaccinations and prompt medical attention for infections.

○ Administer medications as prescribed.

○ Antibiotics are not used to treat asthma, only if a bacterial infection is confirmed.

- Medications
  - Bronchodilators (inhalers)
    - Short-acting beta$_2$-agonists (albuterol [Proventil], levalbuterol [Xopenex], terbutaline [Brethine])
      - Used for acute exacerbations
      - Prevention of exercised-induced asthma
    - Cholinergic antagonists (anticholinergic medications), such as ipratropium (Atrovent), block the parasympathetic nervous system, providing relief of acute bronchospasms.
    - Nursing Considerations
      - Instruct the child and family in the proper use of MDI, DPI, or nebulizer.
      - Watch the child for tremors and tachycardia when taking albuterol.
      - Observe the child for dry mouth when taking ipratropium.
    - Client Education
      - Encourage older children who are taking ipratropium to suck on hard candies to help with dry mouth.
      - Advise children to administer prior to exercise or activity.
  - Anti-inflammatory agents
    - Anti-inflammatory agents decrease airway inflammation.
    - Corticosteroids
      - Methylprednisolone (Solu-Medrol)
      - Prednisone
    - Leukotriene modifiers (montelukast [Singulair]), mast cell stabilizers (cromolyn sodium), and monoclonal antibodies (omalizumab [Xolair])
    - Combination medications
      - Fluticasone/salmeterol (Advair)
      - Inhaled corticosteroid/long-acting beta$_2$-agonist)
    - Nursing Considerations
      - Observe oral mucosa for infection secondary to use of inhaled medication.
      - Monitor weight, blood pressure, electrolytes, glucose, and growth with oral corticosteroid use.
    - Client Education
      - Encourage the child to drink plenty of fluids to promote hydration.
      - Encourage the child to take a oral corticosteroids with food.
      - Instruct the child to rinse her mouth after the use of a corticosteroid inhaler.
      - Instruct the child and family to watch for redness, sores, or white patches in the mouth, and report them to the provider.
      - Instruct the family to follow prescription for medication administration (dosage, tapering off medication, length of time to take).

- Teamwork and Collaboration
  - ○ Consult respiratory services for inhalers and breathing treatments.
  - ○ Contact nutritional services for weight loss or gain related to medications or diagnosis.
  - ○ Consult rehabilitation if the child has prolonged weakness and needs assistance with increasing level of activity.
- Care After Discharge
  - ○ Client Education
    - Instruct the child and family to identify personal triggering agents.
    - Assist the child in avoiding triggering agents.
    - Provide the child and family with an asthma action plan.
    - Instruct the child how to use a peak flow meter.
      - □ Use same time each day.
      - □ Ensure the marker is zeroed.
      - □ Stand up straight.
      - □ Close lips tightly around the mouthpiece (ensure the tongue is not occluding).
      - □ Blow out as hard and as quickly as possible.
      - □ Read the number on the meter.
      - □ Repeat two more times (wait at least 30 seconds between attempts).
      - □ Record highest number.
    - Instruct the child and family how to recognize an asthma exacerbation.
    - Inform the child and family about when to use each of the prescribed medications (rescue vs. maintenance medications).
    - Instruct the child how to properly self-administer medications (nebulizers, inhalers, and spacer).
    - Educate the child and family regarding infection prevention techniques.
      - □ Promote good nutrition.
      - □ Reinforce importance of good hand hygiene.
    - Encourage prompt medical attention for infections.
    - Stress the importance of keeping immunizations, including seasonal influenza and pneumonia vaccines, up to date.
    - Encourage regular exercise as part of asthma therapy.
      - □ Promotes ventilation and perfusion
      - □ Maintains cardiac health
      - □ Enhances skeletal muscle strength
    - Children can require medication before exercise.

Complications

- Status asthmaticus
  - This life-threatening episode of airway obstruction is often unresponsive to common treatment.
  - Manifestations include wheezing, labored breathing, nasal flaring, lack of air movement in lungs, use of accessory muscles, distended neck veins, and risk for cardiac and/or respiratory arrest.
  - Nursing Actions
    - Monitor oxygen saturations continuously.
    - Place on continuous cardiorespiratory monitoring.
    - Position the child sitting upright, standing, or leaning slightly forward.
    - Administer humidified oxygen.
    - Administer three nebulizer treatments of a beta$_2$-agonist 20 to 30 min apart or continuously. Ipratropium bromide can be added to the nebulizer to increase bronchodilation.
    - Obtain IV access.
    - Monitor ABGs and serum electrolytes.
    - Administer corticosteroid.
    - Assist with emergency intubation.
- Respiratory failure
  - Persistent hypoxemia related to asthma can lead to respiratory failure.
  - Nursing Action
    - Monitor oxygenation levels and acid-base balance.

APPLICATION EXERCISES

1. A nurse is checking a child who has asthma. Which of the following are indications of deterioration in the child's respiratory status? (Select all that apply.)

_____ A. Oxygen saturation 95%

_____ B. Wheezing

_____ C. Retraction of sternal muscles

_____ D. Warm extremities

_____ E. Nasal flaring

2. A nurse is reinforcing teaching to an adolescent about the appropriate use of his asthma medications. Which of the following should the client be instructed to take as needed before exercise?

A. Fluticasone/salmeterol (Advair)

B. Montelukast (Singulair)

C. Prednisone

D. Albuterol (Proventil)

3. A nurse is caring for a child who has asthma. Which of the following interventions should be included in the plan of care? (Select all that apply.)

_____ A. Perform chest percussion.

_____ B. Place the child in an upright position.

_____ C. Monitor oxygen saturation.

_____ D. Administer bronchodilators.

_____ E. Administer dornase alfa (Pulmozyme) daily.

4. A nurse is providing instructions to a child who has asthma on how to use a peak flow meter. Which of the following should be included in the teaching? (Select all that apply.)

_____ A. Zero the meter before each use.

_____ B. Record the average of the attempts.

_____ C. Perform three attempts.

_____ D. Deliver a long, slow breath into the meter.

_____ E. Sit in a chair with feet on the floor.

5. A nurse is reinforcing teaching to a child about triggers to asthma. What should be included in the teaching? Use the ATI Active Learning Template: Systems Disorder to complete this item to include Client Education: List at least eight possible triggers to asthma.

APPLICATION EXERCISES KEY

1. A. INCORRECT: Oxygen saturation of 95% is within the expected reference range for a child.

    B. **CORRECT:** Wheezing is an indication of bronchoconstriction and of deterioration in a child's respiratory status.

    C. **CORRECT:** Retractions of sternal muscles are an indication of increased work of breathing and of deterioration in a child's respiratory status.

    D. INCORRECT: Warm extremities are an expected finding in a child.

    E. **CORRECT:** Nasal flaring is an indication of increased work of breathing and of deterioration in a child's respiratory status.

    Ⓝ NCLEX® Connection: Physiological Adaptations, Alterations in Body Systems

2. A. INCORRECT: Fluticasone/salmeterol (Advair) is a combination medication used for maintenance control of asthma.

    B. INCORRECT: Montelukast (Singulair) is a medication used for maintenance control of asthma.

    C. INCORRECT: Prednisone is a medication used for exacerbations of asthma.

    D. **CORRECT:** Albuterol is a beta$_2$-agonist used for bronchodilation and should be administered prior to exercise.

    Ⓝ NCLEX® Connection: Pharmacological Therapies, Expected Actions/Outcomes

3. A. INCORRECT: Chest percussion promotes movement of mucus plugs and is commended for children who have cystic fibrosis.

    B. **CORRECT:** Children who are experiencing an asthma exacerbation have decreased oxygenation. Placing them in an upright position is an appropriate intervention.

    C. **CORRECT:** Children who are experiencing an asthma exacerbation have decreased oxygenation. Monitoring oxygen saturation is an appropriate intervention.

    D. **CORRECT:** Children who are experiencing an asthma exacerbation experience bronchoconstriction. Administering bronchodilators is an appropriate intervention.

    E. INCORRECT: Dornase alfa is a mucolytic and is recommended for children who have cystic fibrosis.

    Ⓝ NCLEX® Connection: Physiological Adaptations, Basic Pathophysiology

4. A. **CORRECT:** The monitor should be zeroed each time it is used to achieve accurate results.

    B. INCORRECT: The highest number achieved is recorded.

    C. **CORRECT:** Three attempts should be performed to achieve accurate results.

    D. INCORRECT: A hard, fast breath should be used for the peak flow meter.

    E. INCORRECT: The child should be standing upright when using a peak flow meter.

    Ⓝ NCLEX® Connection: Reduction of Risk Potential, Therapeutic Procedures

5. *Using the ATI Active Learning Template: Systems Disorder*
    - Client Education
      ○ Allergens
        ▪ Indoor: mold, cockroaches, house dust mites
        ▪ Outdoor: grass, pollen, trees, shrubs, molds, spores, air pollution
      ○ Exercise/activity
      ○ Cold air or changes in weather
      ○ Tobacco smoke
      ○ Infections/colds
      ○ Animal hair or dander
      ○ Medications
      ○ Strong odors
      ○ Emotions
      ○ Gastroesophageal reflux
      ○ Food allergies or additives

    Ⓝ NCLEX® Connection: Physiological Adaptations, Alterations in Body Systems

chapter 17

Overview

- Cystic fibrosis is a respiratory disorder that results from inheriting a mutated gene. It is characterized by:
  - Mucus glands that secrete an increase in the quantity of thick, tenacious mucus, which leads to mechanical obstruction of organs (pancreas, lungs, liver, small intestine, and reproductive system).
  - An increase in organic and enzymatic constituents in the saliva.
  - An increase in the sodium and chloride content of sweat and saliva.
  - Central nervous system abnormalities.

Data Collection

- Risk Factors
  - Both biological parents carry the recessive trait for cystic fibrosis.
- Subjective Data
  - Family history of cystic fibrosis
  - Past medical history, including respiratory infections, failure to thrive
- Objective Data
  - Physical Assessment Findings
    - Meconium ileus at birth manifested as distention of the abdomen, vomiting, and inability to pass stool
    - Respiratory findings
      - Early signs
        - Wheezing
        - Dry, nonproductive cough
      - Increased involvement
        - Dyspnea
        - Paroxysmal cough
        - Mucus plugs and atelectasis on x-ray
      - Advanced involvement
        - Cyanosis
        - Barrel-shaped chest
        - Clubbing of fingers and toes
        - Multiple episodes of bronchitis or bronchopneumonia

- Gastrointestinal findings
  - Large, loose, fatty, sticky, foul-smelling stools
  - Voracious appetite (early), loss of appetite (late)
  - Failure to gain weight or weight loss
  - Delayed growth patterns
  - Distended abdomen
  - Thin arms and legs
  - Deficiency of fat-soluble vitamins
  - Anemia
- Integumentary findings
  - Sweat, tears, and saliva are abnormally salty
- Endocrine and reproductive system findings
  - Viscous cervical mucus
  - Decreased or absent sperm
- Laboratory Tests
  - Blood specimen
    - CBC, CRP, nutritional panel, blood glucose, complete metabolic panel, ABGs
  - Sputum culture for detection of infection
    - *Pseudomonas aeruginosa, Haemophilus influenzae, Burkholderia cepacia, Staphylococcus aureus, Escherichia coli,* or *Klebsiella pneumoniae*
  - Stool analysis
    - For presence of fat and enzymes
    - 72 hr sample with documented food intake
- Diagnostic Procedures
  - Sweat chloride test to diagnose cystic fibrosis
    - A special device stimulates sweat production
    - Collection of sweat from two different sites for adequate sample
    - Expected reference range is the presence of chloride less than 40 mEq/L
    - Diagnostic confirmation of cystic fibrosis: chloride greater than 60 mEq/L for infants less than 3 months of age and a sweat chloride greater than 40 mEq/L is highly suggestive of CF.
  - DNA testing to isolate the mutation
  - Pulmonary function tests (PFTs)
  - Chest x-ray can indicate diffuse atelectasis and obstructive emphysema
  - Abdominal x-ray to detect meconium ileus

Q
EBP

Patient-Centered Care

- Nursing Care
  - Check lung sounds and respiratory status.
  - Obtain vital signs with oxygen saturation.
  - Obtain sputum for culture and sensitivity.
  - Initiate contact isolation for *B. cepacia* and *P. aeruginosa*.
  - Provide support to the child and family.
  - Provide pulmonary management.
    - Perform chest physiotherapy (CPT) with postural drainage (traditional or vest). Avoid CPT before and after meals.
    - Perform airway clearance therapy (flutter mucus clearance device) twice daily.
    - Administer aerosol therapy (bronchodilator, human deoxyribonuclease).
    - Administer IV antibiotics (tobramycin, ticarcillin, or gentamicin).
    - Administer IV antifungal medications.
    - Encourage physical exercise (stationary bicycle).
    - Provide oxygen (check for carbon dioxide retention).
  - Gastrointestinal management
    - Provide a well-balanced diet high in protein and calories.
    - Give three meals a day with snacks.
    - Encourage oral fluid intake.
    - Administer pancreatic enzymes within 30 min of eating.
    - Administer vitamin supplements: multivitamin; vitamins A, D, E, and K.
    - Administer polyethylene-glycol electrolyte solution (GoLYTELY) via nasogastric tube for constipation.
    - Administer histamine-receptor antagonist and motility medications for GERD.
    - Administer possible formula supplements via gastric tube.
    - Consult a dietitian.
  - Endocrine management
    - Monitor blood glucose.
    - Administer insulin.
- Medications
  - Respiratory Medications
    - Short-acting beta$_2$-agonists, such as albuterol (Proventil)
    - Cholinergic antagonists (anticholinergics), such as ipratropium bromide (Atrovent)
    - Fluticasone propionate/salmeterol (Advair)

- Dornase alfa (Pulmozyme)
  - Decreases the viscosity of mucus and improves lung function
  - Nursing Considerations
    - ▸ Monitor sputum thickness and the child's ability to expectorate.
    - ▸ Monitor the child for improvement in PFTs.
  - Client Education
    - ▸ Instruct the child how to use a nebulizer.
    - ▸ Instruct the child to administer once a day.
- Nursing Considerations
  - Instruct the child and family about how to properly use an MDI, DPI, or nebulizer.
  - Monitor the child for tremors and tachycardia when he is taking albuterol.
  - Observe the child for dry mouth when taking ipratropium.
- Client Education
  - Wait 5 min between ipratropium bromide and other inhaled medications.
  - Rinse mouth after fluticasone propionate/salmeterol.
- Antibiotics
  - Administer via IV or aerosol.
  - Specific to treat pulmonary infection – common medications include tobramycin, ticarcillin, or gentamicin.
  - Nursing Considerations
    - Check for allergies.
    - High doses can be prescribed. Collect blood specimens before and after some IV antibiotics to maintain therapeutic levels.
    - Implement special precautions for aerosol antibiotics.
- Pancreatic enzymes – pancrelipase (Pancrease)
  - Treats pancreatic insufficiency associated with cystic fibrosis
  - Nursing Considerations
    - Monitor stools for adequate dosing (increase dose if loose, fatty stools present; decrease dose if constipation present).
    - Administer capsules with all meals and snacks.
    - Client can swallow or sprinkle capsules on food.
- Vitamins
  - Daily multivitamin and vitamins A, E, D, and K

- Teamwork and Collaboration
  - Respiratory and physical therapy, social services, pulmonologists, pharmacists, pediatricians, infectious disease specialists, and dietitians can be involved in the care of the child who has cystic fibrosis.
  - Transplantation of heart, lung, pancreas, and liver for clients who have advanced disease can be a consideration.
- Care After Discharge
  - Ensure that the family has information regarding access to medical equipment and medications.
  - Provide instructions about equipment and medications prior to discharge.
  - Instruct the family about ways to provide CPT and breathing exercises.
  - Promote regular provider visits.
  - Emphasize the need for up-to-date immunizations and a yearly influenza vaccine.
  - Instruct about diet and ways to increase calorie intake.
  - Provide manifestations of infection and when to call the provider.
  - Instruct parents about ways to manage chronic illness in children.
  - Promote regular physical activity.
  - Encourage the family to participate in a support group and use community resources.

Complications

- Respiratory complications
  - Respiratory infections, colonizations
  - Bronchial cysts
  - Emphysema
  - Pneumothorax
  - Nasal polyps
- Gastrointestinal complications
  - Meconium ileus
  - Prolapse of the rectum
  - Distal intestinal obstruction syndrome
  - GERD
- Endocrine complications
  - Diabetes mellitus

APPLICATION EXERCISES

1. A nurse is caring for a child who is suspected of having cystic fibrosis. Which of the following tests should the nurse prepare to administer to confirm this diagnosis?

    A. Sweat chloride

    B. Pulmonary function test

    C. Arterial blood gases

    D. Chest percussion

2. A nurse is assisting with admission of a child who has cystic fibrosis. Which of the following medications should the nurse anticipate including in the plan of care? (Select all that apply.)

_____ A. Tobramycin

_____ B. Solu-Medrol

_____ C. Fat-soluble vitamins

_____ D. Albuterol

_____ E. Dornase alfa

3. A nurse is caring for a child who has cystic fibrosis. Which of the following are expected findings? (Select all that apply.)

_____ A. Wheezing

_____ B. Clubbing of fingers and toes

_____ C. Barrel-shaped chest

_____ D. Thin, watery mucus

_____ E. Rapid growth spurts

4. A nurse is planning care for a child who has cystic fibrosis. Which of the following interventions should be included in the plan of care?

    A. Provide a low-calorie, low-protein diet.

    B. Administer pancreatic enzymes with meals and snacks.

    C. Promote an increase in fluids after 1800.

    D. Restrict physical activity.

5. A nurse is caring for a child who has cystic fibrosis. What nursing interventions should the nurse anticipate providing? Use the Systems Disorder ATI Active Learning Template to complete this item to include:

    A. Nursing Care:
- Describe at least three general nursing actions.
- Describe three nursing actions related to the management of pulmonary function.
- Describe two nursing actions related to gastrointestinal system management.
- Describe two nursing actions related to endocrine system management.

APPLICATION EXERCISES KEY

1. A. **CORRECT:** Children who have cystic fibrosis excrete an abnormal amount of sodium and chloride in their sweat. A sweat chloride test is diagnostic of cystic fibrosis and should be performed.

    B. INCORRECT: Pulmonary function tests evaluate lung function and are used for children who have cystic fibrosis. However, they are not diagnostic of the disease.

    C. INCORRECT: Arterial blood gases are used for children who have cystic fibrosis to determine oxygenation status. However, they are not diagnostic of the disease.

    D. INCORRECT: Chest percussion is used for children who have cystic fibrosis to assist with expectoration of mucus from their lungs, but it is not diagnostic of the disease.

     NCLEX® Connection: Reduction of Risk Potential, Diagnostic Tests

2. A. **CORRECT:** Children who have cystic fibrosis have pulmonary infections. Administering antibiotics should be part of the plan of care.

    B. INCORRECT: Corticosteroid use has been associated with short stature, glucose intolerance, and cataracts. It should not be part of the plan of care.

    C. **CORRECT:** Children who have cystic fibrosis have difficulty absorbing fat. Supplementation of the fat-soluble vitamins should be part of the plan of care.

    D. **CORRECT:** Children who have cystic fibrosis have mucus plugs. Administering a bronchodilator should be part of the plan of care.

    E. **CORRECT:** Children who have cystic fibrosis have mucus plugs. Administering dornase alfa, which decreases the viscosity of the mucus, should be part of the plan of care.

     NCLEX® Connection: Pharmacological Therapies, Expected Actions/Outcomes

3. A. **CORRECT:** Wheezing is a manifestations of cystic fibrosis.

    B. **CORRECT:** Clubbing of fingers and toes is a late manifestation of cystic fibrosis.

    C. **CORRECT:** A barrel-shaped chest is a late manifestation of cystic fibrosis.

    D. INCORRECT: Thick, viscous mucus is a manifestation of cystic fibrosis.

    E. INCORRECT: Delayed growth is a manifestation of cystic fibrosis.

     NCLEX® Connection: Physiological Adaptations, Basic Pathophysiology

4.   A. INCORRECT: Children who have cystic fibrosis should eat a high-calorie, high-protein diet to allow for proper growth.

    B. **CORRECT:** Children who have cystic fibrosis have pancreatic insufficiency. Administering pancreatic enzymes with meals and snacks should be part of the plan of care.

    C. INCORRECT: Children who have cystic fibrosis should increase fluids throughout the day to assist in thinning thick mucus.

    D. INCORRECT: Children who have cystic fibrosis should engage in daily activity to assist with lung expansion and stimulate mucus excretion.

    Ⓝ NCLEX® Connection: Physiological Adaptations, Basic Pathophysiology

5.   *Using the Systems Disorder ATI Active Learning Template*

    A. Nursing Care

- General Nursing Actions
  - Check lung sounds and respiratory status.
  - Obtain vital signs with oxygen saturation.
  - Obtain IV access (peripherally inserted central catheter [PICC]).
  - Obtain sputum for culture and sensitivity.
  - Contact isolation for *B. cepacia* and *P. aeruginosa*.
  - Provide support to the child and family.
- Pulmonary Management
  - Perform chest physiotherapy (CPT) with postural drainage as prescribed (traditional or vest). Avoid immediately before and after meals.
  - Perform airway clearance therapy (flutter mucus clearance device) twice daily.
  - Administer aerosol therapy (bronchodilator, human deoxyribonuclease).
  - Administer IV antibiotics (tobramycin, ticarcillin, or gentamicin).
  - Administer IV antifungals.
  - Encourage physical exercise (stationary bicycle).
  - Provide oxygen (check for carbon dioxide retention).
- Gastrointestinal Management
  - Encourage consuming a well-balanced diet high in protein and calories.
  - Recommend eating three meals a day with snacks.
  - Encourage oral fluid intake.
  - Administer pancreatic enzymes within 30 min of eating.
  - Encourage taking vitamin supplements: multivitamin, vitamins A, D, E, and K.
  - Administer polyethylene-glycol electrolyte solution (GoLYTELY) via nasogastric tube for constipation.
  - Administer histamine-receptor antagonist and motility medications for GERD.
  - Administer possible formula supplements via a gastric tube.
  - Consult a dietitian.
- Endocrine Management
  - Monitor blood glucose.
  - Administer insulin.

    Ⓝ NCLEX® Connection: Physiological Adaptations, Basic Pathophysiology

UNIT 2   Nursing Care of Children with System Disorders

SECTION: CARDIOVASCULAR AND HEMATOLOGIC DISORDERS

› Cardiovascular Disorders
› Hematologic Disorders

NCLEX® CONNECTIONS

When reviewing the chapters in this section, keep in mind the relevant sections of the NCLEX® outline, in particular:

Client Needs: Pharmacological Therapies	Client Needs: Reduction of Risk Potential	Client Needs: Physiological Adaptations
› Relevant topics/tasks include: » Expected Actions/ Outcomes › Reinforce education to client regarding medications. » Medication Administration › Administer a subcutaneous, intradermal or intramuscular medication.	› Relevant topics/tasks include: » Diagnostic Tests › Perform diagnostic testing. » Potential for Complications of Diagnostic Tests/ Treatments/Procedures › Implement measures to prevent complication of client condition or procedure.	› Relevant topics/tasks include: » Alterations in Body Systems › Evaluate achievement of the client treatment goals. › Provide care to correct client alteration in body system. › Reinforce education to client regarding care and condition. » Basic Pathophysiology › Provide the client with strategies to manage decreased cardiac output. › Identify signs and symptoms related to an acute or chronic illness. › Consider general principles of client disease process when providing care.

chapter 18

Overview

- Heart disease can be congenital or acquired.

- Anatomic abnormalities present at birth can lead to congenital heart disease (CHD). These abnormalities result primarily in heart failure and hypoxemia. Congenital disorders that result primarily in heart failure and hypoxemia to be discussed in this chapter include the following.

  - Ventricular defect (VSD)

  - Atrial septal defect (ASD)

  - Patent ductus arteriosus (PDA)

  - Pulmonary stenosis

  - Aortic stenosis

  - Tetralogy of Fallot

  - Coarctation of the aorta

  - Transposition of the great arteries

  - Tricuspid atresia

  - Truncus arteriosus

  - Hypoplastic left heart syndrome

- Acquired cardiovascular disorder

  - Rheumatic fever

  - Hyperlipidemia

- Vascular dysfunction

  - Kawasaki disease

- Heart failure occurs when the heart is unable to pump adequate blood to meet the metabolic and physical demands of the body.

- Due to changing lifestyles and socioeconomic conditions, the incidence of hyperlipidemia is increasing in children. The result is obesity in childhood and leads to heart disease during adulthood.

CONGENITAL HEART DISEASE (CHD)

Overview

- Anatomic defects of the heart prevent normal blood flow to the pulmonary and/or systemic system. Defects are categorized by blood flow patterns in the heart.

  ○ Increased pulmonary blood flow (ASD, VSD, PDA)

  ○ Decreased pulmonary blood flow (Tetralogy of Fallot, tricuspid atresia)

  ○ Obstruction to blood flow (coarctation of the aorta, pulmonary stenosis, aortic stenosis)

  ○ Mixed blood flow (transposition of the great arteries, truncus arteriosus, hypoplastic left heart syndrome)

Data Collection

- Risk Factors

  ○ Maternal factors

    ▪ Infection

    ▪ Alcohol or other substance abuse during pregnancy

    ▪ Diabetes mellitus

  ○ Genetic factors

    ▪ History of congenital heart disease in other family members

    ▪ Certain syndromes such as Trisomy 21 (Down syndrome)

    ▪ Presence of other congenital anomalies or chromosomal abnormalities

- Subjective and Objective Data

M View Images
  › Ventricular Septal Defect   › Coarctation of the Aorta
  › Pulmonary Stenosis   › Tetralogy of Fallot

CONGENITAL HEART DEFECT	MANIFESTATIONS
› Ventricular septal defect (VSD) – a hole in the septum between the right and left ventricle that results in increased pulmonary blood flow (left-to-right shunt)	› Loud, harsh murmur auscultated at the left sternal border › Heart failure › Many VSDs close spontaneously
› Atrial septal defect (ASD) – a hole in the septum between the right and left atria that results in increased pulmonary blood flow (left-to-right shunt)	› Loud, harsh murmur with a fixed split second heart sound › Heart failure › Asymptomatic (possibly)

CONGENITAL HEART DEFECT	MANIFESTATIONS
› Patent ductus arteriosus (PDA) – a condition in which the normal fetal circulation conduit between the pulmonary artery and the aorta fails to close and results in increased pulmonary blood flow (left-to-right shunt)	› Murmur (machine hum) › Wide pulse pressure › Bounding pulses › Asymptomatic (possibly) › Heart failure
› Pulmonary stenosis – a narrowing of the pulmonary valve or pulmonary artery that results in obstruction of blood flow from the ventricles	› Systolic ejection murmur › Asymptomatic (possibly) › Cyanosis varies with defect, worse with severe narrowing › Cardiomegaly › Heart failure
› Aortic stenosis – a narrowing of the aortic valve	› Infants » Faint pulses » Hypotension » Tachycardia » Poor feeding tolerance › Children » Intolerance to exercise » Dizziness » Chest pain » Possible ejection murmur
› Coarctation of the aorta – a narrowing of the lumen of the aorta, usually at or near the ductus arteriosus, that results in obstruction of blood flow from the ventricle	› Elevated blood pressure in the arms › Bounding pulses in the upper extremities › Decreased blood pressure in the lower extremities › Cool skin of lower extremities › Weak or absent femoral pulses › Heart failure in infants › Dizziness, headaches, fainting, or nosebleeds in older children
› Transposition of the great arteries – a condition in which the aorta is connected to the right ventricle instead of the left, and the pulmonary artery is connected to the left ventricle instead of the right a septal defect or a PDA must exist in order to oxygenate the blood	› Murmur depending on presence of associated defects › Severe to less cyanosis depending on the size of the associated defect › Cardiomegaly › Heart failure
› Tricuspid atresia – A complete closure of the tricuspid valve that results in mixed blood flow. An atrial septal opening needs to be present to allow blood to enter the left atrium.	› Infants » Cyanosis » Dyspnea » Tachycardia › Older children » Hypoxemia » Clubbing of fingers

CONGENITAL HEART DEFECT	MANIFESTATIONS
› Tetralogy of Fallot – four defects that result in mixed blood flow » Pulmonary stenosis » Ventricular septal defect » Overriding aorta » Right ventricular hypertrophy	› Cyanosis at birth – progressive cyanosis over the first year of life › Systolic murmur › Episodes of acute cyanosis and hypoxia (blue spells)
› Truncus arteriosus – failure of septum formation, resulting in a single vessel that comes off of the ventricles	› Heart failure › Murmur › Variable cyanosis › Delayed growth › Lethargy › Fatigue › Poor feeding habits
› Hypoplastic left heart syndrome – Left side of the heart is underdeveloped. An ASD or patent foramen ovale allows for oxygenation of the blood.	› Mild cyanosis › Heart failure › Lethargy › Cold hands and feet › Once PDA closes, progression of cyanosis and decreased cardiac output result in eventual cardiac collapse

- Manifestations of heart failure (HF)
  - Impaired myocardial function
    - Sweating, tachycardia, fatigue, pallor, cool extremities with weak pulses, hypotension, gallop rhythm, cardiomegaly
  - Pulmonary congestion
    - Tachypnea, dyspnea, retractions, nasal flaring, grunting, wheezing, cyanosis, cough, orthopnea, exercise intolerance
  - Systemic venous congestion
    - Hepatomegaly, peripheral edema, ascites, neck vein distention, periorbital edema, weight gain
- Manifestations of hypoxemia
  - Cyanosis, poor weight gain, tachypnea, dyspnea, clubbing, polycythemia

View Image: Clubbed Fingers

  - Hypercyanotic spells (blue, or "Tet," spells) manifest as acute cyanosis and hyperpnea.
- Laboratory Tests
  - Hemoglobin (Hgb), hematocrit (Hct), and serum electrolytes

- ○ Diagnostic Procedures
  - ▪ ECG monitoring to identify cardiac dysrhythmias
    - ▢ Nursing Actions
      - ▸ Assist with the application of electrodes.
      - ▸ Assist with maintaining the child in a quiet position.
    - ▢ Client Education – Tell the child that the test will not be painful.
  - ▪ Radiography (chest x-ray) to determine heart size and blood flow
    - ▢ Nursing Actions – Assist with positioning the client.
  - ▪ Echocardiography to determine cardiac defects and heart function
    - ▢ Nursing Actions – Assist with positioning the child.
- ▪ Cardiac catheterization
  - ▢ Cardiac catheterization is an invasive test used for diagnosing, repairing some defects, and evaluating dysrhythmias. A radiopaque catheter is peripherally inserted and threaded into the heart with the use of fluoroscopy. A contrast medium (may be iodine-based) is injected, and images of the blood vessels and heart are taken as the medium is diluted and circulated throughout the body.
  - ▢ Nursing Actions
    - ▸ Preprocedure
      - ▹ Review history and physical examination findings. Evidence of infection, such as a severe diaper rash, can necessitate canceling the procedure if femoral access is required.
      - ▹ Check for allergies to iodine and shellfish.
      - ▹ Provide age-appropriate instruction.
      - ▹ Describe how long the procedure will take, how the child will feel, and what care will be required after the procedure.
      - ▹ Provide for NPO status 4 to 6 hr prior to the procedure. (If the procedure is performed as outpatient, be sure the child and family are given instructions in advance.)
      - ▹ Obtain baseline vital signs, including oxygen saturation.
      - ▹ Locate and mark the dorsalis pedis and posterior tibial pulses on both extremities.
    - ▸ Postprocedure
      - ▹ Provide for continuous cardiac monitoring and oxygen saturation to check for bradycardia, dysrhythmias, hypotension, and hypoxemia.
      - ▹ Check heart rate and respiratory rate for 1 full minute.
      - ▹ Monitor pulses for equality and symmetry.
      - ▹ Monitor temperature and color of extremity. A cool extremity with skin that blanches may indicate arterial obstruction.
      - ▹ Monitor insertion site (femoral or antecubital area) for bleeding and/or hematoma.
      - ▹ Maintain clean dressing.
      - ▹ Prevent bleeding by maintaining the affected extremity in a straight position for 4 to 8 hr.

▷ Monitor I&O for adequate urine output, hypovolemia, or dehydration.

▷ Monitor for hypoglycemia. IV fluids with dextrose can be necessary.

▷ Encourage oral intake, starting with clear liquids.

▷ Encourage the child to void to promote excretion of the contrast medium.

◻ Client Education

▸ Encourage fluid intake to help with the removal of the dye from the body.

▸ Advise the parents and child to monitor the site for infection.

Patient-Centered Care

- Nursing Care
  - General Interventions
    - Remain calm when providing care.
    - Keep the child well-hydrated.
    - Conserve the child's energy by providing frequent rest periods; clustering care; providing small, frequent meals; bathing PRN; and keeping crying to a minimum in cyanotic children.
    - Perform daily weight and I&O to monitor fluid status and nutritional status.
    - Monitor heart rate, blood pressure, serum electrolytes, and renal function for complications.
    - Provide support and resources for parents to promote developmental growth in the child.
    - Monitor family coping and provide support.
    - Administer prescribed medications.
    - Maintain fluid and electrolyte balance.
      ◻ Administer potassium supplements if prescribed. These might not be indicated if the child is concurrently taking an ACE inhibitor.
      ◻ Maintain sodium and fluid restrictions if prescribed.
    - Decrease workload of the heart.
      ◻ Maintain bed rest.
      ◻ Position the infant in a car seat or hold at a 45° angle. Keep safety restraints low and loose on the abdomen.
      ◻ Allow the child to sleep with several pillows and encourage a semi-Fowler's or Fowler's position while awake.
    - Provide for adequate nutrition.
      ◻ Plan to feed the infant using a feeding schedule of every 3 hr. The infant should be rested, which occurs soon after awakening.
      ◻ Use a soft preemie nipple or a regular nipple with a slit to provide an enlarged opening.
      ◻ Hold the infant in a semi-upright position.
      ◻ Allow the infant to rest during feedings, taking approximately 30 min to complete the feeding.

- Gavage feed the infant if he is unable to consume enough formula or breast milk.

- Increase caloric density of formula gradually from 20 to 30 kcal/oz.

- Encourage mothers who are breastfeeding to alternate feedings with high-density formula or fortified breast milk.

  ▪ Increase tissue oxygenation.

  - Provide cool, humidified oxygen via an oxygen hood (or tent), mask, or nasal cannula.

  - Suction the airway as indicated.

  - Monitor oxygen saturation every 2 to 4 hr.

- Medications

  ○ Digoxin (Lanoxin) – improves myocardial contractility

    ▪ Nursing Actions

      - Monitor the pulse and withhold the medication as ordered. Generally, if an infant's pulse is less than 90/min, the medication should be withheld. In children, the medication should be withheld if the pulse is less than 70/min.

      - Monitor for toxicity as evidenced by bradycardia, dysrhythmias, nausea, vomiting, or anorexia.

      - Monitor serum digoxin levels.

  ○ Captopril (Capoten) or enalapril (Vasotec)

    ▪ Angiotensin-converting enzyme (ACE) inhibitors reduce afterload by causing vasodilation, resulting in decreased pulmonary and systemic vascular resistance.

    ▪ Nursing Considerations

      - Monitor blood pressure before and after the medication is administered.

      - Monitor for evidence of hyperkalemia.

    ▪ Client Education – Instruct parents to monitor blood pressure frequently.

  ○ Metoprolol or carvedilol (Coreg) – beta-blockers, which decrease heart rate and blood pressure, and promote vasodilation

    ▪ Nursing Considerations

      - Monitor blood pressure and pulse prior to administration.

      - Monitor for adverse effects such as dizziness, hypotension, and headache.

  ○ Furosemide (Lasix) or chlorothiazide (Diuril) – Potassium-wasting diuretics rid the body of excess fluid and sodium.

    ▪ Nursing Considerations

      - Encourage a diet high in potassium.

      - Monitor I&O.

      - Monitor for adverse affects such as hypokalemia, nausea, vomiting, and dizziness.

      - Monitor weight daily.

- Teamwork and Collaboration

  ○ Dietitians should be consulted to assist the family with appropriate food choices.

- Care After Discharge
  - Client Education
    - Cardiac catheterization
      - Instruct the family to monitor for possible complications (bleeding, infection, thrombosis).
      - Limit activity for 24 hr.
      - Encourage fluids.
    - Digoxin administration
      - Take pulse prior to medication administration. Notify provider if pulse is less than specified rate.
      - Administer digoxin every 12 hr.
      - Direct oral elixir toward the side and back of mouth when administering.
      - Give water following administration to prevent tooth decay if the child has teeth.
      - If a dose is missed, do not give an extra dose or increase the next dose.
      - If the child vomits, do not readminister the dose.
      - Observe for signs of digoxin toxicity (decreased heart rate, decreased appetite, nausea, and/or vomiting). Notify the provider if these occur.
      - Keep the medication in a locked cabinet.
    - Diuretic administration
      - Mix the oral elixir in a small amount of juice to disguise the bitter taste and prevent intestinal irritation.
      - Observe for adverse effects of diuretics, which can include nausea, vomiting, and diarrhea.
      - Observe for manifestations of serum potassium level imbalances (muscle weakness, irritability, excessive drowsiness, and increased or decreased heart rate).
      - Encourage the child to eat foods high in potassium, such as bran cereals, potatoes, tomatoes, bananas, melons, oranges, and orange juice.
      - Instruct the family to monitor weight daily.
    - Instruct the family to report evidence of worsening heart failure, such as increased sweating and decreased urinary output (fewer wet diapers or less frequent toileting).

Complications

- Cardiac catheterization (potential)
  - Nausea, vomiting
  - Low-grade fever
  - Loss of pulse in the catheterized extremity
  - Transient dysrhythmias
  - Acute hemorrhage from entry site

- ○ Nursing Actions

  - Apply direct continuous pressure at 2.5 cm (1 in) above the catheter entry site to localize pressure over the location of the vessel puncture.

  - Position the child flat to reduce the gravitational effect on the rate of bleeding.

  - Notify the provider immediately.

  - Prepare for the possible administration of replacement fluids and/or medication to control emesis.

- ○ Client Education

  - Monitor for infection.

  - Monitor for bleeding.

- Hypoxemia

  - ○ A hypercyanotic spell can result in severe hypoxemia, which leads to cerebral hypoxemia, and should be treated as an emergency.

  - ○ Nursing Actions – Immediately place the child in the knee-chest position, attempt to calm the child, and call for help.

- Bacterial endocarditis or subacute bacterial endocarditis

  - ○ Children who have congenital or acquired heart disease are at increased risk for infection of the valves or lining of the heart.

  - ○ The client should follow the American Heart Association's recommendations for bacterial endocarditis prophylaxis. These include receiving prophylactic antibiotic therapy prior to dental and surgical procedures (dental extractions, endodontic surgery, surgical procedures that involve the respiratory or gastrointestinal mucosa).

  - ○ Causative organisms include *Streptococcus viridans* and *Staphylococcus aureus*.

  - ○ Nursing Actions – Administer antibiotics parenterally for an extended length of time, usually via a peripherally inserted central catheter.

  - ○ Client Education

    - Reinforce teaching with the family about the need for prophylactic antibiotics prior to dental and surgical procedures.

    - Instruct the family about the clinical manifestations of endocarditis (low-grade fever, malaise, decreased appetite with weight loss).

- Heart failure requiring transplant

  - ○ Cardiomyopathy and congenital heart disease are causes of heart failure.

  - ○ Nursing Actions

    - Maintain pharmacological support as prescribed (oxygen, diuretics, digoxin, afterload reducers such as ACE inhibitors).

    - Provide family and child support.

  - ○ Client Education

    - Reinforce the importance of adhering to the medication regimen.

    - Inform the child and family about infection control precautions.

RHEUMATIC FEVER

Overview

- Rheumatic fever is an inflammatory disease that occurs as a reaction to Group A β-hemolytic streptococcus (GABHS) infection of the throat.

Data Collection

- Risk Factors
  - Rheumatic fever usually occurs within 2 to 6 weeks following an untreated or partially treated upper respiratory infection (strep throat) with GABHS.
- Subjective and Objective Data
  - History of recent upper respiratory infection
  - Fever
  - Tachycardia, cardiomegaly, prolonged PR interval, new or changed heart murmur, muffled heart sounds, pericardial friction rub, and report of chest pain, which can indicate carditis
  - Nontender, subcutaneous nodules over bony prominence

  - Large joints (knees, elbows, ankles, wrists, shoulders) with painful swelling, indicating polyarthritis
    - Findings can be present for a few days and then disappear without treatment, frequently returning in another joint.
  - Pink, nonpruritic macular rash on the trunk and inner surfaces of extremities that appears and disappears rapidly, indicating erythema marginatum
  - CNS involvement (chorea) including involuntary, purposeless muscle movements; muscle weakness; involuntary facial movements; difficulty performing fine motor activities; labile emotions; and random, uncoordinated movements of the extremities
  - Irritability, poor concentration, and behavioral problems
  - Laboratory Tests
    - Throat culture for GABHS
    - Serum antistreptolysin-O (ASO) titer – elevated or rising titer, most reliable diagnostic test
    - C-reactive protein (CRP) – elevated in response to an inflammatory reaction
    - Erythrocyte sedimentation rate – elevated in response to an inflammatory reaction
  - Diagnostic Procedures
    - Cardiac function
      - ECG to reveal the presence of conduction disturbances and to evaluate the function of the heart and valves.
      - Nursing Actions – Position the child correctly for the procedure.
      - Client Education – Explain the need for decreased movement during the procedure.

- The diagnosis of rheumatic fever is made on the basis of modified Jones criteria. The child should demonstrate the presence of two major criteria or the presence of one major and two minor criteria following an acute infection with GABHS infection.
  - Major criteria
    - ▸ Carditis
    - ▸ Subcutaneous nodules
    - ▸ Polyarthritis
    - ▸ Rash (erythema marginatum)
    - ▸ Chorea
  - Minor criteria
    - ▸ Fever
    - ▸ Arthralgia

Patient-Centered Care

- Nursing Care
  - Encourage bed rest during the acute illness.
  - Administer antibiotic as prescribed.
  - Encourage nutritionally balanced meals.
  - Check for chorea.
- Medications
  - Antibiotic prophylaxis
    - Follow the prescribed prophylactic treatment regimen, which can include one of the following: two daily oral doses of 200,000 units of penicillin, a monthly IM injection of 1.2 million units of penicillin G, or a daily oral dose of 1 g sulfadiazine (Microsulfon). The length of treatment varies according to residual heart disease, ranging from 5 years to indefinitely.
    - Nursing Considerations
      - Monitor for an allergic response (anaphylaxis, hives, rashes).
      - Check for nausea, vomiting, or diarrhea.
    - Client Education
      - Encourage compliance with medication regimen.
- Care After Discharge
  - Client Education
    - Promote rest during the acute phase.
    - Provide information and reassurance related to the development of chorea and its self-limiting nature.
    - Encourage well-balanced meals.
    - Seek medical care if infection recurrence is suspected.

Complications

- Carditis and heart disease

HYPERLIPIDEMIA

Overview

- Hyperlipidemia is excess lipids (fat) in circulating blood.
- Cholesterol is part of the lipoprotein complex in blood.
- Triglycerides come from two sources: naturally made in the body from carbohydrates, and the end product of fat ingestion.
- Total cholesterol – the sum of all forms of cholesterol.
- High density lipoprotein (HDL) cholesterol – "good" cholesterol, having low level of cholesterol and triglycerides and high level of protein.
- Low density lipoprotein (LDL) cholesterol – "bad" cholesterol, having a high level of cholesterol, low level of triglycerides, and moderate levels of protein.

Data Collection

- Risk Factors
  - Genetic
  - Obesity
  - Lack of exercise
  - History of health condition: diabetes, kidney disease, hypothyroidism
  - Medications: birth control pills, diuretics, beta-blockers
- Subjective and Objective Data
  - Clients who have risk factors should be evaluated.
  - Laboratory Tests
    - Lipid profile – fasting for 12 hr prior to test
    - Fasting blood glucose
- Patient-Centered Care
  - Nursing Care/Client Education
    - Assist in screening clients at risk.
    - Instruct the client to keep a diet history for review by the dietitian.
    - Monitor the client for febrile illness 3 weeks prior to screening (illness will alter results).
    - Instruct about a diet to lower cholesterol: low fat, whole grains, fruit and vegetables.
    - Encourage use of olive oil and canola oil.
    - Assist with an exercise program (60 min per day for 5 days per week of aerobic exercise).

- Medication
  - Cholestyramine (Questran) and colestipol (Colestid)
    - Used in clients who fail conventional treatment
    - Used in children 8 years and older who have a LDL of 190 mg/dL or higher or 160 mg/dL in clients who have risk factors
    - Nursing Considerations
      - Powdered medication mixed in 4 to 6 oz of water or juice, then administered immediately.
      - Monitor for adverse effects: constipation, abdominal pain, flatulence, nausea, and abdominal bloating.
      - Monitor laboratory findings: liver function tests, CBC, creatinine kinase, and fasting lipid profile at 4- and 8-week intervals and with any dosage change.
  - Client Education
    - Instruct the client and family how to administer medications.
    - Instruct the client about adverse effects of medications.
    - Instruct the client to discontinue medication if he exhibits dark urine or muscle aches, and to notify the provider.
- Teamwork and Collaboration
  - Dietary counseling

Complications

- Atherosclerosis and coronary heart disease
  - Nursing Considerations
    - Identify clients who are at risk and promote early screening.
    - Reinforce healthy eating habits to families and clients.

KAWASAKI DISEASE

Overview

- Acute systemic vasculitis

Data Collection

- Risk Factors – etiology unknown
- Subjective and Objective Data
  - Acute phase: onset of high fever that is unresponsive to antipyretics, with development of other clinical manifestations
    - Fever greater than 38.9° C (102° F) lasting 5 days to 2 weeks and unresponsive to antipyretics
    - Irritability
    - Red eyes without drainage
    - Bright red, chapped lips
    - Strawberry tongue with white coating or red bumps on the posterior aspect
    - Red oral mucous membranes
    - Swelling of hand and feet with red palms and soles
    - Nonblistering rash
    - Bilateral joint pain
    - Enlarged lymph nodes
  - Subacute phase: resolution of the fever and gradual subsiding of other clinical manifestations
    - Irritability
    - Peeling skin around the nails, on the palms and soles
  - Convalescent: no clinical manifestations seen except altered laboratory findings. Resolution in about 6 to 8 weeks from onset.
  - Laboratory Tests
    - CBC, CRP, ESR, serum albumin
  - Diagnostic Procedures
    - Chest x-ray
    - Echocardiogram and/or ECG to indicate myocarditis, pericarditis, arthritis, meningitis, inflammation

Patient-Centered Care

- Nursing Care
  - Monitor vital signs and cardiac status. Maintain cardiac monitoring.
  - Monitor client for manifestations of heart failure (decreased urine output, gallop heart rhythm, tachycardia, respiratory distress).
  - Monitor I&O. Obtain daily weight.
  - Administer IV fluids to prevent dehydration. Offer clear liquids and soft foods.
  - Administer IV gamma globulin according to facility policy.
  - Administer aspirin as prescribed.
  - Provide care to promote comfort due to clinical findings.
    - Oral hygiene.
    - Apply cool cloths to skin.
    - Apply skin lotions to maintain hydration.
    - Provide for a calm, quiet environment.
    - Promote rest by clustering care.
- Medication
  - Gamma globulin (IVGG)
    - Nursing Consideration
      - Administer via IV infusion.
      - High dosage: 2 g/kg over 10 to 12 hr.
      - Ideally, administer within the first 7 days of illness.
      - Repeat for clients who remain febrile.
      - Monitor vital signs.
      - Monitor for allergic reaction.
  - Aspirin
    - High dose: 80 to 100 mg/kg/day divided every 6 hr.
    - Once afebrile: 3 to 5 mg/kg/day to continue until platelet count returns to expected range, which can be approximately 6 to 8 weeks.
    - If coronary abnormalities develop, continue aspirin therapy indefinitely.

- Care after discharge
  - Instruct the family about disease progression.
  - Encourage the family to maintain follow-up appointments.
  - Instruct the family that the irritability can last 2 months.
  - Instruct the family that arthritic symptoms can last several weeks.
  - Instruct the family that the skin manifestations are painless but the skin could be tender.
  - Encourage passive ROM exercises in the bathtub.
  - Avoid live immunizations for 11 months.
  - Notify the provider of any fever.
- Ongoing Care
  - Avoid smoking.
  - Maintain a heart-healthy diet.
  - Screen for heart disease as child age.
    - Serum cholesterol testing
    - Blood pressure monitoring
    - Periodic imaging of the heart

Complications

- Coronary artery dilation or aneurysm formation
  - Most common in the subacute phase
  - Echocardiogram to monitor for changes
  - Administer anticoagulation medications as prescribed (enoxaparin [Lovenox])

APPLICATION EXERCISES

1. A nurse is caring for an infant. Which of the following are clinical manifestations of coarctation of the aorta? (Select all that apply.)

_____ A. Weak femoral pulses

_____ B. Cool skin of lower extremities

_____ C. Severe cyanosis

_____ D. Clubbing of the fingers

_____ E. Heart failure

2. A nurse is caring for an infant. Which of the following should the nurse recognize as clinical manifestations of heart failure? (Select all that apply.)

_____ A. Bradycardia

_____ B. Cool extremities

_____ C. Peripheral edema

_____ D. Increased urinary output

_____ E. Nasal flaring

3. A nurse is reinforcing teaching with the mother of an infant who is to start taking digoxin (Lanoxin). Which of the following instructions should the nurse include?

A. "Do not offer your baby fluids after giving the medication."

B. "Digoxin increases your baby's heart rate."

C. "Give the correct dose of medication at regularly scheduled times."

D. "If your baby vomits a dose, you should repeat the dose to ensure that he gets the correct amount."

4. A nurse is caring for a 2-year-old child who is cyanotic and is in the hospital for a cardiac catheterization to repair cardiac defects. Which of the following is an appropriate action for the nurse to take?

A. Place on NPO status for 12 hr prior to the procedure.

B. Check for iodine allergies prior to the procedure.

C. Elevate the affected extremity following the procedure.

D. Limit fluid intake following the procedure

5. A nurse is caring for a child who is suspected of having rheumatic fever. Which of the following manifestations support this diagnosis? (Select all that apply.)

_____ A. Erythema marginatum (rash)

_____ B. Continuous joint pain of the digits

_____ C. Tender, subcutaneous nodules

_____ D. Decreased erythrocyte sedimentation rate

_____ E. Elevated C-reactive protein

6. A nurse is discussing care of a child who has Kawasaki disease with a newly hired nurse. What should be included in this discussion? Use the ATI Active Learning Template: Systems Disorder to complete this item to include:

A. Clinical Manifestations: Identify for the acute, subacute, and convalescent phase.

B. Nursing Care: List seven for this client.

APPLICATION EXERCISES KEY

1. A. **CORRECT:** Narrowing of the lumen of the aorta results in obstruction of blood flow from the ventricle, resulting in weak or absent femoral pulses.

    B. **CORRECT:** Narrowing of the lumen of the aorta results in obstruction of blood flow from the ventricle, resulting in cool skin of the lower extremities.

    C. INCORRECT: A client who has coarctation of the aorta exhibits adequate oxygenation of blood. Therefore, severe cyanosis is not present.

    D. INCORRECT: Clubbing of the fingers is a clinical manifestation of chronic hypoxemia and will not be observed in an infant who has coarctation of the aorta.

    E. **CORRECT:** Heart failure occurs when the heart is unable to meet the body's demands, and is a clinical manifestation of coarctation of the aorta.

    Ⓝ NCLEX® Connection: Physiological Adaptations, Basic Pathophysiology

2. A. INCORRECT: A client who has heart failure will exhibit tachycardia as the heart attempts to meet the body's demands.

    B. **CORRECT:** A client who has heart failure will exhibit cool extremities as the heart is unable to adequately circulate oxygenated blood.

    C. **CORRECT:** A client who has heart failure will exhibit peripheral edema as the heart is unable to adequately circulate blood through the body and back to the heart.

    D. INCORRECT: With heart failure, the heart is unable to keep up with the body's demands. A decrease in urinary output is a clinical manifestation of heart failure.

    E. **CORRECT:** A client who has heart failure will exhibit nasal flaring due to inadequate oxygenation of blood.

    Ⓝ NCLEX® Connection: Physiological Adaptations, Basic Pathophysiology

3.   A. INCORRECT: Digoxin can be given without regard to food or fluids.

    B. INCORRECT: Digoxin slows the heart rate by increasing contractility of the heart.

    C. **CORRECT:** The correct amount of digoxin should be administered at regularly scheduled times to maintain therapeutic blood levels.

    D. INCORRECT: It is not recommended to repeat digoxin following an emesis because it is impossible to determine how much medication was lost.

    Ⓝ NCLEX® Connection: Pharmacological Therapies, Expected Actions/Outcomes

4.   A. INCORRECT: The child should remain NPO 4 to 6 hr prior to the procedure.

    B. **CORRECT:** Iodine-based dyes may be used in this procedure, so the child is checked for allergies to iodine, which could lead to anaphylaxis.

    C. INCORRECT: The affected extremity should be maintained in a straight position following the procedure.

    D. INCORRECT: Fluids should be encouraged after the procedure to maintain adequate urine output and promote excretion of the dye.

    Ⓝ NCLEX® Connection: Reduction of Risk Potential, Potential for Complications of Diagnostic Tests/ Treatments/Procedures

5.   A. **CORRECT:** Rheumatic fever is caused by Group A β-hemolytic streptococcus. An erythema marginatum (rash) is a clinical manifestation.

    B. INCORRECT: A client who has rheumatic fever exhibits migratory joint pain of the large joints.

    C. INCORRECT: A client who has rheumatic fever exhibits nontender subcutaneous nodules of bony prominences.

    D. INCORRECT: Rheumatic fever is caused by Group A β-hemolytic streptococcus, which results in an elevated erythrocyte sedimentation rate.

    E. **CORRECT:** Rheumatic fever is caused by Group A β-hemolytic streptococcus. An increase in C-reactive protein is a clinical manifestation.

    Ⓝ NCLEX® Connection: Physiological Adaptations, Basic Pathophysiology

6. *Using the ATI Active Learning Template: Systems Disorder*

A. Clinical Manifestations

- Acute phase: onset of high fever that is unresponsive to antipyretics, with development of other manifestations
  - Fever greater than 38.9° C (102° F) lasting 5 days to 2 weeks and unresponsive to antipyretics
  - Irritability
  - Red eyes without drainage
  - Bright red, chapped lips
  - Strawberry tongue with white coating or red bumps on the posterior aspect
  - Red oral mucous membranes
  - Swelling of hands and feet with red palms and soles
  - Nonblistering rash
  - Bilateral joint pain
  - Enlarged lymph nodes
- Subacute phase: resolution of the fever and gradual subsiding of other manifestations
  - Irritability
  - Peeling skin around the nails, on the palms and soles
- Convalescent phase: no clinical manifestations seen except altered laboratory findings. Resolution in about 6 to 8 weeks from onset.

B. Nursing Care

- Monitor vital signs, ECG, and cardiac status.
- Monitor for heart failure (decreased urine output, gallop heart rhythm, tachycardia, respiratory distress).
- Monitor I&O. Obtain daily weight.
- Administer IV fluids. Offer clear liquids and soft foods.
- Administer IV gamma globulin according to facility policy.
- Administer aspirin as prescribed.
- Provide care to include oral hygiene, cool cloths to extremities, application of skin lotion. Provide for a quiet environment to promote rest. Cluster nursing care.

Ⓝ NCLEX® Connection: Physiological Adaptations, Basic Pathophysiology

chapter 19

Overview

- Blood disorders that can affect children include the following.

  - Epistaxis

  - Iron deficiency anemia

  - Sickle cell anemia

  - Hemophilia

EPISTAXIS

Overview

- Short, isolated occurrences of epistaxis are common in childhood.

- Although epistaxis is rarely an emergency, it causes the child and the child's caregivers anxiety.

Data Collection

- Risk Factors

  - Trauma, such as picking or rubbing the nose, can cause mucous membranes in the nose, which are vascular and fragile, to tear and bleed.

  - Low humidity, allergic rhinitis, upper respiratory infection, blunt injury, or a foreign body in the nose can all precipitate a nosebleed.

  - Medications that affect clotting factors can increase bleeding.

  - Epistaxis can be the result of underlying diseases (von Willebrand disease, hemophilia, idiopathic thrombocytopenia purpura [ITP], leukemia).

- Subjective Data

  - History of bleeding gums or blood in body fluids and/or stool

  - History of trauma, illness, allergies, or placing foreign bodies in the nose

- Objective Data

  - Physical Assessment Findings

    - Active bleeding from nose

    - Restlessness and agitation

Patient-Centered Care

- Nursing Care
  - Maintain a calm demeanor with the child and family.
  - Have the child sit up with the head tilted slightly forward to prevent aspiration of blood.
  - Apply pressure to the lower nose with the thumb and forefinger for at least 10 min.
  - If needed, cotton or tissue can be packed into the side of the nose that is bleeding.
  - Encourage the child to breathe through her mouth while her nose is bleeding.
  - Apply ice across the bridge of the nose if bleeding continues.
  - Water-soluble jelly or petroleum can be inserted after a nose bleed to prevent crusting of the blood and possible recurrence of bleeding episode.
- Care After Discharge
  - Client Education
    - Keep fingernails short.
    - Use a cool-mist humidifier during the dry winter months.
    - For recurrences, remind the child to sit up and slightly forward so blood does not flow down the throat and cause coughing.
    - Inform the family that bleeding usually stops within 10 min.

Complications

- Hemorrhage
  - Nursing Actions
    - Provide support to the child during cauterization or packing.
  - Client Education
    - Instruct the child and family to seek medical care if bleeding lasts longer than 30 min, and that repeated episodes require further evaluation for bleeding disorders.

IRON DEFICIENCY ANEMIA

Overview

- Iron deficiency anemia is the most common anemia in the U.S.
- Children ages 12 to 36 months are at risk due to consuming a diet high in cow's milk without adequate intake of foods high in iron.
- Adolescents are at risk due to poor diets, menses, obesity, and rapid growth rates.
- The production of Hgb requires iron. Iron deficiency will result in decreased Hgb levels.
- Iron deficiency anemia usually results from an inadequate dietary supply of iron, and is the most preventable mineral disturbance.

Data Collection

- Risk Factors
  - Premature birth resulting in decreased iron stores
  - Excessive intake of cows' milk in toddlers
    - Milk is not a good source of iron.
    - Milk is consumed in place of iron-rich solid foods.
  - Malabsorption disorders due to prolonged diarrhea
  - Poor dietary intake of iron
  - Increased iron requirements (blood loss)
  - Chronic disorders (folate deficiency, sickle cell anemia, hemophilia)
- Subjective and Objective Data
  - Shortness of breath
  - Pallor
  - Brittle, spoon-shaped fingernails
  - Fatigue, irritability, and muscle weakness
  - Systolic heart murmur, enlarged heart, or heart failure
  - Laboratory Tests

EXPECTED REFERENCE RANGES		
AGE	HGB	HCT
2 months	9.0 to 14.0 g/dL	28% to 42%
6 to 12 years	11.5 to 15.5 g/dL	35% to 45%
12 to 18 years	13.0 to 16.0 g/dL (male)	37% to 49% (male)
	12.0 to 16.0 g/dL (female)	36% to 46% (female)

  - CBC – decreased RBC count, Hgb, and Hct
  - RBC indices – decreased, indicating microcytic/hypochromic RBCs
    - Mean corpuscular volume (MVC) – average size of RBC
    - Mean corpuscular Hgb (MCH) – average weight of RBC
    - Mean corpuscular hemoglobin concentration (MCHC) – amount of Hgb relative to size of cell
  - Reticulocyte count – can be decreased (indicates bone marrow production of RBCs)
  - Decreased serum ferritin level (indicator of iron stores)

Patient-Centered Care

- Nursing Care
  - Provide iron supplements for preterm and low-birthweight infants by the age of 2 months.
  - Provide iron supplements to infants who are exclusively breastfed by the age of 4 months.
  - Recommend iron-fortified formula for infants who are not being breastfed.
  - Modify the infant's diet to include high iron, vitamin C, and protein content.
  - Monitor milk intake in toddlers.
    - Limit milk intake to 32 oz (950 mL) per day.
    - Delay giving milk until after a meal.
    - Do not allow toddlers to carry bottles or cups of milk.
  - Allow frequent rest periods.
  - Monitor transfusion of packed RBCs, if required.
- Medications
  - Iron Supplements
    - Nursing Considerations
      - Give 1 hr before or 2 hr after milk or antacid to prevent decreased absorption.
      - Gastrointestinal upset (diarrhea, constipation, nausea) is common at the start of therapy. This will decrease over time.
      - If tolerated, administer iron supplements on an empty stomach. Give with meals, start with reduced dose, and gradually increase if GI distress occurs.
      - Give with vitamin C to increase absorption.
      - Use a straw with liquid preparation to prevent staining of teeth.
      - Use a Z-track into deep muscle for parenteral injections. Do not massage after injection.
    - Client Education
      - Reinforce education to the child and family to expect stools to turn a tarry green color if dose is adequate.
      - Instruct child to brush teeth after oral dose to minimize or prevent staining.
- Care After Discharge
  - Client Education
    - Advise the family that diarrhea, constipation, or nausea can occur at the start of therapy, but these adverse effects are usually self-limiting.
    - Provide information regarding appropriate iron administration.
    - Increase fiber and fluids if constipation develops.
    - Dietary sources of iron
      - Infants – iron-fortified cereals and formula
      - Older children – dried beans and lentils; peanut butter; green, leafy vegetables; iron-fortified breads and flour; poultry; and red meat
    - To prevent overdose, store no more than 1 month's supply in a child-proof bottle, and out of reach of children.

- Encourage parents to allow the child to rest.

- Inform parents that the length of treatment will be determined by the child's response to the treatment. If Hgb levels are not increased after 1 month of therapy, further evaluation is warranted.

- Instruct parents to return for follow-up laboratory tests to determine the effectiveness of treatment.

Complications

- Heart failure
  - Heart failure can develop due to the increased demand on the heart to deliver oxygen to tissues.
  - Nursing Actions
    - Treat anemia.
    - Monitor cardiac rhythm.
    - Give cardiac medications as prescribed.
  - Client Education
    - Reinforce education to the child and family on the manifestations of heart failure.
    - Reinforce how to monitor pulse rates.
- Developmental delay
  - Nursing Actions
    - Check level of functioning.
    - Improve nutritional intake.
    - Assist with referral to appropriate developmental services.
  - Client Education
    - Provide support to the family.

SICKLE CELL ANEMIA

Overview

- Sickle cell disease (SCD) is a group of diseases in which abnormal sickle hemoglobin S (HbS) replaces normal adult hemoglobin (Hgb A).
- Sickle cell anemia (SCA) is the homozygous and most common form of SCD.
- Manifestations and complications of SCA are the result of RBC sickling, which leads to increased blood viscosity, obstruction of blood flow, and tissue hypoxia.
  - Manifestations of SCA are not usually apparent until later in infancy due to the presence of fetal Hgb.
- Tissue hypoxia causes tissue ischemia, which results in pain.
- Increased destruction of RBCs occurs.
- Sickle cell crisis is the exacerbation of SCA.

M View Image: Sickle Cell Anemia

Data Collection

- Risk Factors
  - SCD is an autosomal recessive genetic disorder.
  - SCA primarily affects African-Americans. Other forms of SCD can affect individuals of Mediterranean, Indian, or Middle Eastern descent.
  - Children who have the sickle cell trait do not manifest the disease but can pass the trait to their offspring.
- Subjective and Objective Data
  - Family history of sickle cell anemia or sickle cell trait
  - Reports of pain
  - Shortness of breath/fatigue
  - Pallor/pale mucous membranes
  - Jaundice
  - Hands and feet cool to touch
  - Dizziness
  - Headache

CRISIS	MANIFESTATIONS
Vaso-occlusive (painful episode) › Usually lasts 4 to 6 days	› Acute » Severe pain, usually in bones, joints, and abdomen » Swollen joints, hands, and feet » Anorexia, vomiting, and fever » Hematuria » Obstructive jaundice » Visual disturbances › Chronic » Increased risk of respiratory infections and osteomyelitis » Retinal detachment and blindness » Systolic murmurs » Kidney failure and enuresis » Liver cirrhosis; hepatomegaly » Seizures » Skeletal deformities; shoulder or hip avascular necrosis
Sequestration	› Excessive pooling of blood, primarily in the spleen (splenomegaly) and sometimes in the liver (hepatomegaly) › Reduced circulating blood volume results in hypovolemia and can progress to shock › Hypovolemic shock: irritability, tachycardia, pallor, decreased urinary output, tachypnea, cool extremities, thready pulse, hypotension
Aplastic	› Extreme anemia as a result of decreased RBC production › Typically triggered by an infection
Hyperhemolytic	› Increased rate of RBC destruction leading to anemia, jaundice, and/or reticulocytosis

- ○ Laboratory Tests
  - Screening for SCA in newborns is mandatory in most states.
  - CBC to detect anemia
  - Sickledex (sickle-turbidity) – a screening tool that detects the presence of HbS but will not differentiate the trait from the disease
  - Hemoglobin electrophoresis – separates the various forms of Hgb and is the definitive diagnosis of sickle cell anemia
  - Sickle-cell crisis
    - ▫ Hgb is decreased.
    - ▫ WBC count is elevated.
    - ▫ Bilirubin and reticulocyte levels are elevated.
    - ▫ Peripheral blood smear reveals sickled cells.
- ○ Diagnostic Procedures

  - Transcranial Doppler (TCD) test
    - ▫ Used to assess intracranial vascular flow and detect the risk for cerebrovascular accident (CVA).
    - ▫ A TCD is performed annually on children ages 2 to 16 years who have SCD.

Patient-Centered Care

- Nursing Care
  - ○ Promote rest to decrease oxygen consumption.
  - ○ Administer oxygen as prescribed if hypoxia is present.
  - ○ Maintain fluid and electrolyte balance.
    - Monitor I&O.
    - Give oral fluids.
    - Administer IV fluids with electrolyte replacement.
  - ○ Pain Management
    - Use an interprofessional approach.
    - Treat mild to moderate pain with acetaminophen (Tylenol) or ibuprofen (Advil). Manage severe pain with opioid analgesics.
    - Implement comfort measures, such as warm packs to painful joints.
    - Administer analgesics on a schedule to prevent pain.
  - ○ Assist with monitoring clients who are receiving blood products. Observe for manifestations of hypervolemia and transfusion reaction.
  - ○ Treat and prevent infection.
    - Administer antibiotics.
    - Perform frequent hand hygiene.
    - Give oral prophylactic penicillin.
    - Administer pneumococcal conjugate vaccine (PCV), meningococcal vaccine (MCV4), and yearly seasonal influenza vaccine.
  - ○ Monitor and report laboratory results

- Medications
  - Opioids – codeine, morphine sulfate, oxycodone, hydrocodone (Dilaudid), and methadone (Dolophine)
    - Opioids provide analgesia for pain management.
    - Nursing Considerations
      - Administer orally (immediate- or sustained-release) or IV.
      - Administer on a regular schedule to maintain control, or prevent pain if possible.
      - Assist with clients who are receiving patient-controlled analgesia.
    - Client Education
      - Reinforce the need to avoid activities that require mental alertness.
      - Provide reassurance that analgesics can be necessary in high doses, and that addiction is rare.
- Care After Discharge
  - Client Education
    - Provide emotional support, and assist with referral to social services if appropriate.
    - Reinforce teaching to the child and family about manifestations of crisis and infection.
    - Advise the family of the importance of promoting rest and providing adequate nutrition for the child.
    - Encourage the child and family to maintain good hand hygiene and avoid individuals who have colds/infection/viruses.
    - Give specific directions regarding fluid intake requirements, such as how many bottles or ounces of fluid should be consumed daily.
    - Provide information about genetic counseling.
    - Encourage maintenance of up-to-date immunizations.
    - Advise the child to wear a medical identification wristband or medical identification tags.

Complications

- CVA
  - Nursing Actions
    - Observe for and report manifestations.
      - Seizures
      - Abnormal behavior
      - Weakness of or inability to move an extremity
      - Slurred speech
      - Visual changes
      - Vomiting
      - Severe headache
  - Client Education
    - Blood transfusions are usually performed every 3 to 4 weeks to prevent a repeat CVA.

- Acute chest syndrome
  - Can be life-threatening
  - Nursing Actions
    - Observe for and report manifestations.
      - Chest, back, or abdominal pain
      - Fever of 38.5° C (101.3° F) or greater
      - Cough
      - Tachypnea
      - Dyspnea
      - Retractions
      - Decreased oxygen saturations

HEMOPHILIA

Overview

- Hemophilia is a group of disorders characterized by difficulty controlling bleeding.
- Bleeding time is extended due to lack of a factor required for blood to clot. Bleeding is internal or external.
- Bleeding tendencies are sometimes recognized during infancy following circumcision, but might not become apparent until the infant becomes more active and prone to injuries during the toddler years.
- Hemophilia varies in severity based on the percentage of clotting factor a child's body contains. For example, a child who has mild hemophilia might have up to 49% of the normal factor VIII in his body, while a child with severe hemophilia has very little factor VIII.
- Both hemophilia A and B are X-linked recessive disorders.

TYPES OF HEMOPHILIA	
Hemophilia A	Hemophilia B
› Deficiency of factor VIII	› Deficiency of factor IX
› Referred to as classic hemophilia	› Referred to as Christmas disease
› Accounts for 80% of cases	

Data Collection

- Subjective Data
    - Episodes of bleeding, excessive bleeding, reports of joint pain and stiffness, impaired mobility, easy bruising, and activity intolerance
- Objective Data
    - Physical Assessment Findings
        - Active bleeding, which includes bleeding gums, epistaxis, hematuria, and tarry stools
        - Hematomas or bruising, even with minor injuries
        - Hemarthrosis as evidenced by joint pain, stiffness, warmth, swelling, redness, loss of range of motion, and deformities
        - Headache, slurred speech, and a decreased level of consciousness
    - Laboratory Tests
        - Prolonged partial thromboplastin time (aPTT)
        - Factor-specific assays to determine deficiency
        - Platelets and prothrombin time within expected reference ranges
        - Whole blood clotting time within expected range or prolonged
    - Diagnostic Procedures
        - DNA testing – detects classic hemophilia trait in females

Patient-Centered Care

- Nursing Care
    - Management of bleeding in the hospital
        - Avoid taking temperature rectally.
        - Avoid unnecessary skin punctures. Use surgical aseptic technique.
        - Apply pressure for 5 min after injections, venipuncture, or needle sticks.
        - Monitor urine, stool, and nasogastric fluid for occult blood.
        - Control localized bleeding.
            - Monitor administration of factor replacement.
            - Observe for adverse effects, which include headache, flushing, low sodium, and alterations in heart rate and blood pressure.
            - Encourage the child to rest and immobilize the affected joints.
            - Elevate and apply ice to the affected joints.

- Medications
  - 1-deamino-8-d-arginine vasopressin (DDAVP) is a synthetic form of vasopressin that increases plasma factor VIII (antihemophilic factor [AHF]).
    - Effective for mild, but not severe, hemophilia
    - Not effective for hemophilia B, which involves a factor IX deficiency
    - Nursing Considerations – can be given prior to dental or surgical procedures
  - Factor VIII, products that contain factor VIII, pooled plasma, and recombinant products
    - Used to prevent and treat hemorrhage
    - Nursing Considerations – Assist with the care of children who are receiving an IV infusion.
    - Client Education
      - Instruct the child and family that treatment can require numerous doses.
      - Periodic administration has proven effective for preventing bleeding complications.
  - Corticosteroids
    - Used to treat hematuria, acute episodes of hemarthrosis, and chronic synovitis
    - Nursing Considerations – Monitor for infection and bleeding.
    - Client Education – Encourage the client and family to maintain good hand hygiene and avoid individuals with colds/infection/viruses.
  - Nonsteroidal anti-inflammatory agents
    - Used to treat pain associated with chronic synovitis
    - Nursing considerations – Monitor for infection.
    - Client Education
      - Administer cautiously due to potential inhibition of platelet function.
      - Encourage the client to take the medication with food.
- Teamwork and Collaboration
  - An interprofessional approach includes a pediatrician, hematologist, orthopedist, nurse, physical therapist, and social worker.

- Care After Discharge
  - Client Education
    - Explain to parents how to prevent bleeding at home.
      - Place the infant or child in a padded crib.
      - Provide a safe home and a play environment that is free of clutter. Place padding on corners of furniture.
      - Dress toddlers in extra layers of clothing to provide additional padding.
      - Set activity restrictions to avoid injury. Acceptable activities include low-contact sports (tennis, swimming, golf). While participating in these activities, children should wear protective equipment.
      - Encourage the use of soft-bristled toothbrushes.
    - Encourage regular exercise and physical therapy after active bleeding is controlled.
    - Encourage the family to maintain up-to-date immunizations.
    - Stress the importance of wearing a medical identification wristband or medical identification tags.
    - Explain the manifestations of internal bleeding and hemarthrosis.
    - Discuss ways to control bleeding episodes using the RICE (rest, ice, compression, elevation) method.
    - Encourage the family to participate in a support group.

Complications

- Uncontrolled bleeding (intracranial hemorrhage, airway obstruction from bleeding in mouth, neck, or chest)
  - Nursing Actions
    - Monitor vital signs for evidence of impending shock.
    - Take measures to control bleeding.
    - Monitor the child receiving factor replacement to treat excessive bleeding or hemarthrosis.
    - Monitor blood transfusions, if prescribed.
    - Observe for manifestations of an intracranial bleed.
    - Monitor prophylaxis treatment. Regimens include infusion of factor VIII concentrate:
      - Prior to joint bleed.
      - Three times a week after the first joint bleed.
  - Client Education – Tell the family and child to report signs of bleeding.
- Joint deformity (most often elbows, knees, and ankles)
  - Repeated episodes of hemarthrosis (bleeding into joint spaces) lead to impaired range of motion, pain, tenderness, and swelling, which can develop into joint deformities.
  - Nursing Actions
    - Take appropriate measures to rest, immobilize, elevate, and apply ice to the affected joints during active bleeding.
    - Encourage active range of motion after bleeding is controlled.
    - Encourage maintenance of ideal weight to minimize stress on joints.
    - Encourage maintenance of regular exercise and physical therapy.

APPLICATION EXERCISES

1. A nurse is reinforcing teaching about the management of epistaxis to a child and his family. Which of the following positions should the nurse instruct the child to take when experiencing a nosebleed?

    A. Sit up and lean forward.

    B. Sit up and tilt the head up.

    C. Lie in a supine position.

    D. Lie in a prone position.

2. A nurse is reinforcing teaching about epistaxis to the parent of a school-age child. Which of the following should the nurse include as an appropriate action to take when managing an episode of epistaxis? (Select all that apply.)

    _____ A. Press the nares together at least 10 min.

    _____ B. Breathe through the nose until bleeding stops.

    _____ C. Pack cotton or tissue into the naris that is bleeding.

    _____ D. Apply a warm cloth across the bridge of the nose.

    _____ E. Insert petroleum into the naris after the bleeding stops.

3. A nurse is reinforcing teaching to the parent of a child who has a new prescription for liquid oral iron supplements. Which of the following statements by the parent indicates an understanding of the teaching?

    A. "I should take my child to the emergency department if his stools become dark."

    B. "My child should avoid eating citrus fruits while taking the supplements."

    C. "I should give the iron with milk to help prevent an upset stomach."

    D. "My child should take the supplement through a straw."

4. A nurse is preparing to administer iron dextran (Proferdex) IM to a school-age child who has iron deficiency anemia. Which of the following actions by the nurse is appropriate?

    A. Administer the dose in the deltoid muscle.

    B. Use the Z-track method when administering the dose.

    C. Avoid injecting more than 2 mL with each dose.

    D. Massage the injection site for 1 min after administering the dose.

5. A nurse is caring for an infant whose screening test reveals that he might have sickle cell disease. Which of the following tests should be performed to distinguish if the infant has the trait or the disease?

    A. Sickle solubility test (Sickledex)

    B. Hemoglobin electrophoresis

    C. Complete blood count

    D. Transcranial Doppler

6. A nurse is caring for a child who has a new diagnosis of hemophilia A. Use the ATI Active Learning Template: Systems Disorder to complete this item to include the following:

    A. Objective and Subjective Data: List two physical assessment findings associated with hemophilia.

    B. Client Education: List three concepts to include in the teaching with the family and child.

APPLICATION EXERCISES KEY

1. A. **CORRECT:** The nurse should instruct the child to sit up and lean to prevent aspiration when experiencing a nosebleed.

    B. INCORRECT: Sitting up and tilting the head up could cause aspiration of blood, and is not an appropriate position when experiencing a nosebleed.

    C. INCORRECT: Lying in a supine position could cause aspiration of blood, and is not an appropriate position when experiencing a nosebleed.

    D. INCORRECT: Lying in a prone position could cause aspiration of blood, and is not an appropriate position when experiencing a nosebleed.

    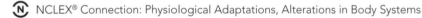 NCLEX® Connection: Physiological Adaptations, Alterations in Body Systems

2. A. **CORRECT:** Pressing the nares together for at least 10 min is an appropriate action to take when managing an episode of epistaxis.

    B. INCORRECT: The child should breathe through the mouth until the bleeding stops.

    C. **CORRECT:** Packing cotton or tissue into the naris that is bleeding is an appropriate action when managing an episode of epistaxis.

    D. INCORRECT: Applying an ice pack across the bridge of the nose is an appropriate action when managing an episode of epistaxis.

    E. **CORRECT:** Inserting petroleum into the naris after the bleeding stops is an appropriate action when managing an episode of epistaxis.

     NCLEX® Connection: Physiological Adaptations, Alterations in Body Systems

3. A. INCORRECT: The child's stools will become a tarry-green color if the iron supplement dose is adequate.

    B. INCORRECT: Vitamin C increases absorption of the iron and should be encouraged while taking the supplement.

    C. INCORRECT: Milk prevents absorption of the iron. The supplement should be given 1 hr before or 2 hr after consuming milk.

    D. **CORRECT:** The child should take the supplement through a straw to prevent or minimize staining of the teeth.

     NCLEX® Connection: Pharmacological Therapies, Expected Actions/Outcomes

4. A. INCORRECT: The nurse should administer the dose in to a large muscle mass.

    B. **CORRECT:** The nurse should use the Z-track method when administering the dose.

    C. INCORRECT: The nurse should avoid injecting more than 1 mL with each dose.

    D. INCORRECT: To reduce irritation and skin staining, the nurse should not massage the injection site after administering the dose.

     NCLEX® Connection: Pharmacological Therapies, Medication Administration

5. A. INCORRECT: The Sickle solubility test is a screening tool that detects the presence of abnormal hemoglobin, but does not distinguish between the trait and the disease.

    B. **CORRECT:** The hemoglobin electrophoresis test is performed to distinguish if the infant has the trait or the disease.

    C. INCORRECT: A complete blood count tests for anemia. It also tells the average size of the red blood cells and the amount of hemoglobin in the red blood cells. It will not distinguish between sickle cell disease and sickle cell trait.

    D. INCORRECT: The transcranial Doppler is performed to assess intracranial vascular flow and detect the risk for cerebrovascular accident. It will not distinguish between sickle cell disease and sickle cell trait.

     NCLEX® Connection: Reduction of Risk Potential, Diagnostic Tests

6. *Using the ATI Active Learning Template: Systems Disorder*

    A. Objective and Subjective Data
    - Active bleeding (possibly from the gums, epistaxis, hematuria, and/or GI tract)
    - Cerebral bleeding can cause headaches, slurred speech, and decreased level of consciousness
    - Hematomas and bruising that occur easily even with minor injuries
    - Joint pain and stiffness, warmth, swelling, redness, loss of range of motion of the joints

    B. Client Education
    - Prevent bleeding at home
      ○ Provide a safe home and a play environment that is free of clutter.
      ○ Place padding on corners of furniture.
      ○ Set activity restrictions to avoid injury. Stress importance of wearing protective equipment during activities.
      ○ Recommend the use of soft-bristled toothbrushes or disposable oral sponges.
    - Encourage regular exercise and physical therapy when not actively bleeding.
    - Encourage that recommended immunizations remain up-to-date.
    - Stress the importance of wearing a medical identification wristband or medical identification tags.
    - Reinforce teaching about the manifestations of internal bleeding and hemarthrosis
    - Inform of the RICE method (rest, ice, compression, elevation) to control active bleeding.

     NCLEX® Connection: Physiological Adaptations, Basic Pathophysiology

UNIT 2   Nursing Care of Children with System Disorders

SECTION: GASTROINTESTINAL DISORDERS

› Acute Infectious Gastrointestinal Disorders
› Gastrointestinal Structural and Inflammatory Disorders

NCLEX® CONNECTIONS

When reviewing the chapters in this section, keep in mind the relevant sections of the NCLEX® outline, in particular:

Client Needs: Reduction of Risk Potential

› Relevant topics/tasks include:
  » Diagnostic Tests
    › Perform diagnostic testing.
  » Potential for Complications of Diagnostic Tests/Treatments/Procedures
    › Identify client response to diagnostic tests/treatments/procedures.

Client Needs: Physiological Adaptations

› Relevant topics/tasks include:
  » Alterations in Body Systems
    › Perform care for client after surgical procedure.
    › Reinforce education to client regarding care and condition.
  » Basic Pathophysiology
    › Identify signs and symptoms related to an acute or chronic illness.
    › Consider general principles of client disease when providing care.
  » Fluid and Electrolyte Imbalances
    › Identify signs and symptoms of client fluid and/or electrolyte imbalances.
    › Provide interventions to restore client fluid and/or electrolyte imbalances.

chapter 20

Overview

- Diarrhea can be mild to severe, and acute or chronic. It can result in mild to severe dehydration.

  - Acute diarrhea is a sudden increase in frequency and change in consistency of stool.

    - It is usually secondary to an infectious agent in the GI tract, upper respiratory infection, urinary tract infection, antibiotic use, or laxative use.

    - Self-resolution occurs in less than 14 days if dehydration does not occur.

  - Acute infectious diarrhea is caused by a variety of viral, bacterial, or parasitic pathogens.

  - Chronic diarrhea is an increase in frequency and change of consistency of stool(s) for more than 14 days.

    - It is caused by chronic conditions such as malabsorption syndrome, food allergies, or inflammatory bowel disease.

  - Chronic nonspecific diarrhea has no identified cause.

- Dehydration is a body fluid disturbance when the output exceeds intake. It results from many causes such as fluid losses through the skin, respiratory tract, urinary tract, or GI tract.

Data Collection

- Risk Factors

  - Lack of clean water, poor hygiene, crowded living environments, poor sanitation, and nutritional deficiency.

- Subjective and Objective Data

  - Reports of fatigue, malaise, change in behavior, change in stool pattern, poor appetite, weight loss, and pain.

  - Observe for clinical manifestations of dehydration.

PATHOGEN	CLINICAL MANIFESTATIONS	TRANSMISSION/INCUBATION
Rotavirus – viral infection	› Most common cause of diarrhea in children younger than 5 years › Affects children of all ages › Fever › Onset of foul-smelling, watery stools, diarrhea for 5 to 7 days › Vomiting for approximately 2 days	› Transmission: fecal-oral › Incubation period: 48 hr
Yersinia enterocolitis – bacterial infection	› Mucoid, possibly bloody diarrhea › Abdominal pain, fever, and vomiting	› Transmission: pets and food › Incubation period: 1 to 3 weeks

PATHOGEN	CLINICAL MANIFESTATIONS	TRANSMISSION/INCUBATION
Escherichia coli (E. coli) – bacterial infection	› Watery diarrhea for 1 to 2 days, followed by abdominal cramping and bloody diarrhea › Could lead to hemolytic uremic syndrome (HUS)	› Transmission: depends on strain of *E. coli* › Incubation period: 3 to 4 days
Salmonella nontyphoidal groups – bacterial infection	› Mild to severe nausea, vomiting, abdominal cramping, bloody diarrhea, and fever (may be afebrile in infants) › Diarrhea can last as long as 2 to 3 weeks › Possible headache, confusion, drowsiness, and seizures › Can lead to meningitis or septicemia	› Transmission: person-to-person, undercooked meats and poultry › Incubation period: 6 to 72 hr
Clostridium difficile (C. difficile) – bacterial infection	› Mild, watery diarrhea for a few days › Possible less severe symptoms in children than adults › Possible leukocytosis, hypoalbuminemia, and high fever in certain children › Possible pseudomembranous colitis	› Transmission: contact with colonized spores, commonly in health care settings › Incubation period: nonspecified
Clostridium botulinum (C. botulinum) – bacterial infection	› Manifestations depend on strain › Abdominal pain, cramping, and diarrhea › Possible respiratory or CNS problems	› Transmission: contaminated food products › Incubation period: 12 to 26 hr
Shigella groups Shigellosis – bacterial infection	› Sick appearance › Fever, fatigue, and anorexia › Cramping abdomen followed by watery or bloody diarrhea lasting 5 to 10 days	› Transmission: contaminated food or water › Incubation period: 1 to 7 days
Norwalk-like organisms Caliciviruses – viral infection	› Abdominal cramps, nausea and vomiting, malaise, watery diarrhea › Lasts 2 to 3 days	› Transmission: contaminated water › Incubation period: 12 to 48 hr
Staphylococcus – bacterial infection	› Diarrhea, nausea, and vomiting	› Transmission: inadequately cooked or refrigerated food › Incubation period: 1 to 8 hr
Enterobius vermicularis (pinworm) – helminthic infection	› Perianal itching, enuresis, sleeplessness, restlessness, and irritability due to itching	› Transmission: fecal-oral › Ingested or inhaled eggs hatch in the upper intestine, and mature. After mating, worms migrate out of the intestine and lay eggs. Eggs can survive for 2 to 3 weeks on surfaces.
Giardia lamblia – parasitic pathogen	› Children 5 years of age or younger » Diarrhea » Vomiting » Anorexia › Older children » Abdominal cramps » Intermittent loose, malodorous, pale, greasy stools	› Transmission: person-to-person, food, animals › The nonmotile stage of protozoa can survive in the environment for months.

○ Laboratory Tests

- Perform a CBC with differential to determine anemia or infection.

- Hct, Hgb, BUN, creatinine, and urine-specific gravity levels are usually elevated with dehydration.

- Stool test for occult blood.

- Perform a urinalysis.

○ Diagnostic Procedures

- Tape test

□ A tape test should be performed to check for *Enterobius vermicularis*.

□ Client Education

▶ Tell the parents to place transparent tape over the child's anus at night. The tape should be removed the following morning prior to the child toileting or bathing. If possible, have the parent apply the tape after the child has gone to sleep and remove it before the child awakens.

▶ Inform the parents that the specimen should be brought to the laboratory for microscopic evaluation.

▶ Remind the parents to use good hand hygiene during this procedure.

- Infectious gastroenteritis

□ Rotavirus – enzyme immunoassay (stool sample)

□ *E. coli* – Sorbitol-MacConkey agar (stool sample)

□ *Salmonella* – Gram stain stool culture

□ *C. difficile* – stool culture

□ *C. botulinum* – blood and stool culture

□ *Staphylococcus* – identification of organism in stool, blood, food, or aspirate

□ *G. lamblia* – enzyme immunoassay (stool sample)

□ Shigellosis – blood and stool culture

□ Caliciviruses – enzyme immunoassay (stool sample)

□ Yersinia enterocolitis – identification of organism in stool, blood, oral secretions, urine, or bile

Patient-Centered Care

- Nursing Care

○ Obtain baseline height and weight.

○ Obtain daily weights at the same time each day.

○ Avoid taking a rectal temperature.

○ Monitor I&O (urine and stool).

○ Administer IV fluids as prescribed.

○ Administer antibiotic as prescribed (*Shigella*, *C. difficile*, and *G. lamblia*).

○ Avoid antibiotics (*C. botulinum*, *E. coli*, *Salmonella*).

○ Avoid antimotility agents (*E. coli*, *Salmonella*, *Shigella*).

○ Administer oral rehydration therapy (ORT).

■ Start replacement with an oral replacement solution (ORS) of 75 to 90 sodium mEq/L at 40 to 50 mL/kg over 4 hr.

■ Determine the need for further rehydration after initial replacement.

□ Initiate maintenance therapy with ORS of 40 to 60 sodium mEq/L and limit to 150 mL/kg/day.

▶ Give ORS alternately with appropriate intake.

▷ Give infants water, breast milk, or lactose-free formula if supplementary fluid is needed.

▷ Older children may resume their regular diets for additional intake.

▶ Replace each diarrheal stool with 10 mL/kg of ORS for ongoing diarrhea.

• Medications

○ Metronidazole (Flagyl) and tinidazole (Tindamax)

■ Indicated for *C. difficile* and *G. lamblia*

■ Nursing Considerations

□ Monitor for allergies.

□ Monitor for GI upset.

■ Client Education

□ Instruct the client to take the medication as prescribed and to report any GI disturbances.

○ Mebendazole, albendazole (Albenza), and pyrantel pamoate (Pin-X) – indicated for *Enterobius vermicularis*

■ Nursing Considerations

□ Administer in a single dose that can need to be repeated in 2 weeks.

□ Administer mebendazole for children older than 2 years of age.

■ Client Education

□ Entire family is treated at the same time.

• Care After Discharge

○ Client Education

■ Have the parents inform the child's school or day care center of the infection/infestation. The child should stay home while the illness is communicable.

■ Instruct the family to use commercially prepared ORS when the child experiences diarrhea. Foods and fluids to avoid include:

□ Fruit juices, carbonated sodas, and gelatin, which all have high carbohydrate content, low electrolyte content, and a high osmolality.

□ Caffeine, due to its mild diuretic effect.

□ Chicken or beef broth, which has too much sodium and not enough carbohydrates.

□ Bananas, rice, applesauce, and toast (BRAT diet).

▶ This diet has low nutritional value, high carbohydrate content, and low electrolytes.

- Reinforce teaching about prevention measures, including immunization for rotavirus.
- Provide frequent skin care to prevent skin breakdown.
- Reinforce teaching to the family about how to avoid the spread of infectious diseases.
  - Change bed linens and underwear daily for several days.
  - Cleanse toys and child care areas thoroughly to prevent further spread or reinfestation.
  - Keep toys separate and avoid shaking linens to prevent the spread of disease.
  - Shower frequently.
  - Avoid undercooked or under-refrigerated food.
  - Perform proper hand hygiene after toileting and after changing diapers.
  - Do not share dishes and utensils. Wash them in hot, soapy water or in the dishwasher.
  - Clip nails. Discourage nail biting and thumb sucking.
  - Clean toilet areas.

Complications

- Dehydration

TYPE	MANIFESTATIONS
Isotonic	› Water and sodium are lost in nearly equal amounts. › Major loss of fluid from extracellular fluid leads to a reduced volume of circulating fluid. › Hypovolemic shock can result. › Serum sodium is within the expected reference range (130 to 150 mEq/L).
Hypotonic	› Electrolyte loss is greater than water loss. › Water moves from extracellular fluid to intracellular fluid. › Physical manifestations are more severe with smaller fluid loss. › Shock is likely. › Serum sodium is less than 130 mEq/L.
Hypertonic	› Water loss is greater than electrolyte loss. › Fluid shifts from intracellular to extracellular. › Shock is less likely. › Neurologic changes (change in level of consciousness, irritability, hyperreflexia) can occur. › Serum sodium concentration is greater than 150 mEq/L.

LEVEL	WEIGHT LOSS	MANIFESTATIONS
Mild	3% to 5% in infants 3% to 4% in children	› Behavior, mucous membranes, anterior fontanel, pulse, and blood pressure are all within normal limits. › Capillary refill is greater than 2 seconds. › Slight thirst can be experienced.
Moderate	6% to 9% in infants 6% to 8% in children	› Capillary refill is between 2 and 4 seconds. › Thirst and irritability can be experienced. › Pulse is slightly increased with normal to orthostatic blood pressure. › Mucous membranes are dry and tears and skin turgor are decreased. › Slight tachypnea. › Normal to sunken anterior fontanel on infants.
Severe	10% or higher in infants 10% in children	› Capillary refill is greater than 4 seconds. › Tachycardia is present and orthostatic blood pressure can progress to shock. › Extreme thirst is present. › Mucous membranes are very dry and skin is tented. › Hyperpnea. › No tearing with sunken eyeballs. › The anterior fontanel is sunken. › Oliguria or anuria is present.

- Nursing Actions
  - Oral rehydration is attempted first for mild and moderate cases of dehydration.
    - Mild: 50 mL/kg rehydration fluid every 4 to 6 hr
    - Moderate: 100 mL/kg rehydration fluid every 4 to 6 hr
    - Replacement of diarrhea losses with 10 mL/kg each stool
  - Monitor parenteral fluid therapy as prescribed.
    - Implemented when a child is unable to drink enough oral fluids to correct fluid losses, and those who have severe dehydration or continued vomiting.
    - Isotonic solution at 20 mL/kg IV bolus with possible repeat for isotonic and hypotonic dehydration.
    - Hypertonic dehydration – Rapid fluid replacement is contraindicated because of the risk of cerebral edema.
    - Administer maintenance IV fluids as prescribed.
    - Avoid potassium replacement until kidney function is verified.
  - Monitor capillary refill.
  - Check vital signs.
  - Monitor weight.
  - Maintain accurate I&O.
- Client Education
  - Encourage oral fluids.
  - Resume normal diet as soon as possible.
  - Monitor and record how many times the child voids.

APPLICATION EXERCISES

1. A nurse is caring for a child who has had watery diarrhea for the past 3 days. Which of the following is an appropriate action for the nurse to take?

    A. Offer chicken broth.

    B. Initiate oral rehydration therapy.

    C. Start hypertonic IV solution.

    D. Keep NPO until the diarrhea subsides.

2. A nurse is caring for a child who is suspected to have *Enterobius vermicularis*. Which of the following is an appropriate action for the nurse to take?

    A. Perform a tape test.

    B. Collect stool specimen for culture.

    C. Test the stool for occult blood.

    D. Initiate IV fluids.

3. A nurse is collecting data on a child who has a rotavirus infection. Which of the following are expected findings? (Select all that apply.)

    _____ A. Fever

    _____ B. Vomiting

    _____ C. Watery stools

    _____ D. Bloody stools

    _____ E. Confusion

4. A nurse is reinforcing teaching to a group of parents about *Salmonella*. Which of the following should be included in the teaching? (Select all that apply.)

    _____ A. Incubation period is nonspecific.

    _____ B. It is a bacterial infection.

    _____ C. Bloody diarrhea is common.

    _____ D. It is diagnosed more frequently in winter months.

    _____ E. Antibiotics are used for treatment.

5. A nurse is reinforcing teaching to a group of parents about *E. coli*. Which of the following should be included in the teaching? (Select all that apply.)

_____ A. Severe abdominal cramping occurs.

_____ B. Watery diarrhea is present for more than 5 days.

_____ C. It can lead to hemolytic uremic syndrome.

_____ D. It is a foodborne pathogen.

_____ E. Antibiotics are given for treatment.

6. A nurse is reinforcing teaching to a parent of a child who has an acute gastrointestinal infection. What should the nurse include in the teaching? Use the ATI Active Learning Template: Systems Disorder to complete this item to include Client Education: Describe at least 10 points to review regarding care after discharge.

APPLICATION EXERCISES KEY

1. A. INCORRECT: Chicken broth is avoided for children who have diarrhea because it contains increased sodium levels and inadequate carbohydrates.

    B. **CORRECT:** Oral rehydration therapy is recommended for children who have diarrhea to replace lost electrolytes.

    C. INCORRECT: Isotonic IV solutions are recommended for children who have severe dehydration.

    D. INCORRECT: Children who have diarrhea are at risk for dehydration. Therefore, keeping them NPO is contraindicated.

    Ⓝ NCLEX® Connection: Physiological Adaptations, Fluid and Electrolyte Imbalances

2. A. **CORRECT:** A tape test is used to check for *Enterobius vermicularis*.

    B. INCORRECT: Stool cultures are obtained to diagnose *Salmonella* or *C. difficile*.

    C. INCORRECT: A clinical manifestation of *E. coli* is bloody stools.

    D. INCORRECT: IV fluids are initiated for children who are dehydrated.

    Ⓝ NCLEX® Connection: Reduction of Risk Potential, Diagnostic Tests

3. A. **CORRECT:** Fever is a clinical manifestation of rotavirus infection.

    B. **CORRECT:** Vomiting for approximately 2 days is a clinical manifestation of rotavirus infection.

    C. **CORRECT:** Foul-smelling, watery stools is a clinical manifestation of rotavirus infection.

    D. INCORRECT: Bloody stools is a clinical manifestation of *E. coli*.

    E. INCORRECT: Confusion is a clinical manifestation of *Salmonella*.

    Ⓝ NCLEX® Connection: Physiological Adaptations, Fluid and Electrolyte Imbalances

4. A. INCORRECT: The incubation period of *Salmonella* is 6 to 72 hr.

    B. **CORRECT:** *Salmonella* is classified as a bacterial infection.

    C. **CORRECT:** *Salmonella* clinical manifestations include bloody diarrhea, nausea, vomiting, and abdominal cramping.

    D. INCORRECT: *Yersinia enterocolitis* is diagnosed more frequently in winter months.

    E. **CORRECT:** *Salmonella* is a bacterial infection. Therefore, antibiotics are recommended for treatment in complicated cases.

    Ⓝ NCLEX® Connection: Physiological Adaptations, Alterations in Body Systems

5. A. **CORRECT:** Severe abdominal cramping is a clinical manifestation of *E. coli*.

    B. INCORRECT: Watery diarrhea lasts 1 to 2 days, then advances to bloody diarrhea.

    C. **CORRECT:** *E. coli* can lead to hemolytic uremic syndrome.

    D. **CORRECT:** *E. coli* is a foodborne pathogen.

    E. INCORRECT: Antibiotics can worsen an *E. coli* infection. Therefore, they are not recommended.

    (N) NCLEX® Connection: Physiological Adaptations, Alterations in Body Systems

6. *Using the ATI Active Learning Template: Systems Disorder*
    - Client Education
        - Have the parents inform the child's school or day care center of the infection/infestation. The child should stay home during the incubation period.
        - Instruct the family to use commercially prepared oral rehydration therapy when the child experiences diarrhea. Foods and fluids to avoid include:
            - Fruit juices, carbonated sodas, and gelatin, which all have high carbohydrate content, low electrolyte content, and a high osmolality.
            - Caffeine, due to its mild diuretic effect.
            - Chicken or beef broth, which has high sodium content and inadequate carbohydrates.
            - Bananas, rice, applesauce, and toast (BRAT diet) due to low nutritional value, high carbohydrate content, and low electrolytes.
        - Reinforce teaching about prevention measures, including immunization for rotavirus.
        - Provide frequent skin care to prevent skin breakdown.
        - Reinforce teaching to the family about how to avoid the spread of infectious diseases.
        - Change bed linens and underwear daily for several days.
        - Cleanse toys and child care areas thoroughly to prevent further spread or reinfestation.
        - Keep toys separate and avoid shaking linens to prevent the spread of disease.
        - Shower frequently.
        - Avoid undercooked or under-refrigerated food.
        - Perform proper hand hygiene after toileting and after changing diapers.
        - Do not share dishes and utensils. Wash them in hot, soapy water or in the dishwasher.
        - Clip nails. Discourage nail-biting and thumb-sucking.
        - Clean toilet areas.

    (N) NCLEX® Connection: Physiological Adaptations, Alterations in Body Systems

chapter 21

Overview

- Gastrointestinal structural disorders
  - Cleft lip and palate
  - Gastroesophageal reflux disease (GERD)
  - Hypertrophic pyloric stenosis
  - Hirschsprung disease
  - Intussusception
- Inflammatory disorders
  - Appendicitis
  - Meckel's diverticulum

CLEFT LIP AND PALATE

Overview

- Cleft lip (CL) results from the incomplete fusion of the oral cavity during intrauterine life. Cleft palate (CP) results from the incomplete fusion of the palatine plates during intrauterine life.

 View Image: Cleft Palate

- A cleft lip and palate can occur together, or either defect can appear alone. The defects can be unilateral (one-sided) or bilateral (two-sided)

Data Collection

- Risk Factors
  - Other syndromes
  - Combination of maternal and environmental factors
    - Family history of cleft lip or palate
    - Exposure to alcohol, cigarette smoke, anticonvulsants, or steroids during pregnancy
    - Folate deficiency during pregnancy

- Objective Data
  - Physical Findings
    - Cleft lip is a visible separation from the upper lip toward the nose.
    - Cleft palate is a visible or palpable opening of the palate connecting the mouth and the nasal cavity.

Patient-Centered Care

- Nursing Care
  - Support and encourage parents in the general care of their child.
  - Promote parent-infant bonding.
  - Promote healthy self-esteem throughout the child's development.
- Teamwork and Collaboration
  - Care of the child who has CL and CP requires care from members of various disciplines (plastic surgeon, orthodontist, ENT specialist, speech and language therapist, occupational therapist, dietitian, social services worker).
- Surgical Interventions
  - Cleft Lip
    - Repair typically is done between 2 to 3 months
    - Infant should be at least 10 weeks old, weigh 10 lb, and have a Hgb of 10 g/dL.
    - Revisions usually are required for severe defects.
  - Cleft Palate
    - Repair typically done is between 6 to 12 months.
    - Majority require a second surgery.
  - Nursing Actions
    - Preoperative
      - Cleft lip and cleft palate repair
        - Inspect the infant's lip and palate using a gloved finger to palpate the palate.
        - Determine the infant's ability to suck.
        - Obtain baseline weight.
        - Observe interaction between the family and infant.
        - Determine family coping and support.
        - Refer the parents to appropriate support groups.
        - Consult with social services to provide needed services (financial, insurance) for the family and infant.
        - Instruct the parents about proper feeding and cares.
        - Observe the ability to feed.

- ▶ Initiate strategies for successful feeding.
  - ▷ For isolated CL
    - ◆ Encourage breast feeding.
    - ◆ Use a wide-based nipple for bottle feeding.
    - ◆ Squeeze the infant's cheeks together during feeding to decrease the gap.
  - ▷ For CP or CL/CP
    - ◆ Position the infant upright while cradling the head during feeding.
    - ◆ Use a specialized bottle with a one-way valve and a specially cut nipple.
    - ◆ Burp the infant frequently.
    - ◆ Syringe feeding can be necessary for the infant who is unsuccessful with other methods.
- ▫ Postoperative
  - ▶ Cleft lip and cleft palate repair
    - ▷ Perform standard postoperative care, including monitoring of vital signs and pain management using an age-appropriate tool.
    - ▷ Keep the infant pain-free to decrease crying and stress on repair.
    - ▷ Administer analgesics as prescribed.
    - ▷ Check the operative sites for signs of crusting and infection.
    - ▷ The child should avoid sucking on a nipple or pacifier.
    - ▷ Avoid hard toys that the infant can bring to their mouth to protect the incision site.
    - ▷ Monitor I&O, and weigh daily.
    - ▷ Observe the family's interaction with the infant.
    - ▷ Observe family coping and support.
  - ▶ Cleft lip repair
    - ▷ Monitor the integrity of the postoperative protective device to ensure proper positioning.
    - ▷ Position the infant upright (infant car seat position), on her back, or on her side in the immediate postoperative period to maintain the integrity of the repair.
    - ▷ Apply elbow restraints to keep the infant from injuring the repair site.
    - ▷ Restraints should be removed periodically to check skin, allow limb movement, and provide for comfort.
    - ▷ Use saline on a sterile swab to clean the incision site. Apply antibiotic ointment if prescribed.
    - ▷ Gently aspirate secretions of mouth and nasopharynx to prevent respiratory complications.

> ▸ Cleft palate repair

  > ▷ Change the infant's position frequently to facilitate breathing. The infant can be placed on the abdomen in the immediate postoperative period.

  > ▷ Maintain IV fluids until the infant is able to eat and drink.

  > ▷ Monitor packing, which usually is removed after 2 to 3 days.

  > ▷ Avoid placing objects (tongue depressor, pacifier) in the infant's mouth.

  > ▷ Elbow restraints can be needed to prevent the infant from injuring the repair.

- Client Education

  □ Inform the parents that the infant can require elbow restraints for 4 to 6 weeks. Instruct the parents in the proper use of the restraints.

  □ Instruct the parents on the postoperative diet and feeding techniques.

  □ Instruct parents in proper care of operative site.

Complications

- Ear infections and hearing loss
  - Related to altered structure and recurrent infections
  - Nursing Actions
    - Feed the infant in an upright position. Monitor temperature.
  - Client Education
    - Describe for parents the manifestations of ear infections.
    - Encourage early intervention.
- Speech and language impairment
  - More common with cleft palate
  - Client Education
    - Refer to early intervention.
    - Refer parents to a speech therapist for care.
- Dental problems
  - Teeth might not erupt normally, and orthodontia usually is necessary later in life.
  - Client Education
    - Instruct the parents and child to promote healthy dental hygiene.
    - Encourage parents to seek early dental care.

GASTROESOPHAGEAL REFLUX DISEASE (GERD)

Overview

- Gastroesophageal reflux (GER) occurs when the gastric contents reflux back up into the esophagus, making esophageal mucosa vulnerable to injury from gastric acid and resulting in gastroesophageal reflux disease (GERD).

- GERD is tissue damage from GER.

- GER is self-limiting and usually resolves by 1 year of age.

Data Collection

- Risk Factors

  ○ GER – prematurity, bronchopulmonary dysplasia, neurological impairments, asthma, cystic fibrosis, cerebral palsy, scoliosis

  ○ GERD – neurologic impairments, hiatal hernia, esophageal atresia, morbid obesity

- Subjective and Objective Data

  ○ Infants

    ▪ Excessive spitting up or forceful vomiting, irritability, excessive crying, blood in stool or vomitus, arching of back, stiffening

    ▪ Respiratory problems

    ▪ Failure to thrive

    ▪ Apnea

  ○ Children

    ▪ Heartburn, abdominal pain, difficulty swallowing, chronic cough, chest pain

- Diagnostic Procedures

  ○ Upper gastrointestinal (GI) test to detect GI structural abnormalities

  ○ 24-hr intraesophageal pH study to measures the amount of gastric acid reflux into the esophagus

  ○ Endoscopy with biopsy to detect esophagitis and strictures

  ○ Scintigraphy to identify the cause of gastric content aspiration

Patient-Centered Care

- Nursing Care

  ○ GER

    ▪ Depends on the severity of the symptoms.

    ▪ Offer small, frequent meals.

    ▪ Thicken the infant's formula with 1 tsp to 1 tbsp rice cereal per 1 oz formula.

- Avoid foods that cause reflux (caffeine, citrus, peppermint, spicy or fried foods).
- Assist with weight control.
- Position the child with the head elevated at 30° for 1 hr after meals.
    ○ GERD
        - Initiate interventions for GER.
        - Administer a proton pump inhibitor such as omeprazole (Prilosec), or an H_2-receptor antagonist such as ranitidine (Zantac).
- Therapeutic Procedures
    ○ Nissen fundoplication
        - Laparoscopic surgical procedure that wraps the fundus of the stomach around the distal esophagus to decrease reflux
        - Used for clients who have severe cases of GERD

Complications

- Recurrent pneumonia, weight loss, and failure to thrive
    ○ Repeated reflux of stomach contents can lead to erosion of the esophagus or pneumonia if stomach contents are aspirated. Esophageal damage can lead to the inability to eat.
    ○ Nursing Actions
        - Follow the prescribed treatment plan.
        - Monitor for clinical manifestations of pneumonia and failure to thrive.
    ○ Client Education
        - Reinforce the plan of care with the family.
        - Instruct the parents about clinical manifestations for pneumonia.

HYPERTROPHIC PYLORIC STENOSIS

Overview

- Hypertrophic pyloric stenosis is the thickening of the pyloric sphincter, which creates an obstruction.
- Usually occurs the first 5 weeks of life.

Data Collection

- Risk Factors – genetic predisposition
- Subjective and Objective Data
    ○ Vomiting that often occurs following a feeding, but can occur up to several hours following a feeding and becomes projectile as obstruction worsens
    ○ Blood-tinged vomit

- ○ Constant hunger

- ○ Olive-shaped mass in the right upper quadrant of the abdomen and possible peristaltic wave that moves from left to right when lying supine

- ○ Failure to gain weight and signs of dehydration, such as skin that is dry and/or pale, cool lips, dry mucous membranes, decreased skin turgor, diminished urinary output, concentrated urine, thirst, rapid pulse, sunken eyes

- Laboratory Tests – serum electrolytes

- Diagnostic Procedures – Ultrasound reveals an elongated, sausage-shaped mass and an elongated pyloric area.

Patient-Centered Care

- Nursing Care – Prepare the child for surgery.

- Therapeutic Procedures

  - ○ Pylorotomy – performed by laparoscope

    - ▪ Preoperative

      - ☐ IV fluids for correction of dehydration and electrolyte imbalances

      - ☐ NG tube for decompression

      - ☐ NPO

      - ☐ I&O

      - ☐ Daily weights

    - ▪ Postoperative

      - ☐ Obtain routine postoperative vital signs.

      - ☐ Administer antiemetic for vomiting.

      - ☐ Provide IV fluids.

      - ☐ Monitor daily weights and I&O.

      - ☐ Administer analgesics for pain.

      - ☐ Monitor for indications of infection.

      - ☐ Start clear liquids 4 to 6 hr after surgery. Advance to breast milk or formula as tolerated.

      - ☐ Document tolerance to feedings.

HIRSCHSPRUNG DISEASE

Overview

- Hirschsprung disease (congenital aganglionic megacolon) is a structural anomaly of the GI tract caused by lack of ganglionic cells in segments of the colon resulting in decreased motility and mechanical obstruction.

Data Collection

- Risk Factor – family history of Hirschsprung disease
- Subjective and Objective Data
  - Newborn
    - Failure to pass meconium within 24 to 48 hr after birth
    - Episodes of vomiting bile
    - Refusal to eat
    - Abdominal distention
  - Infant
    - Failure to thrive
    - Abdominal distention
    - Vomiting
    - Episodes of constipation and watery diarrhea
  - Older child
    - Failure to thrive
    - Abdominal distention
    - Visible peristalsis
    - Palpable fecal mass
    - Constipation
    - Foul-smelling, ribbonlike stool
- Laboratory Tests
  - Serum electrolytes
  - CBC
- Diagnostic Procedures – rectal biopsy to confirm the absence of ganglion cells

Patient-Centered Care

- Nursing Care
  - Prepare family and client for surgery.
  - Assist the family with improving nutritional status until surgery.
    - High-protein, high-calorie, low-fiber diet
    - Total parenteral nutrition in some cases
- Therapeutic Procedures
  - Surgical removal of the aganglionic section of the bowel.
  - Temporary colostomy can be required.
  - Preoperative
    - Prepare the child and family for surgery using developmentally appropriate techniques.
    - Administer electrolyte and fluid replacement as prescribed.
    - Monitor for enterocolitis.
    - Perform bowel prep with saline enemas and oral antibiotics as prescribed.
  - Postoperative
    - Monitor respiratory status and maintain airway.
    - Provide supplemental oxygen as prescribed.
    - Obtain vital signs.
    - Administer analgesics for pain.
    - Inspect surgical site for bleeding or any other abnormalities.
    - Provide Foley catheter care.
    - Check bowel sounds and bowel function.
    - Provide ostomy care if appropriate.
    - Make appropriate referrals.
  - Client Education
    - Instruct the family in ostomy care if indicated.
    - Instruct the family about incision care and how to monitor for infection.
    - Inform the family about the clinical manifestations of dehydration.

Complications

- Enterocolitis – inflammation of the bowel
  - Treatment is aimed at resolving enterocolitis, preventing bowel perforation, maintaining hydration, initiating antibiotic therapy, and performing surgery for colostomy or ileostomy if there is extensive bowel involvement.
  - Nursing Actions
    - Monitor vital signs.
    - Determine and record abdominal girth.
      - Measure abdominal girth with a paper tape measure at the level of the umbilicus or at the widest point of the abdomen.
      - Mark the area with a pen to ensure continuity of future measurements.
    - Monitor for indications of sepsis, peritonitis, or shock caused by enterocolitis.
    - Monitor fluid, electrolyte, and blood product replacement.
    - Administer antibiotics.
- Anal stricture and incontinence
  - Bowel retaining therapy.
  - Can require further procedures such as dilatation.

INTUSSUSCEPTION

Overview

- One part of the intestine telescopes into another part, resulting in lymphatic and venous obstruction that results in edema in the area. With progression, ischemia and increased mucus into the intestine will occur.
- Common in infants and children between the ages of 3 months and 3 years.

Data Collection

- Risk Factors – cystic fibrosis
- Subjective and Objective Data
  - Sudden episodic abdominal pain
  - Screaming with drawing knees to chest during episodes of pain
  - Abdominal mass (sausage-shaped)
  - Stools that are mixed with blood and mucus that resemble the consistency of red currant jelly
  - Vomiting
  - Fever
  - Dehydration
- Diagnostic Procedures – ultrasound

Patient-Centered Care

- Nursing Care
  - Stabilize the child prior to the procedure.
    - IV fluids to correct and prevent dehydration
    - Nasogastric (NG) tube for decompression
  - Instruct the family and child about the nonsurgical procedure.
- Therapeutic Procedures
  - Air enema
    - With or without contrast
    - Performed by a radiologist

Complications

- Reoccurring intussusception
  - Surgery is required for reoccurring cases.

APPENDICITIS

Overview

- Inflammation of the vermiform appendix caused from an obstruction of the lumen of the appendix.
- Average client age is 10 years.

Data Collection

- Subjective and Objective Data
  - Abdominal pain in the right lower quadrant
  - Rigid abdomen
  - Decreased or absent bowel sounds
  - Fever
  - Diarrhea or constipation
  - Lethargy
  - Tachycardia
  - Rapid, shallow breathing
  - Anorexia
  - Possible vomiting

- Laboratory Tests
  - CBC
  - Urinalysis
- Diagnostic Procedures – Computed tomography (CT) scan shows an enlarged diameter of appendix, as well as thickening of the appendiceal wall.

Patient-Centered Care

- Nursing Care
  - Prepare the child and family for surgery using developmentally appropriate techniques.
  - Avoid applying heat to the abdomen.
  - Avoid enemas or laxatives.
- Therapeutic Procedures
  - Laparoscopic Surgery – removal of the nonruptured appendix
    - Preoperative
      - Administer IV fluid replacement as prescribed.
      - Administer IV antibiotic.
    - Postoperative
      - Monitor respiratory status and maintain airway.
      - Provide supplemental oxygen as prescribed.
      - Obtain vital signs.
      - Administer analgesics for pain.
      - Inspect surgical site for bleeding or any other abnormalities.
      - Check bowel sounds and bowel function.
  - Laparoscopic or open surgery – removal of the ruptured appendix.
    - Preoperative
      - Administer electrolyte and fluid replacement.
      - Place NG tube for decompression.
      - Administer IV antibiotics.
    - Postoperative
      - Monitor respiratory status and maintain airway.
      - Provide supplemental oxygen as prescribed.
      - Obtain vital signs.
      - Administer analgesics for pain.
      - Inspect surgical site for bleeding or any other abnormalities.
      - Check bowel sounds and bowel function.
      - Administer IV fluids and antibiotics.

◻ Maintain NPO status.

◻ Maintain NG to low continuous suction.

◻ Provide wound care for open surgical sites with antibacterial solution or saline.

◻ Provide Penrose drain care.

◻ Observe for indications of peritonitis.

▸ Fever

▸ Sudden increase in pain

▸ Irritability

▸ Rigid abdomen

▸ Abdominal distention

▸ Tachycardia

▸ Rapid, shallow breathing

▸ Pallor

▸ Chills

○ Client Teaching

▪ Instruct the family about incision care.

▪ Inform the family about clinical manifestations of infection.

Complications

- Peritonitis – inflammation in the peritoneal cavity

  ○ Nursing Actions

    ▪ Observe for clinical manifestations of peritonitis.

    ▪ Provide pain management.

      ◻ Determine level of pain using a developmentally appropriate tool.

      ◻ Administer analgesics.

    ▪ Monitor IV fluid therapy.

    ▪ Administer IV antibiotics for infection.

    ▪ Regulate NG tube suction.

    ▪ Provide preoperative and postoperative nursing care.

    ▪ Provide surgical wound care with wound irrigation and/or dressings if delayed wound closure is necessary.

    ▪ Provide psychosocial support for the child and family.

  ○ Client Education

    ▪ Reinforce teaching to the child and parents about preoperative care, such as the need to maintain NPO status and the need for pain medication.

    ▪ Reinforce teaching to the child and parent about postoperative care, such as early ambulation, advancement of diet, wound care, and monitoring for infection.

MECKEL'S DIVERTICULUM

Overview

- Meckel's diverticulum is a complication resulting from failure of the omphalomesenteric duct to fuse during embryonic development.

Data Collection

- Subjective and Objective Data
  - Can be asymptomatic
  - Abdominal pain
  - Bloody, mucus stools
- Laboratory Tests – CBC
- Diagnostic Procedures – radionucleotide scan

Patient-Centered Care

- Nursing Care
  - Prepare the child and family for surgery using developmentally appropriate techniques.
- Therapeutic Procedures
  - Surgical removal of the diverticulum
    - Preoperative
      - Carefully monitor blood transfusions to correct hypovolemia.
      - Administer fluid and electrolyte replacement.
      - Provide oxygen as prescribed.
      - Administer IV antibiotics.
      - Maintain bed rest.
      - Closely monitor blood loss in stools.
    - Postoperative
      - Monitor respiratory status and maintain airway.
      - Provide supplemental oxygen as prescribed.
      - Obtain vital signs.
      - Administer analgesics for pain.
      - Inspect surgical site for bleeding or any other abnormalities.
      - Check bowel sounds and bowel function.
      - Administer IV fluids and antibiotics.
      - Maintain NPO status.
      - Maintain NG tube to low continuous suction.
    - Client Teaching – Instruct the family clinical manifestations of infection.

Complications

- GI hemorrhage and bowel obstruction (for untreated Meckel's diverticulum)

APPLICATION EXERCISES

1. A nurse is collecting data on an infant. Which of the following are clinical manifestations of hypertrophic pyloric stenosis? (Select all that apply.)

_____ A. Projectile vomiting

_____ B. Dry mucus membranes

_____ C. Currant jelly stools

_____ D. Sausage-shaped abdominal mass

_____ E. Constant hunger

2. A nurse is caring for a child who has Hirschsprung disease. Which of the following is an appropriate action for the nurse to take?

A. Encourage a high-fiber, low-protein, low-calorie diet.

B. Prepare the family for surgery.

C. Place an NG for decompression.

D. Initiate bed rest.

3. A nursing is caring for an infant who is postoperative following cleft lip and palate repair. Which of the following is an appropriate action for the nurse to take?

A. Remove the packing in the mouth.

B. Place the infant prone.

C. Offer a pacifier with sucrose.

D. Check mouth with a tongue blade.

4. A nurse is reinforcing teaching with a parent of an infant about gastroesophageal reflux disease (GERD). Which of the following should be included in the teaching? (Select all that apply.)

_____ A. Offer frequent feedings.

_____ B. Thicken formula with rice cereal.

_____ C. Use a bottle with a one-way valve.

_____ D. Position baby upright for 1 hr after feedings.

_____ E. Use a wide based nipple for feedings.

5. A nurse is caring for a child who has Meckel's diverticulum. Which of the following are clinical manifestations of Meckel's diverticulum? (Select all that apply.)

_____ A. Abdominal pain

_____ B. Fever

_____ C. Mucus, bloody stools

_____ D. Vomiting

_____ E. Rapid, shallow breathing

6. A nurse is caring for a child who is postoperative open appendectomy following a perforated appendix. Use the ATI Active Learning Template: Systems Disorder to complete this item to include postoperative nursing interventions.

APPLICATION EXERCISES KEY

1. A. **CORRECT:** A client who has a pyloric stricture has thickening of the pyloric sphincter, resulting in projectile vomiting.

    B. **CORRECT:** A client who has a pyloric stricture is unable to consume adequate food and fluid, resulting in dehydration. Dry mucous membranes is a clinical manifestation of hypertrophic pyloric stenosis.

    C. INCORRECT: A client who has intussusception has bloody mucus stools, resulting in currant jelly stools.

    D. INCORRECT: A client who has intussusception has telescoping intestines, resulting sausage shaped abdominal mass.

    E. **CORRECT:** A client who has pyloric stricture is unable to consume adequate food and fluid, resulting in constant hunger.

    Ⓝ NCLEX® Connection: Physiological Adaptations, Basic Pathophysiology

2. A. INCORRECT: A client who has Hirschsprung disease is encouraged to eat a low-fiber, high-protein, high-calorie diet.

    B. **CORRECT:** A client who has Hirschsprung disease requires surgery to remove the affected segment of the intestine.

    C. INCORRECT: A client who has Hirschsprung disease is managed nutritionally. Placing an NG for decompression is not an appropriate action for the nurse to take.

    D. INCORRECT: A client who has Meckel's diverticulum is placed on bed rest to prevent further bleeding.

    Ⓝ NCLEX® Connection: Physiological Adaptations, Basic Pathophysiology

3. A. INCORRECT: The packing in the mouth should stay in place for 2 to 3 days.

    B. **CORRECT:** Placing the infant in prone position will facilitate drainage.

    C. INCORRECT: Objects in the mouth could injure the surgical site and should be avoided.

    D. INCORRECT: Objects in the mouth could injure the surgical site and should be avoided.

    Ⓝ NCLEX® Connection: Reduction of Risk Potential, Potential for Complications of Diagnostic Tests/ Treatments/Procedures

4. A. **CORRECT:** Frequent feeding will assist in decreasing the number of vomiting episodes.

    B. **CORRECT:** Thickened formula will assist in decreasing the number of vomiting episodes.

    C. INCORRECT: A bottle with a one-way valve is used for an infant who has cleft lip and palate.

    D. **CORRECT:** Positioning the infant in an upright position for 1 hr following feedings will assist in decreasing the number of vomiting episodes.

    E. INCORRECT: A wide-based nipple is used for an infant who has cleft lip and palate.

    Ⓝ NCLEX® Connection: Physiological Adaptations, Alterations in Body Systems

5. A. **CORRECT:** Abdominal pain is a clinical manifestation of Meckel's diverticulum.

    B. INCORRECT: Fever is a clinical manifestation of appendicitis.

    C. **CORRECT:** Mucus, bloody stools is a clinical manifestation of Meckel's diverticulum.

    D. INCORRECT: Vomiting is a clinical manifestation of appendicitis.

    E. INCORRECT: Rapid, shallow breathing is a clinical manifestation of appendicitis.

    Ⓝ NCLEX® Connection: Physiological Adaptations, Basic Pathophysiology

6. *Using the ATI Active Learning Template: Systems Disorder*
    - Postoperative Nursing Interventions
        ○ Monitor respiratory status and maintain airway.
        ○ Provide supplemental oxygen as prescribed.
        ○ Obtain vital signs.
        ○ Administer analgesics for pain.
        ○ Inspect surgical site for bleeding or any other abnormalities.
        ○ Check bowel sounds and bowel function.
        ○ Administer IV fluids and antibiotics.
        ○ Maintain NPO status.
        ○ Maintain NG to low continuous suction.
        ○ Provide wound care for open surgical sites with antibacterial solution or saline as prescribed.
        ○ Provide Penrose drain care.
        ○ Monitor for clinical manifestations of peritonitis.

    Ⓝ NCLEX® Connection: Physiological Adaptations, Alterations in Body Systems

UNIT 2   Nursing Care of Children with System Disorders

SECTION: GENITOURINARY AND REPRODUCTIVE DISORDERS

› Enuresis and Urinary Tract Infections
› Structural Disorders of the Genitourinary Tract and Reproductive System
› Renal Disorders

NCLEX® CONNECTIONS

When reviewing the chapters in this section, keep in mind the relevant sections of the NCLEX® outline, in particular:

Client Needs: Pharmacological Therapies

› Relevant topics/tasks include:
  » Dosage Calculation
    › Perform calculations needed for medication administration.
  » Expected Actions/Outcomes
    › Reinforce education to client regarding medications.

Client Needs: Reduction of Risk Potential

› Relevant topics/tasks include:
  » Laboratory Values
    › Notify the primary health care provider about client laboratory test results.

Client Needs: Physiological Adaptations

› Relevant topics/tasks include:
  » Alterations in Body Systems
    › Provide care to correct client alteration in body system.
    › Reinforce education to client regarding care and condition.
  » Basic Pathophysiology
    › Identify signs and symptoms related to an acute or chronic illness.
    › Consider general principles of client disease process when providing care.
    › Apply knowledge of pathophysiology to monitoring client for alterations in body systems.

chapter 22

Overview

- Enuresis is uncontrolled or unintentional urination that occurs after a child is beyond an age at which bladder control is achieved.
- A urinary tract infection (UTI) is an infection in any portion of the urinary tract.

ENURESIS

Overview

- Inappropriate urination must occur at least twice a week for at least 3 months. And, the child must be at least 5 years of age before there's consideration about diagnosing enuresis.
- Rule out organic causes related to genitourinary dysfunction prior to diagnosis of enuresis.
- Primary enuresis: A child has never been free of bedwetting for any extended periods of time.
- Secondary enuresis: A child who started bedwetting after development of urinary control.

Data Collection

- Risk Factors
  - Enuresis has no clear etiology, but it can be related to:
    - Family history of enuresis.
    - Disorders associated with bladder dysfunction.
    - The male gender.
    - Emotional factors.
- Subjective Data
  - History of alterations in toilet training, voiding behaviors, and bowel movement patterns
  - History of chronic or acute illness (UTI, diabetes mellitus, sickle cell disease, neurologic deficits)
  - History of family disruptions or other emotional stressors
  - Family history of enuresis
  - Fluid intake, especially in the evening

Patient-Centered Care

- Nursing Care
  - Determine the child's self-esteem.
  - Determine the child's coping strategies and available support systems.
  - Determine the family's coping.
  - Determine peer and family support groups.
  - Instruct the child and family regarding the management of enuresis.
    - Have the child empty his bladder prior to bedtime.
    - Encourage fluids during the day and restrict fluids in the evening.
    - Avoid fruit and fruit drinks after 1600.
    - Avoid caffeinated or carbonated drinks after 1600.
    - Allow the child to wear regular sleep wear and avoid diapers.
    - Use positive reinforcement. Avoid punishing, scolding, or teasing the child following an incident.
    - Assist the child in keeping a calendar of wet and dry days.
    - Make environmental changes to assist the child to get to the bathroom, such as avoiding the top bunk bed, use of a night light, or a clear path from the bed to the bathroom.
    - Avoid holding urine during the day.
    - Have the child change the bed linens and clothing following an incident.
    - Avoid constipation: increase fiber in diet, encourage regular bowel movements.
    - Wake the child up during the night to void.
    - Administer prescribed medications
    - Offer support to the child and the family.
- Medications
  - Antidiuretic hormone – Desmopressin acetate (DDAVP)
    - Reduces the volume of urine
    - Nursing Considerations
      - Can be prescribed either oral or nasal
      - Monitor I&O
    - Client Education
      - Encourage the family to restrict the child's fluid intake after dinner.
      - Instruct the family to administer the medication at bedtime.
      - Instruct the family to store nasal preparation in the refrigerator.
      - Inform the family of possible adverse reactions.

- ○ Tricyclic antidepressants – Imipramine hydrochloride (Tofranil)
  - ▪ Inhibits urination
  - ▪ Nursing Considerations
    - ▫ Monitor children for an increase in suicidality.
    - ▫ Monitor for therapeutic effectiveness.
    - ▫ Length of treatment is 6 to 8 weeks. Then, plan gradual withdrawal.
    - ▫ Administer with food.
  - ▪ Client Education
    - ▫ Instruct the family to administer the mediation 1 hr before bedtime.
    - ▫ Instruct the family about possible adverse reactions.
    - ▫ Instruct the family to avoid sun exposure.
    - ▫ Instruct the family to avoid using with over-the-counter medications.
- ○ Anticholinergics – Oxybutynin chloride (Ditropan)
  - ▪ Reduces bladder contractions
  - ▪ Nursing Considerations
    - ▫ Monitor for effectiveness of therapy.
  - ▪ Client Education
    - ▫ Instruct the family about possible adverse reactions.

Complications

- • Emotional problems (low self-esteem, altered body image, social isolation, fears)
  - ○ Nursing Actions
    - ▪ Support the child and family by listening to concerns and correcting misperceptions.
    - ▪ Involve the child in the teaching and management.
    - ▪ Make referrals to appropriate resources (support groups, counseling) as necessary.

  - ○ Client Education
    - ▪ Assist the child and family to understand the emotional aspects of the disorder. Early interventions can alleviate long-term emotional issues.

URINARY TRACT INFECTIONS (UTIs)

Overview

- Bacteriuria – bacteria in the urine
- Asymptomatic bacteriuria – bacteriuria with no clinical manifestations of UTI
- Symptomatic bacteriuria – bacteriuria with clinical manifestations of UTI
- Recurrent UTI – multiple occurrences of bacteriuria or symptomatic bacteriuria
- Persistent UTI – unresolved bacteriuria with antibiotic therapy
- Febrile UTI – symptomatic bacteriuria with fever
- Cystitis – inflammation of the bladder
- Urethritis – inflammation of the urethra
- Pyelonephritis – inflammation of the upper urinary tract and the kidneys
- Urosepsis – bacterial illness

Data Collection

- Risk Factors
  - Urinary stasis
  - Urinary tract anomalies
  - Reflux within the urinary tract system
  - Constipation
  - Onset of toilet training
  - Uncircumcised male (inadequate hygiene)
  - Females (urethra in close proximity to rectum)
  - Synthetic, tight underwear and wet bathing suits
  - Sexual activity
- Subjective Data
  - Infants
    - Increase in irritability
    - Screaming with urination
  - Children
    - Abdominal or back pain
    - Pain with urination

- Objective Data
  - Data Collection Findings
    - Infants
      - Poor feeding, vomiting, or failure to gain weight
      - Increase in thirst
      - Frequent urination
      - Straining with urination
      - Foul-smelling urine
      - Fever
      - Diaper rash
      - Dehydration
      - Seizure
      - Pallor
    - Children
      - Poor appetite
      - Vomiting
      - Slowed growth
      - Increase in thirst
      - Enuresis, frequent urination
      - Swelling of the face
      - Seizures
      - Pallor
      - Fatigue
      - Blood in the urine
      - Edema
      - Hypertension
      - Tetany
  - Laboratory Tests
    - Urinalysis and urine culture and sensitivity (C&S)
      - Sterile catheterization and suprapubic aspiration are the most accurate methods for obtaining urine for urinalysis and culture in children less than 2 years of age.
      - Obtain a clean-catch urine sample from children who are able to cooperate.
      - Nursing Actions
        - ► Before performance of a suprapubic aspiration occurs, confirm that informed consent has been obtained.
        - ► To prevent a falsely low bacterial count, avoid having the child drink a large amount of oral fluids prior to obtaining a urine specimen.

- ‣ Send the specimen for culture to the laboratory without delay.
- ‣ Review findings indicative of UTI.
  - ▷ Urine culture – Positive for infecting organisms (*Escherichia coli, Proteus, Pseudomonas, Klebsiella, Haemophilus, Staphylococcus aureus*)
  - ▷ Urinalysis
    - ◆ pH: weak acid or neutral alkaline
    - ◆ Protein: positive
    - ◆ Glucose: positive
    - ◆ Ketones: positive
    - ◆ Leukocytes: positive
    - ◆ Nitrates: positive
- ☐ Client Education
  - ‣ Instruct the child and family about the procedure for collecting a suprapubic aspiration, invasive urinary catheterization, or clean-voided specimen.
- ○ Diagnostic Procedures
  - ▪ Locate the primary infection site or anatomic defects.
    - ☐ Percutaneous kidney tap
    - ☐ Bladder wash outs
    - ☐ Ultrasonography
    - ☐ Voiding cystourethrogram (VCUG)
    - ☐ IV pyelogram (IVP)
    - ☐ Dimercaptosuccinic acid (DMSA) scan
      - ‣ Nursing Actions
        - ▷ Instruct the child and family about the procedure for the diagnostic test prescribed.
        - ▷ Check the child for allergy to iodine or shellfish if a contrast medium is used.
        - ▷ Sedate infants and young children if required. Assist an older child to remain quiet during the examinations.
        - ▷ Maintain the child on NPO status after midnight in preparation for a cystoscopy and IVP. IVP requires bowel preparation.
        - ▷ Prepare the child if catheterization is necessary.
        - ▷ Monitor the child after the procedure, according to facility protocol.

Patient-Centered Care

- Nursing Care
  - Encourage frequent voiding and complete emptying of the bladder.
  - Encourage fluids.
  - Monitor urine output.
  - Prepare the child for diagnostic tests.
  - Administer a mild analgesic (acetaminophen [Tylenol]) for pain management.
- Medications
  - Antibiotics based on findings of urine culture and sensitivity testing (penicillins, sulfonamide, cephalosporins, and nitrofurantoin)
    - Nursing Considerations
      - Monitor for potential allergic response.
    - Client Education
      - Instruct parents to have the child complete all prescribed antibiotics, even if symptoms are no longer present.
- Client Education
  - Instruct the family to watch for signs and symptoms of recurrence of UTIs (dysuria, frequency, urgency).
  - Provide instruction to prevent recurrence.
    - Instruct females to wipe the perineal area from front to back.
    - Tell parents to retract and clean the foreskin of male infants.
    - Instruct the child and parents to keep underwear dry.
    - Suggest the use of cotton underwear.
    - Tell the child to maintain adequate hydration.
    - Instruct avoidance of bubble baths.
    - Encourage frequent voiding.
    - Encourage complete emptying of bladder using double voiding.
    - Advise the child to avoid constipation and straining with bowel movements.
    - Encourage adolescents who are sexually active to void immediately after intercourse.

Complications

- Progressive kidney injury
- Urosepsis
  - Nursing Actions
    - Monitor for clinical manifestations of UTI.
  - Client Education
    - Reinforce teaching about prevention, early identification, and treatment of UTI.

APPLICATION EXERCISES

1. A nurse is collecting data on an infant who has a suspected urinary tract infection. Which of the following are anticipated findings? (Select all that apply.)

_____ A. Increase in hunger

_____ B. Irritability

_____ C. Decrease in urination

_____ D. Vomiting

_____ E. Fever

2. A nurse is collecting data on a child who has a urinary tract infection. Which of the following are clinical manifestations of a urinary tract infection? (Select all that apply.)

_____ A. Night sweats

_____ B. Swelling of the face

_____ C. Pallor

_____ D. Pale-colored urine

_____ E. Fatigue

3. A nurse is reinforcing teaching with the parent of a child who has a urinary tract infection. Which of the following should the nurse include in the teaching? (Select all that apply.)

_____ A. Wear nylon underpants.

_____ B. Avoid bubble baths.

_____ C. Empty bladder completely with each void.

_____ D. Provide information about clinical manifestations of infection.

_____ E. Wipe perineal area back to front.

4. A nurse is assisting with the plan of care for a child who has a urinary tract infection. Which of the following should the nurse include?

A. Administer antidiuretic.

B. Restrict fluids.

C. Determine the child's self-esteem.

D. Encourage frequent voiding.

5. A nurse is caring for a child who has enuresis. Which of the following is a complication of enuresis?

    A. Urinary tract infection

    B. Emotional problems

    C. Urosepsis

    D. Progressive kidney disease

6. A nurse educator is reviewing care of a child who has enuresis with a group of newly hired pediatric nurses. What should she include in the review? Use the ATI Active Learning Template: System Disorder to complete this item to include the following sections:

    A. Description of the Disorder

    B. Client Education: List at least 10 points to review.

APPLICATION EXERCISES KEY

1. A. INCORRECT: An increase in thirst is a clinical manifestation of urinary tract infection in an infant.

   B. **CORRECT:** Irritability is a clinical manifestation of urinary tract infection in an infant.

   C. INCORRECT: An increase in urination is a clinical manifestation of urinary tract infection in an infant.

   D. **CORRECT:** Vomiting is a clinical manifestation of urinary tract infection in an infant.

   E. **CORRECT:** Fever is a clinical manifestation of urinary tract infection in an infant.

   Ⓝ NCLEX® Connection: Physiological Adaptations, Basic Pathophysiology

2. A. INCORRECT: Night sweats are not a clinical manifestation in a child who has a urinary tract infection.

   B. **CORRECT:** Swelling of the face is a clinical manifestation in a child who has a urinary tract infection.

   C. **CORRECT:** Pallor is a clinical manifestation in a child who has a urinary tract infection.

   D. INCORRECT: Bloody urine is a clinical manifestation in a child who has a urinary tract infection.

   E. **CORRECT:** Fatigue is a clinical manifestation in a child who has a urinary tract infection.

   Ⓝ NCLEX® Connection: Physiological Adaptations, Basic Pathophysiology

3. A. INCORRECT: The nurse should discuss the use of cotton underwear.

   B. **CORRECT:** The nurse should discuss avoiding bubble baths.

   C. **CORRECT:** The nurse should discuss the need to completely empty the bladder with each void.

   D. **CORRECT:** The nurse should review the clinical manifestations of infection.

   E. INCORRECT: The nurse should discuss the importance of wiping the perineal area from front to back.

   Ⓝ NCLEX® Connection: Physiological Adaptations, Alterations in Body Systems

4. A. INCORRECT: An antidiuretic is not indicated for a child who has a urinary tract infection.

    B. INCORRECT: The nurse should encourage fluids for a child who has a urinary tract infection.

    C. INCORRECT: The nurse should determine self-esteem in a child who has enuresis.

    D. **CORRECT:** The nurse should encourage frequent voiding, which assists in flushing bacteria through the urinary system.

    ⓝ NCLEX® Connection: Physiological Adaptations, Basic Pathophysiology

5. A. INCORRECT: Urinary tract infections can occur in children, but they are not a complication of enuresis.

    B. **CORRECT:** Emotional problems are a complication of enuresis.

    C. INCORRECT: Urosepsis is a complication of urinary tract infections.

    D. INCORRECT: Progressive kidney disease is a complication of urinary tract infections.

    ⓝ NCLEX® Connection: Physiological Adaptations, Basic Pathophysiology

6. *Using the ATI Active Learning Template: System Disorder*

    A. Description of the Disorder

    - Inappropriate urination must occur at least twice a week for at least 3 months, and the child must be at least 5 years of age before consideration of diagnosing enuresis

    B. Client Education

    - Have the child empty his bladder prior to bedtime.

    - Encourage fluids during the day, and restrict fluids in the evening.

    - Instruct the child to avoid fruit and fruit drinks after 1600.

    - Instruct the child to avoid caffeinated or carbonated drinks after 1600.

    - Allow the child to wear regular sleep wear and avoid diapers.

    - Use positive reinforcement. Avoid punishing, scolding, or teasing the child following an incident.

    - Assist the child in keeping a calendar of wet and dry days.

    - Make environmental changes to assist the child to get to the bathroom, such as avoiding the top bunk bed, providing a night light, and clearing a path from the bed to the bathroom.

    - Instruct the child to avoid holding urine during the day.

    - Have the child change bed linens and clothing following an incident.

    - Avoid constipation: increase fiber in the diet and encourage regular bowel movements.

    - Wake the child during the night to void.

    - Instruct the child to take all medications as prescribed.

    ⓝ NCLEX® Connection: Physiological Adaptations, Alterations in Body Systems

chapter 23

CHAPTER 23   Structural Disorders of the Genitourinary Tract and Reproductive System

Overview

- Various structural disorders can be evident at birth and can affect normal genitourinary and reproductive function. These disorders include:

  - Obstructive uropathy: Structural or functional obstruction in the urinary system.

  - Inguinal hernia: Protrusion of abdominal organs through the inguinal canal into the scrotum.

  - Chordee: Ventral curvature of the penis.

  - Bladder exstrophy: Eversion of the posterior bladder through the anterior bladder wall and lower abdominal wall.

  - Hypospadias: Urethral opening located behind the glans of the penis or on the ventral surface of the penile shaft.

  - Epispadias: Meatal opening located on the dorsal surface of the penis.

  - Phimosis: Narrowing of the preputial opening of the foreskin.

  - Cryptorchidism: Undescended testes.

  - Hydrocele: Fluid in the scrotum.

  - Varicocele: Elongation, dilatation, and tortuosity of the veins superior to the testicle.

  - Testicular torsion: Testicle hangs free from the vascular structures.

  - Ambiguous genitalia: Erroneous or abnormal sexual differentiation.

- Children become aware of and are very interested in the genital area, normality of genital function, and gender differences between 3 and 6 years of age. Due to this, repair of structural defects ideally should be done between 6 to 15 months of age, but before 3 years of age, to minimize impact on body image and to promote healthy development.

Data Collection

- Risk Factor – possible genetic link
- Objective and Subjective Data
  - Obstructive uropathy
    - Hydronephrosis
    - Partial obstructions can go undetected.
    - Possible other genetic disorders (prune belly syndrome, chromosomal anomalies, anorectal malformation, defects of the pinna of the ear)

- Inability to concentrate urine
- Urinary tract infections
- Increased urine flow
- Metabolic acidosis
○ Inguinal hernia – painless inguinal swelling varying in size
○ Chordee – ventral curvature of the penis
○ Bladder exstrophy
  - Epispadias present
  - Exposed bladder, urethra, and ureteral orifices through the suprapubic area
○ Hypospadias
  - Meatus opening below the glans penis
  - Meatus opening along the ventral surface of the penis, scrotum, or perineum
  - Possible chordee present
○ Epispadias
  - Male
    □ Widened pubic symphysis
    □ Broad, spadelike penis
    □ Urethra opened on dorsal surface of the penis
    □ Possible exstrophy of the bladder
  - Female
    □ Wide urethra
    □ Bifid clitoris
    □ Possible exstrophy of the bladder
○ Phimosis – inability to retract foreskin of penis
○ Cryptorchidism – inability to palpate testes within the scrotum
○ Hydrocele
  - Enlarged scrotal sac
  - Possible pain
○ Varicocele
  - Bulge above the testicle when bearing down
  - Mild to moderate pain
○ Testicular torsion
  - Enlargement of affected testicle
  - Sudden, severe onset of pain

- ○ Ambiguous genitalia
  - Possible congenital adrenal hypoplasia
  - Enlarged clitoral hood
  - Enlarged clitoris
  - Micropenis
  - Bifid scrotum
- Diagnostic/Therapeutic Procedures
  - ○ Obstructive uropathy – surgical procedures that divert the flow of urine to bypass the obstruction
  - ○ Inguinal hernia
    - Can resolve spontaneously.
    - Surgery is indicated for defects that have not closed by 1 year of age.
  - ○ Chordee – surgical release of fibrous band
  - ○ Bladder exstrophy – immediate surgery
  - ○ Hypospadias/Epispadias
    - Surgery performed during the first year of life.
    - Male circumcision not performed.
  - ○ Phimosis – Circumcision in severe cases
  - ○ Cryptorchidism
    - Surgical orchiopexy
    - Older children: administration of human chorionic gonadotropin
  - ○ Hydrocele
    - Can resolve spontaneously
    - Surgical repair if not resolved in 1 year
  - ○ Varicocele – percutaneous embolization
  - ○ Testicular torsion – immediate surgery
  - ○ Ambiguous genitalia
    - Chromosomal analysis to determine genetic karyotype
    - Gonad biopsy and surgery
    - Plan for gender assignment
    - Radiographic contrast studies
    - Endoscopy
    - Ultrasonography
    - Biochemical tests

- ○ Nursing Actions
  - ▪ Provide support for parents during the diagnosis.
  - ▪ Administer sedation, and assist with the procedure as needed.
- ○ Client Education
  - ▪ Advise the family and/or child about the procedure and what to expect.
  - ▪ If NPO status is necessary, explain the parameters to the family and/or child.

Patient-Centered Care

- Nursing Care
  - ○ Nursing care should focus on education and support of the family and child.
    - ▪ Determine the family's perception of the child's defect, family support, and coping.
    - ▪ Assist parents to identify ways to help the child maintain a positive self-image.
    - ▪ Promote healthy growth and development.
    - ▪ Assist child with maintaining self-image.
  - ○ Obstructive uropathy – surgical repair with insertion of percutaneous nephrostomy or cutaneous ureterostomy tubes
  - ○ Bladder exstrophy
    - ▪ Cover the exposed bladder with sterile, nonadherent dressing.
    - ▪ Prepare for immediate surgery.
  - ○ Phimosis – Retract foreskin and perform cleansing, if prescribed, for mild cases.
  - ○ Ambiguous genitalia
    - ▪ Obtain detailed family history.
    - ▪ Collaborate with genetic counseling services in preparing parents for evaluation, testing, diagnostic procedures, discussion of gender assignment, and surgery as indicated.
- Surgical Interventions
  - ○ Structural defects are treated with surgical intervention. The goal of most structural defect repairs is to preserve or create normal urinary and sexual function. Early intervention minimizes emotional trauma.
  - ○ Nursing Actions
    - ▪ Preoperative
      - ▫ Provide explanations to the child and family related to the procedure and expectations for postoperative care.
      - ▫ Provide emotional support to the child and family.
      - ▫ Encourage parents to express concerns and fears related to the surgical procedure and outcomes.

- Postoperative
  - □ Determine pain using an appropriate pain assessment tool.
  - □ Administer pain medication. An antispasmodic, such as oxybutynin (Ditropan), can be prescribed to treat painful bladder spasms.
  - □ Monitor I&O.
  - □ Monitor urinary catheters, drains, tubes, or stents.
  - □ Provide wound and dressing care.
  - □ Monitor for signs of infection, such as redness, warmth, drainage, or edema at surgical site. Monitor for fever, lethargy, and foul-smelling urine.
  - □ Do not provide tub baths for at least 1 week or as prescribed.
  - □ Limit activity as prescribed.
- Client Education
  - Explain measures to prevent infection to include good hand hygiene, and care of wounds, drains, and urinary catheters.
  - Explain procedures at the appropriate level for child and/or parents.
  - Use age-appropriate interventions to allay fears and anxiety.
  - Help the child understand that surgery is not a punishment, and it will not mutilate the body.

Complications

- Infection
  - Nursing Action
    - Observe for signs of infection including fever, skin inflammation, foul urine odor, cloudy urine, and/or urinary frequency.
  - Client Education
    - Instruct the family to observe for signs of infection and report them immediately.
- Emotional problems (poor self-esteem, altered body image, social isolation, fears)
  - Nursing Actions
    - Support the child and family by listening to concerns and correcting misperceptions.
    - Use play therapy for toddlers and preschoolers.
    - Encourage peer-to-peer social networking for older children.
  - Client Education
    - Provide information to the child and family regarding support groups.

APPLICATION EXERCISES

1. A nurse is caring for an infant who has a hydrocele. Which of the following is an appropriate action for the nurse to take?

    A. Prepare for immediate surgery.

    B. Explain to the parents that this will self-resolve.

    C. Retract the foreskin and cleanse properly.

    D. Refer the family for counseling.

2. A nurse is caring for a male infant. Which of the following are clinical manifestations of an epispadias? (Select all that apply.)

    _____ A. Bladder exstrophy

    _____ B. Inability to retract foreskin

    _____ C. Widened pubic symphysis

    _____ D. Broad, spade-like penis

    _____ E. Pain

3. A nurse is caring for an infant who has ambiguous genitalia. Which of the following are appropriate actions for the nurse to take? (Select all that apply.)

    _____ A. Prepare for surgery.

    _____ B. Obtain a detailed family history.

    _____ C. Plan for a circumcision.

    _____ D. Refer to genetic counseling.

    _____ E. Explain the need for a chromosomal analysis.

4. A nurse is caring for an infant. Which of the following are clinical manifestations of obstructive uropathy? (Select all that apply.)

_____ A. Decreased urine flow

_____ B. Urinary tract infection

_____ C. Metabolic alkalosis

_____ D. Concentrated urine

_____ E. Hydronephrosis

5. A nurse is reinforcing teaching with a newly licensed nurse about structural disorders of the genitourinary tract and reproductive system. What should be included in the instruction? Use the ATI Active Learning Template: Basic Concept to complete this item to include the following:

A. Related Content/Underlying Principles: Describe six structural disorders of the genitourinary tract and reproductive system.

APPLICATION EXERCISES KEY

1. A. INCORRECT: Hydroceles are surgically repaired if they have not resolved spontaneously in 1 year.

    B. **CORRECT:** Hydrocele is fluid in the scrotum and resolves spontaneously in the majority of cases.

    C. INCORRECT: Retracting foreskin and cleansing properly is done when an infant has phimosis.

    D. INCORRECT: A referral for genetic counseling is recommended for families who have an infant with ambiguous genitalia.

    (N) NCLEX® Connection: Physiological Adaptations, Alterations in Body Systems

2. A. **CORRECT:** Bladder exstrophy is a clinical manifestation of a male infant who has epispadias.

    B. INCORRECT: Inability to retract foreskin is a clinical manifestation of phimosis.

    C. **CORRECT:** Widened pubic symphysis is a clinical manifestation of a male infant who has epispadias.

    D. **CORRECT:** Broad, spade-like penis is a clinical manifestation of a male infant who has epispadias.

    E. INCORRECT: Pain is a clinical manifestation of testicular torsion, varicocele, and hydrocele.

    (N) NCLEX® Connection: Physiological Adaptations, Basic Pathophysiology

3. A. **CORRECT:** Infants who have ambiguous genitalia will need surgery.

    B. **CORRECT:** A detailed family history is used for gender assignment.

    C. INCORRECT: Circumcision is not recommended for an infant who has ambiguous genitalia.

    D. **CORRECT:** Families who have an infant who has ambiguous genitalia will need ongoing support. Referring to genetic counseling is an appropriate action for the nurse to take.

    E. **CORRECT:** Chromosomal analysis is used for gender assignment.

    (N) NCLEX® Connection: Physiological Adaptations, Basic Pathophysiology

4. A. INCORRECT: Increased urine flow is a clinical manifestation of obstructive uropathy.

   B. **CORRECT:** Urinary tract infection is a clinical manifestation of obstructive uropathy.

   C. INCORRECT: Metabolic acidosis is a clinical manifestation of obstructive uropathy.

   D. INCORRECT: Inability to concentrate urine is a clinical manifestation of obstructive uropathy.

   E. **CORRECT:** Hydronephrosis is a clinical manifestation of obstructive uropathy.

   (N) NCLEX® Connection: Physiological Adaptations, Basic Pathophysiology

5. *Using the ATI Active Learning Template: Basic Concept*

   A. Related Content/Underlying Principles
   - Obstructive Uropathy: Structural or functional obstruction in the urinary system.
   - Inguinal hernia: Protrusion of abdominal organs through the inguinal canal into the scrotum.
   - Chordee: Ventral curvature of the penis.
   - Bladder exstrophy: Eversion of the posterior bladder through the anterior bladder wall and lower abdominal wall.
   - Hypospadias: Urethral opening located behind the glans of the penis or on the ventral surface of the penile shaft.
   - Epispadias: Meatal opening located on the dorsal surface of the penis.
   - Phimosis: Narrowing of the preputial opening of the foreskin.
   - Cryptorchidism: Undescended testes.
   - Hydrocele: Fluid in the scrotum.
   - Varicocele: Elongated, dilated, and tortuosity of the veins superior to the testicle.
   - Testicular torsion: Testicle hangs free from the vascular structures.
   - Ambiguous genitalia: Erroneous or abnormal sexual differentiation.

   (N) NCLEX® Connection: Physiological Adaptations, Basic Pathophysiology

chapter 24

Overview

- Acute glomerulonephritis (AGN)
- Nephrotic syndrome

ACUTE GLOMERULONEPHRITIS

Overview

- Acute glomerulonephritis – The glomeruli are inflamed, which impairs the kidney's ability to filter the urine properly.
- Acute poststreptococcal glomerulonephritis (APSGN) is an antibody-antigen disease that occurs as a result of certain strains of the Group A ß-hemolytic streptococcal infection and is most commonly seen in children between the ages of 2 and 7 years.

Data Collection

- Risk Factors
  - APSGN: streptococcal infection with a specific strain of group A ß-hemolytic streptococcus
- Subjective Data
  - Recent upper respiratory infection or streptococcal infection
- Objective Data
  - Physical Findings
    - Cloudy, tea-colored urine
    - Decreased urine output
    - Irritability
    - Ill appearance
    - Lethargy
    - Anorexia
    - Vague reports of discomfort (headache, abdominal pain, dysuria)
    - Periorbital edema
    - Facial edema that is worse in the morning but then spreads to extremities and abdomen with progression of the day
    - Mild to severe hypertension

○ Laboratory Tests

- Throat culture to identify possible streptococcus infection (usually negative by the time of diagnosis)

- Urinalysis – proteinuria, smoky or tea-colored urine, hematuria

- Renal function – elevated BUN and creatinine

- Antistreptolysin O (ASO) titer – positive indicator for the presence of streptococcal antibodies

- Antihyaluronidase (AHase), antideoxyribonuclease B (ADNase-B), streptozyme antibodies – can be present

- Serum complement (C3) – decreased initially; increases as recovery takes place; returns to normal at 8 weeks post-glomerulonephritis

○ Diagnostic Procedures

- Chest x-ray to identify pulmonary edema, cardiac enlargement, or pleural effusion

  □ Nursing Actions

  ▸ Ensure that adolescents are not pregnant.

  ▸ Assist with proper positioning.

  □ Client Education

  ▸ Explain the procedure to the child and family.

Patient-Centered Care

- Nursing Care

  ○ Clients who have normal blood pressure and urine output can be managed at home.

  ○ Monitor I&O.

  ○ Monitor daily weights. Weigh the child on the same scale with the same amount of clothing daily.

  ○ Monitor vital signs.

  ○ Monitor neurologic status and observe for behavior changes, especially in children who have edema, hypertension, and gross hematuria. Implement seizure precautions if the condition indicates.

  ○ Encourage adequate nutritional intake.

  - Possible restriction of sodium and fluid.

  - Restrict foods high in potassium during periods of oliguria.

  - Provide small, frequent meals of favorite foods due to a decrease in appetite.

  - Refer the child for dietary consultation if indicated.

  - Avoid added salt and salty foods such as chips.

  ○ Manage fluid restrictions during periods of edema and hypertension.

  ○ Monitor skin for breakdown.

  - Encourage frequent turning and repositioning.

  - Keep skin dry.

  - Pad bony prominences, and use a specialty mattress.

  - Elevate edematous body parts.

- ○ Check tolerance for activity. Provide for frequent rest periods.
- ○ Provide for age-appropriate diversional activities.
- ○ Cluster care to facilitate rest and tolerance of activity.
- ○ Monitor and prevent infection.
  - ▪ Advise the child to turn, cough, and deep breathe to prevent pulmonary involvement.
  - ▪ Monitor vital signs, especially temperature, for changes secondary to infection.
  - ▪ Maintain good hand hygiene.
  - ▪ Administer antibiotic therapy.
- ○ Provide emotional support.
- • Medications
  - ○ Diuretics and antihypertensives to remove accumulated fluid and manage hypertension
    - ▪ Nursing Considerations
      - ▫ Monitor blood pressure.
      - ▫ Monitor I&O.
      - ▫ Monitor for electrolyte imbalances, such as hypokalemia.
      - ▫ Observe for adverse effects of medications.
    - ▪ Client Education
      - ▫ Inform the client and family that dizziness can occur with the use of antihypertensives.
      - ▫ Instruct the client and family to take the medication as prescribed and to notify the provider if adverse effects occur. Give instructions to continue the medication unless instructed otherwise.
- • Teamwork and Collaboration
  - ○ Obtain a dietary consult.
- • Ongoing Care
  - ○ Client Education
    - ▪ Encourage the child to verbalize feelings related to body image.
    - ▪ Instruct the child regarding appropriate dietary management.
    - ▪ Encourage adequate rest.
    - ▪ Instruct the family about the need for follow-up care.
    - ▪ Instruct the family how to monitor blood pressure and daily weight.
    - ▪ Explain to the family about administration and side effects of diuretics and antihypertensive medications.
    - ▪ Encourage the child and family to avoid contact with others who might be ill.

NEPHROTIC SYNDROME

Overview

- In nephrotic syndrome, alterations in the glomerular membrane allow proteins (especially albumin) to pass into the urine, resulting in decreased serum osmotic pressure.

- It can be primary, secondary, or congenital.

Data Collection

- Risk Factors
  - Minimal change nephrotic syndrome (MCNS)
    - Peak incidence is between 2 and 7 years of age.
    - Cause is unknown, but it can have a multifactorial etiology (immune-mediated, biochemical).
  - Secondary nephrotic syndrome (occurs after or is associated with glomerular damage due to a known cause)
  - Congenital nephrotic syndrome (an inherited disorder)
- Subjective and Objective Data
  - Physical Findings
    - Weight gain over days or weeks
    - Facial and periorbital edema – decreased throughout the day
    - Ascites
    - Edema in the legs or ankles
    - Anorexia
    - Diarrhea
    - Irritability
    - Lethargy
    - Decreased frothy urine
    - Blood pressure within expected reference range or slightly below
  - Laboratory Tests
    - Urinalysis/24-hr urine collection
      - Proteinuria – protein greater than 2+ on dipstick
      - Hyaline casts
      - Few RBCs
      - Oval fat bodies

- Serum chemistry
  - □ Hypoalbuminemia – reduced serum protein and albumin
  - □ Hyperlipidemia – elevated serum lipid levels
  - □ Hemoconcentration – elevated Hgb, Hct, and platelets
  - □ Possible hyponatremia – reduced sodium level
  - □ Glomerular filtration rate – normal or high
- Diagnostic Procedures
  - Kidney biopsy is indicated only if nephrotic syndrome is unresponsive to steroid therapy.
    - □ Biopsy will show damage to the epithelial cells lining the basement membrane of the kidney.

Patient-Centered Care

- Nursing Care
  - Provide rest.
  - Monitor I&O. Monitor urine for protein.
  - Monitor vital signs.
  - Monitor daily weights. Weigh the child on the same scale with the same amount of clothing.
  - Monitor edema and measure abdominal girth daily. Measure at the widest area, usually at or above the umbilicus. Check degree of pitting, color, and texture of skin.
  - Monitor and prevent infection.
    - Assist the client to turn, cough, and deep breathe to prevent pulmonary involvement.
    - Monitor vital signs, especially temperature, for changes secondary to infection.
    - Maintain good hand hygiene.
    - Administer antibiotic therapy.
  - Encourage nutritional intake within restriction guidelines. Salt and fluids can be restricted during the edematous phase.
  - Cluster care to provide for rest periods.
  - Observe skin for breakdown areas.
    - Avoid use of urinary collection bags in very young children.
    - Pad bony prominences or use a specialty mattress to reduce breakdown of skin.
    - Encourage frequent turning and repositioning.
    - Keep the client's skin dry.
    - Elevate edematous body parts.

- Medications
    - Corticosteroid – prednisone
        - Nursing Considerations
            - 2 mg/kg/day for 6 weeks followed by 1.5 mg/kg every other day for 6 weeks.
            - Monitor for adverse effects such as hirsutism, slowed linear growth, hypertension, GI bleeding, infection, and hyperglycemia.
            - Administer with meals.
        - Client Education
            - Instruct the client and family to avoid large crowds (to decrease the risk of infection).
            - Inform the client and family that using corticosteroids can increase appetite, cause weight gain (especially in the face), and cause mood swings.
            - Instruct the client and the family about the medication regime.
            - Instruct the client and the family about adverse effects and when to notify the provider.
    - Diuretic – furosemide (Lasix)
        - Eliminates excess fluid from the body
        - Nursing Considerations
            - Encourage the child to eat foods that are high in potassium.
            - Monitor serum electrolyte levels periodically.
    - 25% albumin
        - Increases plasma volume and decreases edema
        - Nursing Considerations
            - Assist with administration per protocol.
            - Monitor I&O.
            - Monitor for anaphylaxis.
    - Cyclophosphamide
        - Administer for children who cannot tolerate prednisone or who have repeated relapses of MCNS.
- Teamwork and Collaboration
    - Obtain a dietary consult.
- Ongoing Care
    - Client Education
        - Encourage the client to verbalize feelings related to body image.
        - Instruct the client regarding appropriate dietary management.
        - Encourage adequate rest.
        - Instruct the family about the need for follow-up care.
        - Inform the family of strategies to decrease the risk of infection (good hand hygiene, up-to-date immunizations, avoidance of infected people).

- Explain to the family how to monitor blood pressure, daily weight, and protein in urine. Instruct the family to notify the provider if symptoms worsen, which indicates relapse.

- Instruct the family about administration and side effects of medication.

- Provide support to families and make appropriate referrals as needed. Relapses can cause physical, emotional, and financial stress for the client and family.

Complications

- Sepsis/Infection
  - Steroid therapy increases the risk for infection.
    - Common infections seen in children with nephrotic syndrome include pneumonia, peritonitis, and cellulitis.

  - Nursing Actions
    - Keep the child away from potential infection sources.
    - Monitor for signs of infection.
  - Client Education
    - Reinforce teaching about the importance of completing the full dose of antibiotic.
    - Remind about the need for performing frequent hand hygiene.
    - Explain about clinical manifestations of infection and when to contact the provider.
    - Reinforce teaching about potential infection sources (live plants, sick family members).
- Circulation insufficiency
- Thromboembolism

APPLICATION EXERCISES

1. A nurse is caring for a child. Which of the following are clinical manifestations of nephrotic syndrome? (Select all that apply.)

_____ A. Dipstick protein of 1+

_____ B. Edema in the ankles

_____ C. Hyperlipidemia

_____ D. Weight loss

_____ E. Anorexia

2. A nurse is caring for a child. Which of the following are clinical manifestations of acute poststreptococcal glomerulonephritis (APSGN)? (Select all that apply.)

_____ A. Frothy urine

_____ B. Periorbital edema

_____ C. Ill appearance

_____ D. Decreased creatinine

_____ E. Hypertension

3. A nurse is caring for a 10-year-old child who has acute glomerulonephritis (AGN). Which of the following findings should the nurse report to the provider?

A. Serum BUN 8 mg/dL

B. Serum creatinine 1.3 mg/dL

C. Blood pressure 100/74 mm Hg

D. Urine output 550 mL over 24 hr

4. A nurse is caring for a 10-year-old child who has nephrotic syndrome. Which of the following findings should the nurse report to the provider?

A. Serum protein 5.0 g/dL

B. Hgb 14.5 g/dL

C. Hct 40%

D. Platelets 200,000 mm^3

5. A nurse is caring for a child who has a prescription for prednisone 2 mg/kg/day. The child weighs 35 kg. How many mg should the nurse administer per day? (Round the answer to the nearest whole number.)

6. A nurse is reinforcing teaching with the parent of a child who has a new prescription for prednisone for nephrotic syndrome. Use the Active Learning Template: Medication to complete this item to include the following:

    A. Nursing Considerations: List three.

    B. Client Education: List four teaching points.

APPLICATION EXERCISES KEY

1. A. INCORRECT: A client who has nephrotic syndrome will exhibit proteinuria of 2+ or greater due to the kidneys' inability to filter urine.

    B. **CORRECT:** A client who has nephrotic syndrome will exhibit edema in the ankles due to the decreasing colloidal osmotic pressure in the capillaries.

    C. **CORRECT:** A client who has nephrotic syndrome will exhibit hyperlipidemia due to the increased hepatic synthesis of proteins and lipids.

    D. INCORRECT: A client who has nephrotic syndrome will exhibit weight gain due to the decreasing colloidal osmotic pressure in the capillaries, which causes edema.

    E. **CORRECT:** A client who has nephrotic syndrome will exhibit anorexia due to the edema of the intestinal mucosa.

    (N) NCLEX® Connection: Physiological Adaptations, Basic Pathophysiology

2. A. INCORRECT: A client who has APSGN will exhibit cloudy, tea-colored urine because of blood and protein in the urine.

    B. **CORRECT:** A client who has APSGN will exhibit periorbital edema because of decrease in plasma filtration.

    C. **CORRECT:** A client who has APSGN will exhibit an ill appearance because of the manifestations experienced from the inadequate functioning of the kidneys.

    D. INCORRECT: A client who has APSGN will exhibit increased creatinine because of impaired glomerular filtration of the kidneys.

    E. **CORRECT:** A client who has APSGN will exhibit hypertension because of inadequate function of the kidneys and possibly edema.

    (N) NCLEX® Connection: Physiological Adaptations, Basic Pathophysiology

3. A. INCORRECT: Serum BUN 8 mg/dL is within the reference range for a 10-year-old child.

    B. **CORRECT:** Serum creatinine 1.3 mg/dL is out of the reference range for a 10-year-old child.

    C. INCORRECT: Blood pressure of 100/74 mm Hg is within the reference range for a 10-year-old child.

    D. INCORRECT: Urine output of 550 mL over 24 hr is within the reference range for a 10-year-old child.

    (N) NCLEX® Connection: Reduction of Risk Potential, Laboratory Values

4. A. **CORRECT:** Serum protein 5.0 g/dL is out of reference range for a 10-year-old child and should be reported to the provider.

   B. INCORRECT: Hgb 14.5 g/dL is within reference range for a 10-year-old child.

   C. INCORRECT: Hct 40% is within reference range for a 10-year-old child.

   D. INCORRECT: Platelet 200,000 mm³ is within reference range for a 10-year-old child.

   Ⓝ NCLEX® Connection: Reduction of Risk Potential, Laboratory Values

5. **70** mg

Using Ratio and Proportion, Desired Over Have, and Dimensional Analysis		
STEP 1: *What is the unit of measurement to calculate?* mg	STEP 2: *Set up an equation and solve for X.* mg x kg/day = X 2 mg x 35 kg/day = 70 mg/day STEP 3: *Round if necessary.*	STEP 4: *Reassess to determine whether the amount makes sense.* If the prescribed amount is 2 mg/kg/day and the client weighs 35 kg, it makes sense to give 70 mg/day.

   Ⓝ NCLEX® Connection: Pharmacological Therapies, Dosage Calculation

6. *Using the Active Learning Template: Medication*

   A. Nursing Considerations
   - Administer 2 mg/kg/day for 6 weeks followed by 1.5 mg/kg every other day for 6 weeks.
   - Monitor for adverse effects such as hirsutism, slowed linear growth, hypertension, GI bleeding, infection, and hyperglycemia.
   - Administer with meals.

   B. Client Education
   - Instruct the client and family to avoid large crowds (to decrease the risk of infection).
   - Inform the client and family that using corticosteroids can increase appetite, cause weight gain (especially in the face), and cause mood swings.
   - Instruct the client and the family on the medication regime.
   - Reinforce teaching with the client and the family on adverse effects and when to notify the provider.

   Ⓝ NCLEX® Connection: Pharmacological Therapies, Expected Actions/Outcomes

UNIT 2   Nursing Care of Children with System Disorders

SECTION: MUSCULOSKELETAL DISORDERS

› Fractures
› Musculoskeletal Congenital Disorders
› Chronic Neuromusculoskeletal Disorders

NCLEX® CONNECTIONS

When reviewing the chapters in this section, keep in mind the relevant sections of the NCLEX® outline, in particular:

Client Needs: Basic Care and Comfort

› Relevant topics/tasks include:
  » Mobility/Immobility
    › Provide care to an immobilized client.

Client Needs: Pharmacological and Parenteral Therapies

› Relevant topics/tasks include:
  » Expected Actions/Outcomes
    › Apply knowledge of pathophysiology when addressing client pharmacological agents.

Client Needs: Reduction of Risk Potential

› Relevant topics/tasks include:
  » Potential for Complications of Diagnostic Tests/Treatments/Procedures
    › Implement measures to prevent complication of client condition or procedure.
  » Potential for Complications of Diagnostic Tests/Treatments/Procedures
    › Provide care for client before surgical procedure including reinforcing teaching.
  » Therapeutic Procedures
    › Assist with the performance of a diagnostic or invasive procedure.

Client Needs: Physiological Adaptations

› Relevant topics/tasks include:
  » Alterations in Body Systems
    › Reinforce education to client regarding care and condition.
  » Basic Pathophysiology
    › Identify signs and symptoms related to an acute or chronic illness.
    › Consider general principles of client disease process when providing care.
    › Apply knowledge of pathophysiology to monitoring client for alterations in body systems.

chapter 25

Overview

- A fracture occurs when the resistance between a bone and an applied stress yields to the applied stress, resulting in a disruption to the integrity of the bone.

- Bone healing and remodeling is faster in children than in adults, due to a thicker periosteum and good blood supply.

- Epiphyseal plate injuries can result in altered bone growth.

- Radiographic evidence of previous fractures in various stages of healing or in infants may be the result of physical abuse or osteogenesis imperfecta.

Data Collection

- Risk Factors

  - Obesity

  - Poor nutrition

  - Developmental characteristics, ordinary play activities, and recreation place children at risk for injury (falls from climbing or running; trauma to bones from skateboarding, skiing, or playing soccer or basketball)

- Subjective and Objective Data

  - Physical Assessment Findings

    - Common types of fractures in children

      - Plastic deformation (bend) – The bone is bent no more than 45°.

      - Buckle (torus) – Compression of the bone resulting in a bulge or raised area at the fracture site.

      - Greenstick – Incomplete fracture of the bone.

      - Transverse – Break is straight across the bone.

      - Oblique – Break is diagonal across the bone.

      - Spiral – Break spirals around the bone.

      - Growth plate – Injury to the end of the long bone on the growth plate.

      - Stress – Tiny cracks in the bone.

M View Image: Fractures

      - Complete – Bone fragments are separated.

      - Incomplete – Bone fragments are still attached.

- □ Closed or simple – The fracture occurs without a break in the skin.

- □ Open or compound – The fracture occurs with an open wound and bone protruding.

- □ Complicated fracture – The fracture results in injury to other organs and tissues.

- Pain

- Crepitus

- Deformity

- Edema

- Ecchymosis

- Warmth or redness

○ Diagnostic Procedures

- Radiograph

- □ Nursing Actions

- ▸ Instruct and assist the client to remain still during the procedure.

- □ Client Education

- ▸ Inform the client and parents about what to expect during the procedure.

- ▸ Provide emotional support.

Patient-Centered Care

- Nursing Care

○ Provide emergency care at the time of injury.

- Maintain ABCs.

- Monitor vital signs, pain, and neurologic status.

- Check the neurovascular status of the injured extremity.

- Position the client in a supine position.

- Stabilize the injured area, avoiding unnecessary movement.

- Elevate the affected limb and apply ice packs.

- Administer analgesics as prescribed.

- Keep the client warm.

○ General nursing interventions

- Check pain frequently using an age-appropriate pain tool. Use appropriate pain management, both pharmacological and nonpharmacological.

- Monitor neurovascular status on a regular schedule. Report any change in status.

- □ Neurovascular Assessment

- ▸ Sensation – Check the client for numbness or a tingling sensation of the extremity. Loss of sensation can indicate nerve damage.

- ▸ Skin temperature – Check the temperature of the extremity. The extremity should be warm, not cool, to the touch.

- ▶ Skin color – Observe the color of the affected extremity. Check distal to the injury and look for changes in pigmentation.

- ▶ Capillary refill – Press the nail beds of the affected extremity until blanching occurs. Blood return should be within 3 seconds.

- ▶ Pulses – Pulses should be palpable and strong. Pulses should also be equal to the pulses of the unaffected extremity.

- ▶ Movement – The client should be able to move the affected extremity in passive motion.

  - ■ Maintain proper alignment.

  - ■ Promote range of motion of fingers, toes, and unaffected extremities.

  - ■ Instruct the client and family regarding activity restrictions.

- • Medications

  - ○ Analgesics

    - ■ Administer analgesics for pain.

    - ■ Nursing Considerations (for use of opioid analgesia)

      - ▢ Monitor for respiratory depression and constipation.

    - ■ Client Education

      - ▢ Instruct the client and parents about the need for adequate pain relief.

- • Teamwork and Collaboration

  - ○ Orthopedic specialists are generally consulted for fracture care in children.

  - ○ Notify social services in situations in which abuse is suspected.

- • Therapeutic Procedures

  - ○ Casting

    - ■ Types of casts: long-leg, short-leg, bilateral long-leg, long-arm, short-arm, full spica, and single spica

    - ■ Plaster of Paris casts are heavy, not water-resistant, and can take 10 to 72 hr to dry. Synthetic fiberglass casts are light, water-resistant, and dry very quickly (in 5 to 20 min).

    - ■ Prior to casting, the skin area should be observed for integrity, cleaned, and dried. Bony prominences should be padded to prevent skin breakdown. The casting material is then applied by the provider.

    - ■ Nursing Actions

      - ▢ Provide atraumatic care prior to cast application by demonstrating the procedure on a doll or toy.

      - ▢ Monitor neurovascular status.

      - ▢ Elevate the cast above the level of the heart during the first 24 to 48 hr to prevent swelling.

      - ▢ Apply ice for the first 24 hr to decrease swelling.

      - ▢ Turn and position the client every 2 hr so that dry air circulates around and under the cast for faster drying. This also will prevent pressure from changing the shape of the cast.

        - ▶ Do not use heat lamps or warm hair dryers.

      - ▢ Turn the client frequently while supporting all extremities and joints.

  □ Instruct the client to keep the affected extremity supported (with a sling) or elevated when sitting.

  □ Check for increased warmth or hot spots on the cast surface, which could indicate infection.

  □ If a wound is present, monitor the skin through the window that has been placed in an area of the cast to allow for skin inspection.

  □ Monitor for drainage on the cast. Outline any drainage on the outside of the cast with a marker (and note date and time) so it can be monitored for any additional drainage.

  □ Inspect the general skin condition and the area around the cast edges.

  □ Provide routine skin care and thorough perineal care to maintain skin integrity.

  □ Plaster casts: Use palms of hands to avoid denting, expose the case to air to promote drying.

  □ Use moleskin over any rough area of the cast that may rub against the client's skin.

  □ Prevent soiling the cast with urine or feces by covering necessary areas with plastic during elimination.

  □ Assist with proper crutch-fitting, and reinforce proper use.

- Client Education

  □ Inform the client and parents that when the cast is applied it will feel warm, but it will not burn the client.

  □ Instruct the parents and client to report pain that is extremely severe or is not relieved 1 hr after the administration of pain medication.

  □ Show the parents and client how to perform neurovascular checks and when to contact the provider.

  □ Reinforce instructions for the proper use of crutches for lower-extremity casts.

  □ Reinforce skin and perineal care with a spica cast.

  □ Instruct the client not to place any foreign objects inside the cast to avoid trauma to the skin.

  □ Reinforce use of proper restraints when transporting the client in any vehicle.

  □ Tell the client and parents about cast removal and cast cutter.

  □ Instruct the client to soak the extremity in warm water and then apply lotion after the cast has been removed

Traction care – Traction, countertraction, and frictional force are used to align, immobilize, and reduce muscle spasms associated with certain fractures. Through the use of a forward-pulling force and a backward force, adding or removing weight controls the degree of force applied to maintain traction and alignment. The type of traction used depends on the fracture, age of the client, and associated injuries.

- Skin traction uses a pulling force that is applied by weights (may be used intermittently). Using tape and straps applied to the skin along with boots and/or cuffs, weights are attached by a rope to the extremity (Buck, Russell, Bryant traction).

- Skeletal traction uses a continuous pulling force that is applied directly to the skeletal structure and/or specific bone. A pin or rod is inserted through or into the bone. Force is applied through the use of weights attached by rope. Skeletal traction (90°/90° traction) allows the client to change positions without interfering with the pull of the traction and decreases complications associated with immobility and traction.

- Balanced suspension traction suspends the leg in a flexed position. The hip and hamstring muscles are relaxed.
- Halo traction (cervical traction) uses a halo-type bar that encircles the head. Screws are inserted into the outer table of the skull. The halo is attached to either bed traction or rods that are secured to a vest worn by the client.

View Images
- › Balanced Suspension Skeletal Traction
- › Halo Traction

- Nursing Actions
  - Maintain body alignment.
  - Provide pharmacological and nonpharmacological interventions for the management of pain and muscle spasms.
  - Notify the provider if the client experiences severe pain from muscle spasms that is unrelieved with medications and/or repositioning.
  - Monitor neurovascular status.
  - Routinely monitor the client's skin integrity and document findings.
  - Inspect pin sites for pain, redness, swelling, drainage, or odor. Provide pin care per facility protocol.
  - Check for changes in elimination, and maintain usual patterns of elimination.
  - Ensure that all the hardware is tight and that the bed is in the correct position.
  - Maintain weights so that they hang freely and the ropes are free of knots. Do not lift or remove weights unless prescribed and supervised by the provider.
  - Ensure that the wrench to release the rods is attached to the vest when using halo traction in the event that CPR is necessary.
  - Move the client in halo traction as a unit without applying pressure to the rods. This will prevent loosening of the pins and pain.
  - Consult with the provider for an overbed trapeze to assist the client to move in bed.
  - Provide range of motion and encourage activity of nonimmobilized extremities to maintain mobility and prevent contractures.
  - Encourage deep breathing and use of incentive spirometry.
  - Promote frequent position changing within restrictions of traction.
  - Remove sheets from the head of the bed to the foot of the bed, and remake the bed in the same manner.
- Client Education
  - Instruct about the need to provide adequate hydration and nutrition while in traction.
  - Reinforce education about the use of and need for stool softeners.
  - Tell the client and parents to report signs of infection.
  - Tell the client to report any signs of compartment syndrome immediately.

- Surgical Interventions
  - Depending on the type of fracture, surgical intervention can be required. The most common fractures requiring surgery include supracondylar fractures and fractures of the humerus and femur.
  - Surgical reduction is achieved by either a closed (no incision) or open (with incision) reduction with or without pinning.
    - Nursing Actions
      - Monitor for indications of infection at the incision site.
      - Encourage mobilization as soon as prescribed.
      - Medicate for pain as needed.
    - Client Education
      - Reinforce teaching to the client and parents about what to expect before and after the procedure, including NPO status.
      - Discuss the need for pain medication.
  - Care After Discharge
    - Reinforce proper cast care, as well as pin care if indicated.
    - Reinforce how to perform neurovascular checks, and explain when to call or return to the provider.
    - Instruct the client and parents about the need for and use of antipruritic medications if prescribed.
    - Instruct the parents to maintain physical restrictions as prescribed.
    - Instruct the parents in appropriate pain management.
    - Instruct the parents to report increasing pain, redness, inflammation, or fever to the provider.
    - Instruct the parents regarding the importance of follow-up care as instructed.

Complications

- Compartment syndrome
  - Compression of nerves, blood vessels, and muscle inside a confined place.
  - If untreated, tissue necrosis can result.
  - Findings
    - Increased pain that is unrelieved with elevation or analgesics
    - Intense pain when passively moved
    - Paresthesia or numbness
    - Pulselessness distal to the fracture
    - Inability to move digits
    - Warm digits with skin that is tight and shiny
    - Pallor

✗ Nursing Actions

- Inspect the extremity at frequent intervals. Notify the provider if compartment syndrome is suspected.

- Prevention

  □ Loosen the constrictive dressing or cut the bandage or tape.

  □ Elevate the extremity and apply ice.

- Prepare the client for fasciotomy.

○ Client Education

- Instruct the client to report pain that is not relieved by analgesics, pain that continues to increase in intensity, numbness or tingling, or a change in color of the extremity.

- Osteomyelitis

  ○ Infection within the bone secondary to a bacterial infection from an outside source, such as with an open fracture (endogenous) or from a bloodborne bacterial source (hematogenous)

  ○ Clinical Manifestations

    - Appearing ill

    - Irritability

    - Fever

    - Tachycardia

    - Edema

    - Pain

    - Not wanting to use the affected extremity

    - Site of infection tender, and bone pain worsens with movement

  ○ Nursing Actions

    - Assist in diagnostic procedures, such as obtaining skin, blood, and bone cultures.

    - Assist with joint or bone biopsy.

    - Administer IV and oral antibiotic therapy.

    - Assist with proper positioning to promote comfort.

    - Administer pain medication as prescribed.

    - Consult with the parents and provider regarding home care needs.

  ○ Client Education

    - Inform the client and parents about the length of treatment that may be needed and long-term antibiotic therapy.

    - Remind the client and parents to avoid bearing any weight until cleared by the provider.

    - Advise the parents to provide for diversional activities consistent with the client's level of development.

    - Inform the client about the need for proper nutrition.

APPLICATION EXERCISES

1. A nurse is caring for a child who is in a plaster spica cast. Which of the following is an appropriate action for the nurse to take?

    A. Use a heat lamp to facilitate drying.

    B. Avoid turning the child until the cast is dry.

    C. Assist the client with crutch walking after the cast is dry.

    D. Apply moleskin to the edges of the cast.

2. A nurse is reinforcing teaching with a group of parent about fractures. Which of the following should be included in the teaching?

    A. "Children need a longer time to heal from a fracture than an adult."

    B. "Epiphyseal plate injuries may result in altered bone growth."

    C. "A greenstick fracture is a complete break in the bone."

    D. "Bones are unable to bend, so they break."

3. A nurse is caring for a child who sustained a fracture. Which of the following are appropriate actions for the nurse to take? (Select all that apply.)

    _____ A. Place a heat pack on the site of injury.

    _____ B. Elevate the affected limb.

    _____ C. Check neurovascular status frequently.

    _____ D. Encourage ROM of the affected limb.

    _____ E. Stabilize the injury.

4. A nurse is caring for a child who has a fracture. Which of the following are clinical manifestations of a fracture? (Select all that apply.)

    _____ A. Crepitus

    _____ B. Edema

    _____ C. Pain

    _____ D. Fever

    _____ E. Ecchymosis

5. A nurse is caring for a child who is in Russell traction. Which of the following are appropriate actions for the nurse to take? (Select all that apply.)

_____ A. Remove the boots once a day for a bath.

_____ B. Check the child's position frequently.

_____ C. Check pin sites every 4 hr.

_____ D. Ensure the weights are hanging freely.

_____ E. Ensure the buttocks are raised off of the bed.

6. A nurse is caring for a client who has a newly placed cast. Use the ATI Active Learning Template: Systems Disorder to complete this item to include clinical manifestations of compartment syndrome.

APPLICATION EXERCISES KEY

1. A. INCORRECT: A cool fan can be used to facilitate drying of a plaster cast.

    B. INCORRECT: The child should be turned every 2 hr to expose all areas of the cast to facilitate drying.

    C. INCORRECT: A client who has a spica cast is non-weight-bearing until the cast is removed.

    D. **CORRECT:** The nurse should apply moleskin to the edges of the cast to prevent the cast from rubbing on the client's skin.

    Ⓝ NCLEX® Connection: Basic Care and Comfort, Mobility/Immobility

2. A. INCORRECT: Children heal from fractures quicker than adults due to a thicker periosteum and good blood supply.

    B. **CORRECT:** Detection and early treatment is crucial for an epiphyseal plate injury to prevent altered bone growth.

    C. INCORRECT: A greenstick fracture is a partial break in the bone.

    D. INCORRECT: Children's bones are soft and pliable and can bend up to 45° before breaking.

    Ⓝ NCLEX® Connection: Physiological Adaptations, Alterations in Body Systems

3. A. INCORRECT: The nurse should place a cold pack on the site of injury to decrease swelling.

    B. **CORRECT:** Elevating the affected limb can decrease swelling at the injury site.

    C. **CORRECT:** Checking neurovascular status assists the nurse in determining if the affected limp has adequate blood supply.

    D. INCORRECT: The nurse should encourage ROM of the nonaffected limb.

    E. **CORRECT:** Stabilizing the injury will prevent further injury and damage.

    Ⓝ NCLEX® Connection: Physiological Adaptations, Basic Pathophysiology

4. A. **CORRECT:** A fracture can leave bone fragments that will exhibit a grating sound. Crepitus is a clinical manifestation of a fracture.

    B. **CORRECT:** Swelling at the site occur related to the trauma. Edema is a clinical manifestation of a fracture.

    C. **CORRECT:** A child who has a fracture will experience pain from the trauma.

    D. INCORRECT: A child who has a fracture will not exhibit a fever related to the fracture.

    E. **CORRECT:** Bleeding under the skin can occur related to the trauma. Ecchymosis is a clinical manifestation of a fracture.

    Ⓝ NCLEX® Connection: Physiological Adaptations, Basic Pathophysiology

5. A. INCORRECT: The boots should only be removed by the provider or in an emergency situation.

    B. **CORRECT:** Hip flexion must be maintained in Russell traction. The nurse should check the child's position frequently.

    C. INCORRECT: Russell traction is a skin traction. The client will not have pin sites to check.

    D. **CORRECT:** The nurse should ensure that the weights are hanging freely to allow for prescribed traction.

    E. INCORRECT: The buttocks are raised off of the bed when Bryant traction is used.

    Ⓝ NCLEX® Connection: Basic Care and Comfort, Mobility/Immobility

6. *Using the ATI Active Learning Template: Systems Disorder*
    - Clinical Manifestations of Compartment Syndrome
        ○ Increased pain that is unrelieved with elevation or analgesics
        ○ Intense pain when passively moved
        ○ Paresthesia or numbness
        ○ Pulselessness distal to the fracture
        ○ Inability to move digits
        ○ Warm digits with skin that is tight and shiny
        ○ Pallor

    Ⓝ NCLEX® Connection: Physiological Adaptations, Basic Pathophysiology

chapter 26

Overview

- Clubfoot

- Legg-Calve-Perthes

- Developmental dysplasia of the hip (DDH)

- Osteogenesis imperfecta

- Scoliosis

CLUBFOOT

Overview

- A complex deformity of the ankle and foot

- Can affect one or both feet, and occur as an isolated defect or in association with other disorders, such as cerebral palsy and spinal bifida

- Categorized as positional clubfoot (occurs from intrauterine crowding), syndromic (occurs in association with other syndromes), or congenital (idiopathic)

M ⬦   View Images

    › Clubfoot   › Developmental Dysplasia of the Hip (DDH)

Data Collection

- Risk Factors – presence of other syndromes

- Subjective and Objective Data

  ○ Talipes varus – inversion (bending inward)

  ○ Talipes valgus – eversion (bending outward)

  ○ Talipes calcaneus – dorsiflexion (toes are higher than the heel)

  ○ Talipes equinus – plantar flexion (toes are lower than the heel)

  ○ Talipes equinovarus – toes face inward and are lower than the heel

- Diagnostic Procedures

  ○ Prenatal – ultrasound can identify the deformity

Patient-Centered Care

- Nursing Care
  - Encourage parents to hold and cuddle the child.
  - Encourage parents to meet the developmental needs of the child.
  - Perform neurovascular and skin integrity checks.
- Therapeutic Procedures
  - Castings
    - A series of castings starts shortly after birth and continues until maximum correction is accomplished.
    - Nursing Care
      - Check neurovascular status.
      - Perform cast care.
    - Client Education
      - Instruct the family about cast care.
      - Instruct the family on follow-up care for cast changes.
- Surgical Interventions (congenital clubfoot and syndromic clubfoot)
  - Osteotomy – removing part of the bone
  - Fusion – fusing two or more bones together
  - Tendon lengthening or shortening
- Complications
  - Growth and development delays
    - Nursing Care – Monitor growth and development.
    - Client Education – Give the family strategies to enhance normal growth and development.
  - Effects of casting
    - Skin breakdown
    - Neurovascular alterations

LEGG-CALVE-PERTHES DISEASE

Overview

- Aseptic necrosis of the femoral head can be unilateral or bilateral

Data Collection

- Risk Factors
  - Trauma, inflammation to the femoral head
  - Coagulation defects

- Subjective and Objective Data
  - Intermittent painless limp
  - Hip stiffness
  - Limited ROM
  - Thigh pain
  - Shortening of the affected leg
- Diagnostic Procedures – radiographs of the hip and pelvis

Patient-Centered Care

- Nursing Care
  - Treatment varies with the child's age and the appearance of the femoral head.
  - Administer NSAIDs.
  - Maintain rest and nonweightbearing.
    - Abduction brace
    - Casts
    - Leather harness sling
    - Traction
  - Advance to active motion as prescribed.
- Surgical Interventions
  - Total hip resurfacing
    - Replace the hip joint.
- Client Education
  - Instruct about the nonweightbearing treatment prescribed.
  - Offer developmental appropriate strategies for learning and activities during the nonweightbearing periods.

DEVELOPMENTAL DYSPLASIA OF THE HIP (DDH)

Overview

- A variety of disorders resulting in abnormal development of the hip structures that can affect infants or children
- Acetabular dysplasia – delay in acetabular development
- Subluxation – incomplete dislocation of the hip
- Dislocation – femoral head does not have contact with the acetabulum

Data Collection

- Risk Factors
  - Birth order
  - Family history
  - Intrauterine position
  - Delivery type
  - Joint stability
- Subjective and Objective Data
  - Infant
    - Asymmetry of gluteal and thigh folds
    - Limited hip abduction
    - Shortening of the femur
    - Positive Ortolani test (hip is reduced by abduction)
    - Positive Barlow test (hip is dislocated by adduction)
  - Child
    - One leg shorter than the other
    - Positive Trendelenburg sign (while bearing weight on the affected side, the pelvis tilts downward)
    - Walking on toes on one foot
    - Walk with a limp
- Diagnostic Procedures
  - Ultrasound – should be performed at 2 weeks of age to determine the cartilaginous head of the femur
  - X-ray – can diagnose DDH in infants older than 4 months of age

Patient-Centered Care

- Nursing Care
  - Treatment starts as soon as DDH is diagnosed and depends on the child's age and the extent of the dysplasia.
  - Encourage parents to hold and cuddle the infant/child.
  - Encourage parents to meet the developmental needs of the infant/child.
  - Newborn to 6 months
    - Pavlik harness
      - Maintain harness placement for 6 to 12 weeks.
      - Check straps every 1 to 2 weeks for adjustment.
      - Perform neurovascular and skin integrity checks.
      - Removing the harness is dependent on the client.

- □ Client Teaching
  - ▸ Instruct the family not to adjust the straps.
  - ▸ Instruct the family how to place the harness if removal is prescribed.
  - ▸ Instruct the family about skin care (use an undershirt and knee socks, check skin, gently massage skin under straps, avoid lotions and powders, place diaper under the straps).
- Bryant traction or hip spica cast (when adduction contracture is present)
  - □ Bryant traction
    - ▸ Skin traction
    - ▸ Hips flexed at a 90° angle with the buttock raised off of the bed
    - ▸ Nursing Actions
      - ▷ Neurovascular checks
      - ▷ Maintain traction (ropes, boots, pulleys, and weights)
      - ▷ Ensure the client maintains alignment
      - ▷ Skin care
  - □ Hip spica cast
    - ▸ Needs to be changed to accommodate growth
    - ▸ Nursing Actions
      - ▷ Check and maintain the hip spica cast.
      - ▷ Perform frequent neurovascular checks.
      - ▷ Perform range of motion with the unaffected extremities.
      - ▷ Perform frequent inspection of skin integrity, especially in the diaper area.
      - ▷ Determine need for pain control using an age-appropriate pain tool. Intervene as indicated.
      - ▷ Monitor hydration status frequently.
      - ▷ Check and record elimination status daily.
    - ▸ Client Education
      - ▷ Reinforce teaching regarding positioning, turning, neurovascular assessments, and care of the cast.
      - ▷ Position casts on pillows.
      - ▷ Keep casts elevated until dry.
      - ▷ Encourage frequent position changes to allow for drying.
      - ▷ Handle casts with the palm of the hand until dry.
      - ▷ Note color and temperature of toes on casted extremity.
      - ▷ Give sponge baths to avoid wetting the cast.
      - ▷ Use a waterproof barrier around the genital opening of the spica cast to prevent soiling with urine or feces.
      - ▷ Instruct the family regarding care after discharge with emphasis on using appropriate equipment (stroller, wagon, car seat) for maintaining mobility.

- ○ 6 months to 2 years
  - ■ Surgical closed reduction with placement of hip spica cast
    - □ Nursing Actions
      - ▸ Prepare family and client for surgery
      - ▸ Perform neurovascular checks
      - ▸ Manage postoperative pain
      - ▸ Skin care
      - ▸ Cast care
    - □ Client Education
      - ▸ Instruct the family about spica cast and home cares.
- ○ Older children
  - ■ Surgical reduction with presurgical traction
  - ■ Femoral osteotomy, reconstruction, and tenotomy are often needed

Complications

- Postoperative complications (atelectasis, ileus, infection)
- Effects of immobilization (decreased muscle strength, bone demineralization, altered bowel motility)
- Effects of casting (skin breakdown, neurovascular alterations)
- Infection
  - ○ Infection can be caused by bacteria, such as *Staphylococcus aureus*.
  - ○ Nursing Actions
    - ■ Monitor vital signs. Observe changes in temperature that could be associated with complications of infection.
    - ■ Keep the cast dry and intact.
    - ■ Monitor for changes in neurovascular status (numbness; tingling; decreased mobility, sensation, or capillary refill).
    - ■ Reposition the child frequently.
    - ■ Maintain a high-fiber diet and promote adequate hydration.
    - ■ Monitor bowel and bladder elimination. Report any changes, especially the decrease or absence of bowel sounds or distention.
    - ■ Report any foul odor from cast or urine.
    - ■ Observe changes in behavior, especially increasing irritability in infants.
  - ○ Client Education
    - ■ Reinforce expected complications of specific treatment or procedure with the child and/or family.
    - ■ Reinforce the need to notify the provider with any concerns or signs of complications.
    - ■ Instruct the child and/or family about follow up.

OSTEOGENESIS IMPERFECTA (OI)

Overview

- Heterogeneous, autosomal dominant disorder of the bones resulting in fractures and deformity
- Several classifications of OI

Data Collection

- Risk Factors
  - Parent who has OI
- Subjective and Objective Data
  - Classic manifestations
    - Multiple bone fractures
    - Blue sclera
    - Early hearing loss
  - More severe manifestations
    - Bowed legs and arms
    - Kyphosis
    - Scoliosis
- Diagnostic Procedures
  - Bone biopsy
    - Nursing Actions
      - □ Prepare the client for the procedure.
      - □ Assist with positioning the client.

Patient-Centered Care

- Nursing Care
  - Treatment is supportive.
  - Medication
    - Pamidronate (Aredia)
      - □ Increase bone density
      - □ Nursing Actions
        - ▸ Assist with IV administration.
        - ▸ Monitor for adverse effects (hypokalemia, hypomagnesemia, hypocalcemia, hypophosphatemia, general malaise).
      - □ Client Education
        - ▸ Inform about adverse effects and when to call the provider.

- Instruct the family and client about low-impact exercises.
- Explain to the family about the prescribed medication regime.
- Consult with physical therapy.
- Assist with braces and splints.
- Assist client with meeting developmental milestones.
- Reinforce teaching to the parents on the client's limitations.
- Encourage support groups.
- Surgical Interventions (for severe cases)
  - Correct bone deformities, placement of rods.

Complications

- Disuse osteoporosis
  - Limit time in casts.
  - Encourage activity.
- Hearing loss
- Permanent deformities

SCOLIOSIS

Overview

- Scoliosis is a complex deformity of the spine that also affects the ribs.
- It is characterized by a lateral curvature of the spine and spinal rotation that causes rib asymmetry.
- A curve needs to be at least 10° for diagnosis, and mild curves (less than 25°) are monitored.
- Idiopathic or structural scoliosis is the most common form of scoliosis and can be seen in isolation or associated with other conditions.
  - Bracing and exercise

 View Image: Brace for Scoliosis

Data Collection

- Risk Factors
  - Genetic tendency
- Subjective and Objective Data
  - Asymmetry in scapula, ribs, flanks, shoulders, and hips
  - Improperly fitting clothing (one leg shorter than the other)

- Diagnostic Procedures
  - ○ Screen during preadolescence for boys and girls.
    - Observe the child, who should be wearing only underwear, from the back.
    - Have the child bend over at the waist with arms hanging down, and observe for asymmetry of ribs and flank.
    - Measure truncal rotation with a scoliometer.
  - ○ Radiographs
    - Use the Cobb technique to determine the degree of curvature.
    - Use the Risser scale to determine the skeletal maturity.

Patient-Centered Care

- Nursing Care
  - ○ Treatment depends on the degree, location, and type of curvature.
- Therapeutic Procedures
  - ○ Bracing
    - Customized braces that slow the progression of the curve
    - Nursing Actions
      - □ Assist with fitting the client with a brace.
      - □ Inspect skin.
      - □ Assist the client with self-image.
    - Client Education
      - □ Instruct the client how to apply the brace.
- Surgical Interventions
  - ○ Spinal fusion with rod placement
  - ○ Used for curvatures greater than 45°
  - ○ Nursing Actions
    - Preoperative
      - □ Inform and assist the adolescent to obtain autologous (self-donated) blood donations.
      - □ Obtain routine laboratory studies, including a type and cross match for blood.
      - □ Orient the adolescent and family to the ICU.
      - □ Inform the adolescent and family about what can be expected during the postoperative period, such as monitoring equipment, NG tube, chest tubes, indwelling urinary catheters, and patient-controlled analgesia (PCA) pump.
    - Postoperative
      - □ Assist with monitoring the adolescent initially in the intensive care unit.
      - □ Perform standard postoperative care to prevent complications.
      - □ Monitor pain using an age-appropriate pain tool.

☐ Assist with analgesia management using a PCA pump.

☐ Perform frequent neurovascular checks.

☐ Turn the adolescent frequently by log rolling to prevent damage to the spinal fusion.

☐ Inspect skin for pressure areas, especially if a brace has been prescribed.

☐ Provide skin care by keeping skin clean and dry.

☐ Monitor surgical and drain sites for signs of infection. Provide wound care.

☐ Auscultate bowel sounds and monitor, observing for paralytic ileus.

☐ Monitor for decreases in Hgb and Hct. Observe for indications of bleeding.

☐ Assist with the monitoring of blood transfusion. The adolescent can have self-donated blood available for transfusion.

☐ Encourage mobility as soon as tolerated.

☐ Observe for signs of infection.

☐ Perform range of motion on unaffected extremities.

☐ Provide age-appropriate activities and opportunities to visit with friends and family during the hospital stay.

○ Client Education

  ▪ Preoperative

   ☐ Reinforce teaching (use of incentive spirometer, turning, coughing, deep breathing) to prevent complications.

   ☐ Reinforce preoperative teaching to educate the adolescent and/or family and to promote cooperation and participation in recovery.

   ☐ Demonstrate the use of a patient-controlled analgesic pump if age-appropriate.

   ☐ Demonstrate log rolling that will be used after surgery.

   ☐ Demonstrate the respiratory therapy techniques that will be used postoperatively to reduce complications of anesthesia.

   ☐ Discuss medical terms that are unfamiliar to the adolescent and/or family.

  ▪ Postoperative

   ☐ Emphasize the importance of physical therapy and proper positioning of the spine.

   ☐ Encourage independence following surgery for the adolescent who has a brace.

   ☐ Encourage the adolescent to contact friends when able.

   ☐ Emphasize the necessity of follow-up care.

○ Care After Discharge

  ▪ Client Education

   ☐ Reinforce the expected course of treatment and recovery.

   ☐ Suggest that the family arrange the environment to facilitate the adolescent's ability to be as independent as possible (keep favorite items within reach).

   ☐ Emphasize the necessity of follow-up care.

Complications

- Breathing difficulties (with severe curvatures)
- Lower self-esteem
  - ○ Assist the client with age-appropriate actions with self-esteem.
- Infection following surgery
  - ○ Infection can be caused by bacteria, such as *Staphylococcus aureus*.
  - ○ Nursing Actions
    - Monitor vital signs. Observe changes in temperature that could be associated with complications of infection.
    - Monitor for changes in neurovascular status (numbness; tingling; decreased mobility, sensation, or capillary refill).
    - Reposition the child frequently.
    - Maintain a high-fiber diet and promote adequate hydration.
  - ○ Client Education
    - Reinforce expected complications of specific treatment or procedure with the child and family.
    - Reinforce the need to notify the provider with any concerns or signs of complications.
    - Inform the child and/or family about follow up.
- Spine or nerve damage (uncorrected scoliosis)

APPLICATION EXERCISES

1. A nurse is caring for a toddler who has hip dysplasia and is in a hip spica cast. The child's mother asks the nurse why a Pavlik harness is not being used. Which of the following responses by the nurse appropriately addresses the mother's question?

    A. "The Pavlik harness is used for children with scoliosis, not hip dysplasia."

    B. "The Pavlik harness is used for school-age children."

    C. "The Pavlik harness cannot be used for your child because her condition is too severe."

    D. "The Pavlik harness is used for infants less than 6 months of age."

2. A nurse is reinforcing preoperative teaching with an adolescent client who is going to receive spinal instrumentation for scoliosis. Which of the following information should the nurse include in the instructions?

    A. "You will go home the same day of surgery."

    B. "You will have minimal pain."

    C. "You will need to receive blood."

    D. "You will not be able to eat until the day after surgery."

3. A nurse is collecting data on a child. Which of the following are clinical manifestations of Legg-Calve-Perthes disease? (Select all that apply.)

    _____ A. Longer affected leg

    _____ B. Hip stiffness

    _____ C. Intense pain

    _____ D. Limited ROM

    _____ E. Limp with walking

4. A nurse is caring for a preschool-age child. Which of the following techniques should the nurse use to check for developmental dysplasia of the hip?

    A. Barlow test

    B. Trendelenburg sign

    C. Manipulation of foot and ankle

    D. Ortolani test

5. A nurse is caring for a child. Which of the following diagnostic procedures should the nurse prepare the child for to determine if the child has Legg-Calve-Perthes disease?

    A. Bone biopsy

    B. Genetic testing

    C. MRI

    D. Radiographs

6. A nurse is caring for a child in a hip spica cast. What should the nurse include in the care of this client? Use the ATI Active Learning Template: Therapeutic Procedure to complete this item to include the following:

    A. Nursing Actions: List seven.

    B. Client Education: List eight instructions.

APPLICATION EXERCISES KEY

1. A. INCORRECT: The Pavlik harness is for infants who have hip dysplasia.

    B. INCORRECT: The Pavlik harness is for infants who have hip dysplasia.

    C. INCORRECT: The Pavlik harness is for infants who have hip dysplasia.

    D. **CORRECT:** The Pavlik harness is a soft brace designed for infants younger than 6 months of age.

     NCLEX® Connection: Physiological Adaptations, Basic Pathophysiology

2. A. INCORRECT: Clients who have spinal instrumentation for scoliosis are hospitalized for approximately 1 week.

    B. INCORRECT: Clients who have spinal instrumentation for scoliosis experience intense pain that requires a PCA pump.

    C. **CORRECT:** Clients who have spinal instrumentation for scoliosis have a lengthy surgery with blood loss and require blood replacements.

    D. INCORRECT: Clients who have spinal instrumentation for scoliosis are allowed to advance their diet as tolerated.

     NCLEX® Connection: Reduction of Risk Potential, Potential for Complications from Surgical Procedures and Health Alterations

3. A. INCORRECT: A child who has Legg-Calve-Perthes exhibits shortening of the affected leg.

    B. **CORRECT:** A child who has Legg-Calve-Perthes exhibits hip stiffness due to the necrosis of the femoral head.

    C. INCORRECT: A child who has Legg-Calve-Perthes exhibits a painless intermittent limp.

    D. **CORRECT:** A child who has Legg-Calve-Perthes exhibits limited ROM because of necrosis of the femoral head.

    E. **CORRECT:** A child who has Legg-Calve-Perthes exhibits a limp with walking because of necrosis of the femoral head.

     NCLEX® Connection: Physiological Adaptations, Basic Pathophysiology

4. A. INCORRECT: The Barlow test is used to assess developmental dysplasia of the hip for infants.

    B. **CORRECT:** The Trendelenburg sign is used to assess for developmental dysplasia of the hip. The preschooler bears weight on the affected leg while holding on to something for balance. The examiner observes from behind for abnormal downward tilting of the pelvis on the unaffected side.

    C. INCORRECT: Manipulation of the foot and ankle is used to assess for clubfoot.

    D. INCORRECT: The Ortolani test is used to assess developmental dysplasia of the hip for infants.

     NCLEX® Connection: Physiological Adaptations, Basic Pathophysiology

5. A. INCORRECT: A bone biopsy is used to diagnosis cancer, infection, and other bone disorders. It is not indicated to diagnose Legg-Calve-Perthes.

    B. INCORRECT: Legg-Calve-Perthes is necrosis of the femoral head and is not genetic.

    C. INCORRECT: An MRI is used to visualize structures inside the body. Legg-Calve-Perthes is necrosis of the femoral head. An MRI is not indicated to diagnose Legg-Calve-Perthes.

    D. **CORRECT:** A child who has Legg-Calve-Perthes exhibits necrosis of the femoral head that can be diagnosed by radiographs of the hip and pelvis.

    Ⓝ NCLEX® Connection: Reduction of Risk Potential, Therapeutic Procedures

6. *Using the ATI Active Learning Template: Therapeutic Procedure*

    A. Nursing Actions
    - Check and maintain the hip spica cast.
    - Perform frequent neurovascular checks.
    - Perform range of motion with the unaffected extremities.
    - Perform frequent assessment of skin integrity, especially in the diaper area.
    - Check for pain control using an age-appropriate pain tool. Intervene as indicated.
    - Evaluate hydration status frequently.
    - Check elimination status daily.

    B. Client Education
    - Reinforce teaching regarding positioning, turning, neurovascular assessments, and care of the cast.
    - Position casts on pillows.
    - Keep casts elevated until dry.
    - Encourage frequent position changes to allow for drying.
    - Handle casts with the palm of the hand until dry.
    - Note color and temperature of toes on the casted extremity.
    - Give sponge baths to avoid wetting the cast.
    - Use a waterproof barrier around the genital opening of spica cast to prevent soiling with urine or feces.
    - Instruct regarding care after discharge with emphasis on using appropriate equipment (stroller, wagon, car seat) for maintaining mobility.

    Ⓝ NCLEX® Connection: Reduction of Risk Potential, Potential for Complications of Diagnostic Tests/ Treatments/Procedures

UNIT 2 NURSING CARE OF CHILDREN WITH SYSTEM DISORDERS
SECTION: MUSCULOSKELETAL DISORDERS

CHAPTER 27 Chronic Neuromuscuskeletal Disorders

Overview

- Chronic neuromusculoskeletal disorders affect the brain, muscles, joints, and skeletal structures of the body.
  - Cerebral palsy (CP)
  - Spina bifida
  - Down syndrome
  - Juvenile idiopathic arthritis (JIA)
  - Muscular dystrophy (MD)

CEREBRAL PALSY

Overview

- Cerebral palsy (CP) is a nonprogressive impairment of motor function, especially that of muscle control, coordination, and posture.
- CP can cause abnormal perception and sensation; visual, hearing, and speech impairments; seizures; and cognitive disabilities.
- CP manifests differently in each child. Developmental outcomes vary and depend on the severity of the injury.

Data Collection

- Risk Factors
  - The exact cause of CP is not known. Prenatal, perinatal, and postnatal risk factors known to be associated with CP include the following.
    - Existing brain anomalies, cerebral infections, head trauma (shaken baby syndrome), and/or anoxia to the brain
    - Maternal chorioamnionitis
    - Premature birth and postterm birth (42 weeks or later)
    - Multiple births
    - Extremely low or very low birth weights in newborns
    - Inability of the placenta to provide the developing fetus with oxygen and nutrients
    - Interruption of oxygen delivery to the fetus during birth
    - Kernicterus as a result of high levels of bilirubin in the neonatal period

- Subjective Data
  - Parents may describe concerns with development.
- Objective Data
  - Physical Assessment Findings
    - Failure to meet developmental milestones
    - Persistent primitive reflexes (Moro or tonic neck)
    - Gagging or choking with feeding, poor suck reflex
    - Tongue thrust
    - Poor head control
    - Rigid posture and extremities, abnormal posturing
    - Asymmetric crawl
    - Hyperreflexia
    - Vision or hearing impairments
    - Seizures
    - Impaired social relationships
    - Assessment findings associated with specific types of CP
      - Spastic (Pyramidal)
        - Hypertonicity (muscle tightness or spasticity); increased deep-tendon reflexes; clonus; and poor control of motion, balance, and posture.
        - Impairments of fine and gross motor skills.
        - Can present in all extremities (quadriplegia), similar parts of the body (diplegia), three limbs (triplegia), one limb (monoplegia), or one side of the body (hemiplegia); often causes affected limbs to be shorter and thinner.
        - Gait can appear crouched with a scissoring motion of the legs with intoeing and use of primarily the balls of the feet in a tip-toe fashion.
      - Dyskinetic (Nonspastic, Extrapyramidal)
        - Athetoid: Findings include involuntary jerking movements that appear slow, writhing, and wormlike. These movements involve the trunk, neck, face, and tongue.
        - Dystonic: Slow, twisting movements affect the trunk and extremities with abnormal posturing from muscle contractions.
      - Ataxic (Nonspastic, Extrapyramidal)
        - Evidence of wide-based gait and difficulty with coordination
        - Poor ability to do repetitive movements
        - Difficulty with quick or precise movements (writing or buttoning a shirt)
        - Shakiness
        - Low muscle tone

- ○ Diagnostic Procedures
  - ▪ Collect data related to neurological function.
  - ▪ MRI
    - □ Used to evaluate structures or abnormal areas located near bone, and sedation may be necessary.
    - □ Nursing Actions
      - ‣ Assist the child to stay still during the procedure.
      - ‣ Sedate the child if prescribed.
    - □ Client Education
      - ‣ Provide emotional support.
  - ▪ Metabolic and genetic testing

Patient-Centered Care

- Nursing Care
  - ○ Individualize care to meet a client's needs.
  - ○ Monitor developmental milestones.
  - ○ Evaluate the need for hearing and speech evaluations.
  - ○ Promote independence with self-care activities as much as possible. Assist the client to maintain a positive self-image and a high level of self-esteem.
  - ○ Determine the extent of family coping and support.
  - ○ Determine the family's awareness of available resources.
  - ○ Determine the client's developmental level.
  - ○ Structure interventions and communications around the client's developmental level, rather than chronological age.
  - ○ Communicate with the child directly, but include parents as needed.
  - ○ Help the child to use augmented communication, such as electronic devices for speech and other types of communication tools.
  - ○ Include the family in physical care during hospitalization.
    - ▪ Ask the family about routine care, and encourage them to provide it if appropriate.
    - ▪ Encourage the family to help verify the client's needs if communication is impaired.
  - ○ Maintain an open airway by elevating the head of the child's bed. (This is especially important if the child has increased oral secretions.)
  - ○ Ensure suction equipment is available if required. Suction oral secretions as needed.
  - ○ Monitor for pain (especially with muscle spasms) using a developmentally appropriate pain tool.
  - ○ Administer medication for pain and/or spasms as prescribed.
  - ○ Ensure adequate nutrition.
    - ▪ Monitor for the possibility of aspiration for children who are severely disabled.
    - ▪ Determine the child's ability to take oral nutrition.
    - ▪ Ascertain the correct positioning for feeding the child. Use head positioning and manual jaw control methods as needed.

- Provide foods that are similar to foods eaten at home when possible. Administer supplements as prescribed.

- Administer feedings by gastric tube as prescribed.

- Maintain weight/height chart.

- Provide skin care.

    □ Monitor skin under splints and braces if applicable.

    □ Maintain skin integrity by turning the child to keep pressure off bony prominences.

    □ Keep skin clean and dry.

- Provide rest periods as needed.

- Medications

    ○ Baclofen (Lioresal)

        - Used as a centrally acting skeletal muscle relaxant that decreases muscle spasm and severe spasticity

        - Nursing Considerations

            □ Administer orally or intrathecally via a specialized, surgically implanted pump.

            □ Monitor effectiveness of the medication.

            □ Monitor for muscle weakness, increased fatigue, or less-common adverse effects (diaphoresis, constipation).

        - Client Education

            □ Reinforce teaching with the family about expected responses of medications.

            □ Reinforce with the family the adverse effects of medications and when to call the provider.

    ○ Diazepam (Valium)

        - Skeletal muscle relaxant used to decrease muscle spasms and severe spasticity

        - Nursing Considerations

            □ Use in older children and adolescents.

            □ Monitor for drowsiness and fatigue.

        - Client Education

            □ Reinforce teaching with the family about expected responses to medications.

            □ Reinforce with the family the adverse effects of the medication and when to call the provider.

    ○ Botulinum toxin A (Botox)

        - Reduces spasticity in specific muscle groups

        - Used primarily for client's with spasticity only in the lower extremities

        - Nursing Considerations – Monitor for temporary weakness.

        - Client Education – Explain to the family that onset of the medication is 24 to 72 hr, with a peak of 2 weeks, lasting 3 to 6 months.

    ○ Antiepileptics

        - Control seizure activity

- Teamwork and Collaboration
  - Coordinate care with other professionals such as speech, physical and recreational therapists, and education and/or medical specialists.
  - Initiate referral for technical aids that can assist with coordination, speaking, mobility, and an increased level of independence. This may be achieved with the use of a voice-activated wheelchair.
  - Surgical intervention may be needed for tendon release to correct contractures or other spastic deformities.
  - Care after Discharge
    - Client Education
      - Reinforce the therapeutic plan of care.
      - Reinforce the need for rest periods.
      - Reinforce feeding schedule and feeding techniques if changes were made during hospitalization.
      - Reinforce adherence to medication regimen.
      - Encourage regular dental care.
      - Encourage parents to provide developmental stimulation.
      - Explain wound care if needed.
      - Explain to the family and client about ankle-foot orthoses if prescribed.
      - Reinforce teaching about self-urinary catheterization if needed.
      - Explain pulmonary hygiene techniques.
      - Coordinate interdisciplinary team with cares.
      - Help the family identify resources needed (respite care).
      - Suggest participation in a support group for CP.

Complications

- Aspiration
  - Nursing Actions
    - Keep the child's head elevated.
    - Keep suction available if copious oral secretions are present or the child has difficulty with swallowing foods and/or fluids.
  - Client Education
    - Reinforce teaching with the family about feeding techniques to decrease the risk of aspiration.
    - Encourage the family to take CPR classes.

- Potential for injury
  - Nursing Actions
    - Make sure the child's bed rails are raised to prevent falls from the bed.
    - Pad side rails and wheelchair arms to prevent injury.
    - Secure the child in mobility devices, such as wheelchairs.
    - Encourage the child to receive adequate rest to prevent injury at times of fatigue.
    - Encourage the use of helmets, seat belts, and other safety equipment.
  - Client Education
    - Review safety precautions with the child and family.

SPINA BIFIDA

Overview

- Spinal bifida is failure of the osseous spine to close.
- Neural tube defects (NTDs) are present at birth and affect the CNS and osseous spine.
  - Spina bifida occulta – Mostly affects the lumbosacral area and is not visible.
  - Spina bifida cystica – Has a visual sac protrusion.
    - Meningocele – The sac contains spinal fluid and meninges.
    - Myelomeningocele – The sac includes meninges, spinal fluid, and nerves.

 View Image: Spina Bifida

Data Collection

- Risk Factors
  - Medications/drugs taken during pregnancy
  - Maternal malnutrition
  - Insufficient folic acid intake during pregnancy
  - Exposure to radiation or chemicals during pregnancy
  - Prepregnancy obesity, diabetes mellitus, hyperthermia, or low vitamin B_{12}
- Subjective Data
  - Evaluate prenatal history.
  - Determine family history of neural tube defects.
- Objective Data
  - Physical Assessment Findings
    - Protruding sac midline of the osseous spine
    - Dimpling in the lumbosacral area

Q
EBP

- ○ Laboratory Tests
  - ▪ Maternal blood tests – Maternal serum alpha-fetoprotein (MSAFP) test between 16 and 18 weeks of gestation indicates possible NTD.
  - ▪ Infant blood tests – Blood cultures to determine causative pathogen if appropriate.
- ○ Diagnostic Procedures
  - ▪ Prenatal
    - □ Ultrasound may show visual defect.
    - □ Amniocentesis is done following elevated alpha-fetoprotein levels to detect anencephaly or myelomeningocele.
  - ▪ Infant following birth
    - □ MRI, ultrasonography, and CT to evaluate the spinal cord and brain

Patient-Centered Care

- • Nursing Care
  - ○ Monitor for infant-parent attachment.
  - ○ Check the sac.
  - ○ Perform a routine newborn examination.
  - ○ Determine the level of neurologic involvement.
  - ○ Obtain accurate output measurements.
  - ○ Obtain head circumference and check fontanels.
- • Teamwork and Collaboration
  - ○ Neurosurgery, neurology, urology, orthopedics, physical therapy, occupational therapy, and social services
- • Surgical Interventions
  - ○ Closure of a myelomeningocele sac is done as soon as possible to prevent complications of injury and infection.
  - ○ Nursing Actions
    - ▪ Preoperative
      - □ Prepare the family for surgery (within the first 24 to 48 hr after birth).
      - □ Protect the sac from injury.
      - □ Place infant in a warmer, without clothing.
      - □ Apply a sterile, moist, nonadhering dressing with 0.9% sodium chloride on the sac, changing it every 2 hr.
      - □ Inspect the sac closely for leaks and irritation.
      - □ Monitor for signs of infection (fever, irritability, and lethargy).
      - □ Place infant in the prone position with hips flexed and legs abducted.
      - □ Monitor the IV site and administration of IV antibiotic as prescribed.
      - □ Avoid rectal temperatures.
      - □ Avoid cuddling or putting pressure on the sac.

- Postoperative
  - Monitor vital signs.
  - Monitor I&O.
  - Monitor for signs of infection.
  - Provide pain management as prescribed.
  - Provide incision care as prescribed.
  - Determine presence of CSF leakage.
  - Maintain prone position until other positions are prescribed.
  - Resume oral feedings.
  - Provide range of motion (ROM) to extremities.
- Care After Discharge
  - Provide teaching on postoperative care at home.
  - Depending on disability teach ROM techniques.
  - Ongoing care
    - Obtain head circumference.
    - Determine skin integrity.
    - Determine allergies, such as latex allergy.
    - Determine cognitive development.
    - Determine bladder and bowl functioning.
    - Determine motor development.
    - Monitor for infections.
    - Address body image concerns.
    - Offer support to the family.
    - Assist the client with independence through lifespan.
    - Assist the family with obtaining medical equipment/services needed at home.

Complications

- Skin ulceration
  - Caused by prolonged pressure in one area
  - Nursing Actions
    - Monitor skin for breakdown.
    - Reposition frequently to prevent pressure on bony prominences.
    - Monitor skin under splints and braces.
  - Client Education
    - Reinforce teaching to child and family related to monitoring skin integrity.

- Latex allergy
  - The child has a high risk of allergy to latex. Allergy responses range from urticaria to wheezing, which may progress to anaphylaxis. There also can be an allergy to certain foods (bananas, avocados, kiwi, and chestnuts).
  - Nursing Actions
    - Assist with testing for allergy.
    - Reduce exposure.
  - Client Education
    - Reinforce teaching with the parents to avoid exposing the child to latex.
    - Provide the family with a list of household items that may contain latex (disposable diapers, cleaning or kitchen gloves, elastic found in clothing).
    - Reinforce teaching with the family about how to identify signs and symptoms of allergic reaction and report them to the provider.
    - Reinforce instruction about the use of epinephrine (EpiPen).
- Increased intracranial pressure
  - Caused by shunt malfunction or hydrocephalus.
  - Prepare for surgery for shunt or shunt revision.
  - Clinical manifestations
    - Infants – high-pitched cry, lethargy, vomiting, bulging fontanels, and/or widening cranial suture lines, increased head circumference
    - Children – headache, lethargy, nausea, vomiting, double vision, decreased school performance of learned tasks, decreased level of consciousness, seizures
    - Nursing Actions
      - Use gentle movements when performing ROM exercises.
      - Minimize environmental stressors (noise, frequent visitors).
      - Monitor and manage pain.
    - Client Education
      - Reinforce teaching regarding the clinical manifestation of shunt malfunction and hydrocephalus and when to notify the provider.
- Bladder surgery
  - Can be performed to manage bladder dysfunction (either spasms or flaccidity)
  - Nursing Actions
    - Monitor for signs of bladder dysfunction.
    - Monitor for signs of bladder infection.
    - Monitor for bleeding.
    - Prepare the family and client for surgery if needed.
    - Explain to the child and family care of stoma (vesicostomy) if applicable.

- Orthopedic issues
  - Corrections of associated potential problems, such as clubfoot, scoliosis, and other malformations of the feet and legs
  - Nursing Actions
    - Monitor for signs of infection.
    - Administer pain medications.
    - Prepare the family and client for surgery if needed.
    - Provide cast care if cast is present.
    - Monitor for neurosensory deficits.
  - Client Education
    - Reinforce teaching with the family about signs and symptoms of infection.
    - Reinforce teaching with the family about cast and splint care if indicated.

DOWN SYNDROME

Overview

- Down syndrome is a chromosomal abnormality.
- Many medical conditions (congenital heart malformation, hypotonicity, dysfunction of the immune system, thyroid dysfunction, leukemia) accompany Down syndrome.

Data Collection

- Risk Factors
  - Maternal age greater than 35
- Objective Data
  - Physical Assessment Findings
    - Separated sagittal suture
    - Enlarged anterior fontanel
    - Small round head
    - Flattened forehead
    - Upward, outward slant to eyes
    - Small nose with depressed nasal bridge
    - Small ears with short pinna
    - High-arched narrow palate
    - Protruding tongue
    - Short, broad neck

- Shortened rib cage

- Possible congenital heart defect

- Protruding abdomen

- Broad, short feet and hands with stubby toes and fingers

- Transverse palmar crease

- Large space between big and second toes with plantar crease

- Short stature

- Hyperflexibility and hypotonia

- Diagnostic Procedures

- Prenatal – maternal serum alpha-fetoprotein (MSAFP) test

- Infant – chromosome analysis and echocardiography

Patient-Centered Care

- Nursing Care

  - Support family at the time of diagnosis.

  - Make appropriate referrals.

  - Assist the parents in holding and bonding with the infant.

  - Manage secretions and prevention of upper respiratory infections.

- Surgical Interventions – depend on the associated congenital anomalies, which can include cardiac defects or strabismus.

- Teamwork and Collaboration

  - Social work, home health, school early intervention, genetic counseling, speech therapy, physical therapy, occupational therapy

  - Nursing Actions

    - Listen to the concerns of the parents, and discuss ethical dilemmas regarding treatment for physical defects.

    - Provide standard postoperative care with emphasis on wound care, respiratory care, and pain management.

  - Client Education

    - Reinforce education about postoperative and home-care management.

    - Reinforce the therapeutic plan of care.

- Ongoing Care

  - Reinforce teaching with the family about how to aspirate nasal secretions.

  - Reinforce teaching with the family to rinse the mouth after feedings.

  - Reinforce instruction with the family to use cool mist in the room to assist in moistening secretions.

  - Encourage the family to change the infant's position frequently.

  - Explain to the family pulmonary hygiene by performing postural drainage with percussion.

○ Explain to the family feeding strategies to accommodate for the protruding tongue.

○ Explain to the family skin care and the need for moisturizing creams daily.

○ Encourage a diet high in fiber and fluid to prevent constipation, and to monitor calorie intake to prevent obesity.

○ Encourage regular health care visits.

○ Monitor developmental milestones.

○ Monitor height and weight by plotting growth on a Down syndrome growth chart.

○ Prepare for surgery for cardiac problems or strabismus if indicated.

○ Monitor eyesight and hearing frequently.

○ Perform frequent thyroid functioning tests.

○ Monitor for atlantoaxial instability (neck pain, weakness, and torticollis).

○ Reinforce education to the family regarding prevention of complications.

Complications

- Respiratory infections

  ○ Respiratory infections are common due to decreased muscle tone and poor drainage of mucus due to hypotonicity and associated underdeveloped nasal bone.

  ○ Nursing Actions

    ▪ Rinse the child's mouth with water after feeding and at other times of the day when it is dry. Mucous membranes are dry due to constant mouth breathing, which also increases the risk for respiratory infection.

    ▪ Provide cool mist humidification and clearing of the nasal passages with a bulb syringe as needed.

    ▪ Encourage exercise in older children.

  ○ Client Education

    ▪ Reinforce teaching to the parents and child about good hand hygiene. Encourage frequent repositioning of the child to promote respiratory function.

    ▪ Reinforce instruction to the parents to perform postural drainage and percussion if needed.

    ▪ Reinforce the need for routine immunizations.

    ▪ Reinforce instruction to the parents to seek health care at the earliest sign of infection.

    ▪ Reinforce the need to follow the antibiotic schedule if prescribed.

JUVENILE IDIOPATHIC ARTHRITIS

Overview

- Juvenile idiopathic arthritis (JIA) is a chronic autoimmune inflammatory disease affecting joints and other tissues.

- The chronic inflammation of the synovium of the joints leads to wearing down and damage to the articular cartilage.

- JIA is rarely life-threatening, and it may subside over time, but it can result in residual joint deformities and altered joint function.

- There are multiple classifications of JIA with or without a rheumatoid factor.

Data Collection

- Risk Factors
  - Immunogenic susceptibility
  - Environmental triggers
- Subjective and Objective Data
  - Physical Assessment Findings
    - Joint swelling, stiffness, redness, and warmth that tend to be worse in the morning or after naps
    - Mobility limitations
    - Fever
    - Rash
    - Limp in the morning
    - Enlarged lymph nodes
    - Delayed growth

  - Laboratory Tests
    - Anticyclic citrullinated peptide (anti-CCP) antibodies can be detected before symptoms of disease occur.
    - Erythrocyte sedimentation rate (ESR) may or may not be elevated.
    - CBC with differential can demonstrate elevated WBCs, especially during exacerbations.
    - Antinuclear antibodies (ANA) indicate an increased risk for uveitis.
    - Rheumatoid factor is rarely detected in children.
  - Diagnostic Procedures
    - Radiographic studies can be used for baseline comparison. X-rays can demonstrate increased synovial fluid in the joint, which causes soft tissue swelling or widening of the joint. Later findings can include osteoporosis and narrowed joint spaces.
    - Slit-lamp eye examination is used to diagnosis uveitis.

Patient-Centered Care

- Nursing Care

  - Care is primarily in an outpatient setting.

  - Assist the client with an exercise program.

  - Reinforce teaching to the client about relaxation techniques and nonpharmacological pain management.

  - Monitor the child's pain and response to prescribed analgesics.

  - Encourage a support group.

  - Encourage the child to participate in a physical therapy program to increase mobility and prevent deformities.

  - Encourage activity as tolerated.

  - Reinforce teaching to parents to apply splints for nighttime sleep. Splints should be applied to knees, wrists, and hands to decrease pain and prevent flexion deformities.

  - Encourage proper positioning with sleep. Encourage the use of electric blankets or sleeping bags for extra warmth.

  - Provide firm mattress and discourage use of pillows under knees. Use no pillow or a flat pillow for the head.

  - Encourage full ROM exercises.

  - Apply heat or warm moist packs to the child's affected joints prior to exercise.

  - Encourage warm baths.

  - Identify alternate ways for the child to meet developmental needs, especially during periods of exacerbation.

  - Encourage self-care by allowing adequate time for completion.

  - Encourage a well-balanced diet with adequate fluid intake.

  - Encourage participation in school and contact with peers.

  - Assist in collaborative efforts with the school nurse and teachers to arrange for care during the school day (medication administration, rest periods, extra time to get to classes, extra sets of books, split days).

  - Remind the family that exacerbation worsens with illnesses.

  - Reinforce instruction to the family about routine follow up with provider and regular eye exams.

- Medications

  - Nonsteroidal anti-inflammatory medications (NSAIDs)

    - Ibuprofen (Motrin), naproxen (Naprelan), and tolmetin (Tolectin)

    - Control pain and inflammation

    - Nursing Considerations

      - Instruct the child and family to administer NSAIDs as prescribed.

      - Instruct the child and family that NSAIDs should be taken with food to minimize gastric irritation.

- Client Education
  - Explain to the child and family to report changes in stool, GI discomfort, or increase in bruising immediately.

Q
EBP

- Methotrexate
  - A cytotoxic disease-modifying antirheumatic drug (DMARD) that slows joint degeneration and progression of rheumatoid arthritis when NSAIDs do not work alone
  - Nursing Considerations
    - ▸ Monitor liver function tests and CBC regularly.
  - Client Education
    - ▸ Reinforce teaching to adolescents to avoid alcohol.
    - ▸ Discuss the use of effective birth control to avoid birth defects while taking this medication.
- Corticosteroids: prednisone
  - Provide symptomatic relief of inflammation and pain. They are reserved for life-threatening complications, severe arthritis, and uveitis.
  - Nursing Considerations
    - ▸ Administer as eye solution or orally.
    - ▸ Administer at the lowest effective dose for short-term therapy, and then discontinue by tapering the dose.
  - Client Education
    - ▸ Advise the child and family that weight gain, especially in the face, is a common adverse effect.
    - ▸ Monitor height and weight.
    - ▸ Advise the family that an alteration in growth is a possible long-term complication of corticosteroids.
    - ▸ Advise the child to avoid exposure to potentially infectious agents.
    - ▸ Advise the child and family to practice healthy eating habits.
  - ○ Etanercept (Enbrel)
    - Etanercept is a tumor necrosis factor alpha-receptor blocker, another DMARD, that is used when methotrexate is not effective for immunosuppressive action.
    - Nursing Considerations
      - Administer etanercept once or twice each week by subcutaneous injection.
    - Client Education
      - Reinforce teaching about the potential for allergic reactions.
      - Explain to the child and family to avoid exposure to infectious agents.
- Teamwork and Collaboration
  - ○ Physical therapist, occupational therapist, ophthalmologist, dentist, dietitian, social worker, school nurse

Complications

- Joint deformity and functional disability
  - Nursing Actions
    - Reinforce the individualized therapeutic plan of care.
    - Advocate for the child when treatments are not producing expected results.
  - Client Education
    - Encourage the child and family to adhere to the treatment regimen.
    - Encourage self-care and active participation in an exercise program.

MUSCULAR DYSTROPHY

Overview

- Muscular dystrophy (MD) is a group of inherited disorders with progressive degeneration of symmetric skeletal muscle groups.
- Onset of disease, pace of progression, and muscle group affected depend on the type of MD.
  - Duchenne (pseudohypertrophic) muscular dystrophy (DMD) is the most common form of MD. Inherited as an X-linked recessive trait, DMD has an onset between 3 and 7 years of age. A progressive disease, life expectancy with current technology for DMD reaches into early adulthood.
  - Facioscapulohumeral muscular dystrophy is an autosomal dominant inherited disorder. Progression is slow with normal life span.
  - Limb-girdle muscular dystrophy (LGMD) is an autosomal dominant and recessive, heterogeneous disorder. It appears later in childhood with a slow progression.

DUCHENNE MUSCULAR DYSTROPHY

Data Collection

- Risk Factors
  - Family genetic history
- Subjective and Objective Data
  - Physical Assessment Findings
    - Fatigue
    - Muscle weakness beginning in the lower extremities
    - Unsteady gait, with a waddle
    - Lordosis
    - Delayed motor skill development
    - Frequent falling

- Difficulty getting out of bed, rising from a seated position, or climbing stairs
- Learning difficulties
- Mild cognitive delays that do not worsen with disease
- Progressive difficulty walking with possible loss of ability to walk by the age of 12 years
- Progressive muscle atrophy
- Respiratory and cardiac difficulties usually start by age 20
  - ○ Laboratory Tests
    - Serum polymerase chain reaction (PCR) to detect the dystrophin gene mutation
    - Serum creatine kinase (CK) – elevated and can be elevated prior to clinical manifestations
  - ○ Diagnostic Procedures
    - Muscle biopsy
    - EMG

Patient-Centered Care

- Nursing Care
  - ○ Encourage and provide for genetic counseling.
  - ○ Monitor the following.
    - The child's ability to perform ADLs
    - The child's respiratory function, including depth, rhythm, and rate of respirations during sleep and daytime hours
    - The child's cardiac function
    - The child and parent's understanding of long-term effects
    - The child and parent's coping and support
  - ○ Maintain optimal physical function for as long possible.
    - Encourage the child to be independent for as long as possible and to perform ADLs.
    - Perform ROM exercises and provide appropriate physical activity. Include stretching exercises, strength and muscle training, and breathing exercises.
    - Maintain proper body alignment and encourage the child to reposition self frequently to avoid skin breakdown.
    - Assist with splints and braces as prescribed.
  - ○ Maintain respiratory functioning.
    - Encourage the use of incentive spirometry.
    - Position the child to enhance expansion of lungs.
    - Reinforce teaching to the client on how to use a mechanical cough device.
    - Provide oxygen as prescribed.
    - Provide noninvasive ventilation as prescribed.

- ○ Encourage adequate fluid intake.
- ○ Monitor and encourage adequate nutritional intake.
- ○ Encourage routine physical exams and immunizations.
- ○ Facilitate discussion of end-of-life decisions when appropriate.
- • Medications
  - ○ Corticosteroids – prednisone
    - ■ Increases muscle strength
    - ■ Nursing Considerations
      - □ Monitor for infection.
      - □ Monitor for adverse effects.
    - ■ Client Education
      - □ Reinforce instruction to the child and parents to avoid potentially infectious agents.
      - □ Encourage the child and family to practice healthy eating habits.
      - □ Reinforce teaching to the family about adverse effects and when to notify the provider.
  - ○ Other medications can include bronchodilators, amino acids, vitamins, and mineral supplements.
- • Teamwork and Collaboration
  - ○ Neurologist; genetic counselor; physical, occupational, and respiratory therapists; dietitian; social worker; school teacher.
  - ○ Encourage parents to consider assistance with care as disease progresses (respite care, long-term care, and home-health care).
  - ○ Provide information to the child and parents about support groups for MD.
- • Surgical Interventions
  - ○ Surgery may be indicated for release or repair of contractures or for insertion of a gastrostomy tube or tracheostomy.

Complications

- • Respiratory compromise
  - ○ The child's respiratory muscles are unable to maintain adequate respirations.
  - ○ Nursing Actions
    - ■ Help the child turn hourly or more frequently.
    - ■ Have the child use deep breathing and coughing.
    - ■ Suction as needed.
    - ■ Administer oxygen as prescribed.
    - ■ Use intermittent positive pressure ventilation and mechanically-assisted cough devices if indicated.
    - ■ Administer antibiotics as prescribed.
  - ○ Client Education
    - ■ Discuss mechanical ventilation options with the child and parents.

APPLICATION EXERCISES

1. A nurse is caring for a child who has cerebral palsy. Which of the following medications should the nurse expect to administer to treat painful muscle spasms? (Select all that apply.)

_____ A. Baclofen (Lioresal)

_____ B. Diazepam (Valium)

_____ C. Oxybutynin chloride (Ditropan)

_____ D. Methotrexate

_____ E. Prednisone

2. A nurse is caring for a school-age child who has juvenile idiopathic arthritis. Which of the following are appropriate home care recommendations? (Select all that apply.)

_____ A. Sleep on a firm mattress.

_____ B. Use cold compresses for joint pain.

_____ C. Take ibuprofen (Motrin) on an empty stomach.

_____ D. Take frequent rest periods throughout the day.

_____ E. Perform range-of-motion exercises.

3. A nurse is reinforcing teaching with a group of parents about possible manifestations of Down syndrome. Which of the following should she include in the explanation? (Select all that apply.)

_____ A. Large head with bulging fontanelles

_____ B. Larger ears that are set back

_____ C. Protruding abdomen

_____ D. Broad, short feet and hands

_____ E. Hypotonia

4. A nurse is caring for a child who has muscular dystrophy. The nurse should monitor for which of the following findings? (Select all that apply.)

_____ A. Purposeless, involuntary, abnormal movements

_____ B. Spinal defect and saclike protrusion

_____ C. Muscular weakness in lower extremities

_____ D. Unsteady, wide-based, or waddling gait

_____ E. Upward slant to the eyes

5. A nurse is caring for an infant who has a myelomeningocele. Which of the following should the nurse contribute to the plan of care?

A. Assist the mother with breastfeeding.

B. Check the infant's temperature rectally.

C. Place the infant in a supine position.

D. Apply a moist dressing on the sac.

6. A nurse is caring for a child who has a new prescription for baclofen (Lioresal). Use the ATI Active Learning Template: Medication to complete this item to include the following sections:

A. Therapeutic Uses

B. Nursing Administration

C. Adverse Effects

D. Client Education

APPLICATION EXERCISES KEY

1. A. **CORRECT:** Baclofen is a centrally acting skeletal muscle relaxant that decreases muscle spasm and severe spasticity.

    B. **CORRECT:** Diazepam is a skeletal muscle relaxant that decreases muscle spasms and severe spasticity.

    C. INCORRECT: Oxybutynin chloride is an antispasmodic, anticholinergic medication that decreases bladder spasms.

    D. INCORRECT: Methotrexate is a cytotoxic disease-modifying antirheumatic drug (DMARD) that slows joint degeneration and progression of rheumatoid arthritis. It is used for children with juvenile idiopathic arthritis (JIA).

    E. INCORRECT: Prednisone is a corticosteroid that increases muscle strength for children who have muscular dystrophy. It decreases inflammation in children with JIA.

    Ⓝ NCLEX® Connection: Pharmacological Therapies, Expected Actions/Outcomes

2. A. **CORRECT:** A firm mattress can help prevent joint deformities and maintain body alignment.

    B. INCORRECT: Using a warm compresses or moist packs can provide comfort and relieve stiffness.

    C. INCORRECT: Ibuprofen should be taken with food to prevent GI distress.

    D. **CORRECT:** Frequent rest periods are necessary to conserve energy.

    E. **CORRECT:** Range of motion will assist in maintaining function of the joints.

    Ⓝ NCLEX® Connection: Physiological Adaptations, Basic Pathophysiology

3. A. INCORRECT: A child with hydrocephalus will exhibit a large head with bulging fontanelles because of the increased CSF in the head.

    B. INCORRECT: A child with Down syndrome will exhibit small features, such as small ears with a short pinna.

    C. **CORRECT:** A child with Down syndrome will exhibit small features, such as short stature. The child will exhibit a protruding abdomen.

    D. **CORRECT:** A child with Down syndrome will exhibit small features, such as broad, short feet and hands.

    E. **CORRECT:** A child with Down syndrome will exhibit hyperflexibility and hypotonia.

    Ⓝ NCLEX® Connection: Physiological Adaptations, Alterations in Body Systems

4. A. INCORRECT: A child who has cerebral palsy will exhibit purposeless, involuntary, abnormal movements.

    B. INCORRECT: An infant who has the spinal defect myelomeningocele will exhibit a saclike protrusion.

    C. **CORRECT:** A child who has MD will exhibit muscular weakness in the lower extremities as one of the first clinical signs.

    D. **CORRECT:** A child who has MD will exhibit an unsteady, wide-based, or waddling gait because of the progressive muscle weakness.

    E. INCORRECT: A child with Down syndrome may exhibit an upward slant to the eyes.

    (N) NCLEX® Connection: Physiological Adaptations, Basic Pathophysiology

5. A. INCORRECT: Breastfeeding could cause pressure on the sac, which could cause rupture.

    B. INCORRECT: Rectal temperatures could cause irritation or rectal prolapse.

    C. INCORRECT: Placing the infant in supine position could cause pressure on the sac, which could cause rupture.

    D. **CORRECT:** A sterile, moist, nonadhering dressing is placed on the sac to keep it moist until surgery.

    (N) NCLEX® Connection: Physiological Adaptations, Basic Pathophysiology

6. *Using the ATI Active Learning Template: Medication*

    A. Therapeutic Uses
    - Used as a centrally acting skeletal muscle relaxant that decreases muscle spasm and severe spasticity.

    B. Nursing Administration
    - Provider administers orally or intrathecally via a specialized, surgically implanted pump.
    - Monitor effectiveness of the medication.

    C. Adverse Effects
    - Muscle weakness
    - Increased fatigue
    - Less-common adverse effects (diaphoresis, constipation)

    D. Client Education
    - Explain to the family about expected responses of medications.
    - Reinforce with the family the adverse effects of medications and when to call the provider.

    (N) NCLEX® Connection: Pharmacological Therapies, Expected Actions/Outcomes

UNIT 2   Nursing Care of Children with System Disorders

SECTION: INTEGUMENTARY DISORDERS

› Skin Infections and Infestations
› Dermatitis and Acne
› Burns

NCLEX® CONNECTIONS

When reviewing the chapters in this section, keep in mind the relevant sections of the NCLEX® outline, in particular:

Client Needs: Reduction of Risk Potential	Client Needs: Physiological Adaptation

› Relevant topics/tasks include:
» Laboratory Values
  › Monitor diagnostic or laboratory test results.
	› Relevant topics/tasks include:
	» Alterations in Body Systems
	  › Identify signs and symptoms of an infection.
	  › Provide care to correct client alteration in body system.
	  › Reinforce education to client regarding care and condition.
	» Basic Pathophysiology
	  › Apply knowledge of pathophysiology when caring for the client with fluid and electrolyte imbalances.
	  › Identify signs and symptoms related to an acute or chronic illness.
	  › Consider general principles of client disease process when providing care.
	  › Apply knowledge of pathophysiology to monitoring client for alterations in body systems.

chapter 28

Overview

- Skin infections can be bacterial, viral, or fungal.

- Arthropod bites and stings can be due to flies, mosquitoes, chiggers, bees, fire ants, mites, ticks, spiders, and scorpions.

- Skin infestations include scabies and lice.

SKIN INFECTION

Overview

- Bacterial infections include impetigo contagiosa, pyoderma, folliculitis, furuncle, carbuncle, cellulitis, and staphylococcal scalded skin syndrome.

- Viral infections include verruca, verruca plantaris, herpes simplex virus, varicella-zoster virus, and molluscum contagiosum.

- Fungal infections include tinea capitis, tinea corporis, tinea cruris, tinea pedis, and candidiasis.

Data Collection

- Risk Factors
  - Bacterial
    - Congenital or acquired immunodeficiency disorders
    - Immunosuppression
    - Generalized malignancy
  - Viral
    - Contact with infected person
  - Fungal
    - Geographic area
- Subjective Data
  - History of causative agent/exposure

- Objective Data
  - History of causative agent/exposure

BACTERIAL INFECTION/CAUSATIVE AGENTS CLINICAL MANIFESTATIONS	
Impetigo contagiosa – *Staphylococcus*	
› Reddish macule becomes vesicular	› Spreads peripherally and by direct contact
› Erupts easily, leaving moist erosion on the skin; dries leaving crusty secretions	› Pruritus common
Pyoderma – *Staphylococcus, Streptococcus*	
› Deeper infection into the dermis	› Possible systemic effects (fever, lymphangitis)
Folliculitis (pimple) – *Staphylococcus aureus*	
› Infection of a hair follicle	
Furuncle (boil) – *Staphylococcus aureus*	
› Larger swollen, red lesion of a single hair follicle	
Carbuncle (multiple boils) – *Staphylococcus aureus*	
› More extensive swollen, red lesions involving multiple hair follicles	
Cellulitis – Streptococcus, *Staphylococcus, Haemophilus influenzae*	
› Firm, swollen, red area of the skin and subcutaneous tissue	› Possible systemic effects (fever, malaise)
Staphylococcal scalded skin syndrome – *Staphylococcus aureus*	
› Rough-textured skin with macular erythema	› Epidermis becomes wrinkled within 2 days, with large bullae appearing

VIRAL INFECTION/CAUSATIVE AGENTS CLINICAL MANIFESTATIONS	
Verruca (warts) – Human papillomavirus	
› Elevated, rough, gray-brown firm papules	› Can be single or in groups
› Can occur anywhere on the skin	
Verruca plantaris (plantar warts)	
› Flat warts on the plantar surface of the feet	› Possibly surrounded by hyperkeratosis
Herpes simplex virus – Type I: cold sore, fever blister; Type II: genital	
› Near a mucocutaneous area (lips, nose, buttock, genitalia)	› After drying, form a crusty area followed by exfoliation
› Group of vesicles that itch and burn	› Healing occurs in 8 to 10 days
	› Possible lymphadenopathy
Varicella-zoster virus (herpes zoster, shingles)	
› Neurologic pain, hyperesthesias, or itching	› Same virus as chicken pox
Molluscum contagiosum (pox virus)	
› Asymptomatic flesh-colored papules on stalks	

FUNGAL INFECTION/CAUSATIVE AGENTS CLINICAL MANIFESTATIONS	
Tinea capitis – *Trichophyton tonsurans, Microsporum audouinii, Microsporum canis*	
› Scaly, circumscribed lesion with alopecia on the scalp	
Tinea corporis – *Trichophyton rubrum, Trichophyton mentagrophytes, Microsporum canis*	
› Round erythematous scaling patch	› Spreads peripherally and clears centrally
Tinea cruris (jock itch) – *Epidermophyton floccosum, Trichophyton rubrum, Trichophyton mentagrophytes*	
› Medial and proximal aspect of the thigh and crural folds › May include the scrotum	› Pruritic › Round erythematous scaling patch › Spreads peripherally and clears centrally
Tinea pedis (athlete's foot) – *Trichophyton rubrum, Trichophyton interdigitale, Epidermophyton floccosum*	
› Between toes or on the plantar surface of the feet	› Maceration and fissuring lesions between the toes and patches with tiny vesicles on the plantar surface of the foot
Candidiasis (moniliasis) – *Candida albicans*	
› Found in moist areas of the skin surface › White exudate, peeling inflamed areas that bleed easily	› Pruritic

- ○ Laboratory Tests
  - ▪ Cultures (bacterial, viral, fungal)

Patient-Centered Care

- Nursing Care
  - ○ Collect data related to the general condition of the affected area.
  - ○ Collect data for evidence of associated infection.
  - ○ Assist in preventing the child to itch or touch the affected areas.

BACTERIAL INFECTION/CAUSATIVE AGENTS MANAGEMENT	
Impetigo contagiosa – *Staphylococcus*	
› Use compresses of 1:20 aluminum acetate in water (Burow's solution) to remove crusted exudate.	› Use topical antibacterial ointment. › Oral or parenteral antibiotics for severe cases.
Pyoderma – *Staphylococcus, Streptococcus*	
› Cleanse with soap and water. › Apply wet compresses. › Bathe using antibacterial soap.	› Launder washcloths and towels to prevent bacterial spread. › Apply mupirocin (Bactroban) to lesions as prescribed. › Systemic antibiotics, as prescribed in severe cases.
Folliculitis (pimple) – *Staphylococcus aureus* **Furuncle (boil) –** *Staphylococcus aureus* **Carbuncle (multiple boils) –** *Staphylococcus aureus*	
› Apply warm moist compresses. › Clean skin often. › Topical antibiotic medications.	› Systemic antibiotics for severe cases. › Incision, draining, and irrigation of severe lesions.
Cellulitis – *Streptococcus, Staphylococcus, Haemophilus influenzae*	
› Oral or parenteral antibiotics, as prescribed. › Rest and immobilize affected area.	› Apply warm, moist compresses.
Staphylococcal scalded skin syndrome – *Staphylococcus aureus*	
› Use systemic antibiotics.	› Clean gently with saline, Burow's solution, or 0.25% silver nitrate compresses.

VIRAL INFECTION/CAUSATIVE AGENTS MANAGEMENT	
Verruca (warts) – Human papillomavirus	
› Individualized destructive therapy such as surgical removal, electrocautery, cryotherapy, laser.	
Verruca plantaris (plantar warts)	
› Apply caustic solution to wart. › Wear insoles with holes to decrease pressure for 2 to 3 days.	› Soak affected area for 20 min. › Repeat treatment until wart falls off.
Herpes simplex virus – Type I: cold sore, fever blister; Type II: genital	
› Apply Burow's solution during weeping stage. › Apply penciclovir (Denavir) cream to oral lesion.	› Oral antiviral (acyclovir) to reduce duration. › Oral antiviral (valacyclovir) for genital herpes.
Varicella-zoster virus (herpes zoster, shingles)	
› Use oral or topical analgesics. › Apply moist compresses.	› Oral antiviral (acyclovir).
Molluscum contagiosum (pox virus)	
› Resolves spontaneously in 18 months.	› Complicated cases: remove pox.

FUNGAL INFECTION/CAUSATIVE AGENTS MANAGEMENT	
Tinea capitis – *Trichophyton tonsurans, Microsporum audouinii, Microsporum canis*	
› Use selenium sulfide shampoos. › Topical antifungal medications (clotrimazole). › Oral griseofulvin.	› Complicated cases: oral ketoconazole. › Treat infected pets, if necessary.
Candidiasis (moniliasis) – *Candida albicans*	
› Topical antifungal ointment (Amphotericin B, nystatin).	
Tinea corporis – *Trichophyton rubrum, Trichophyton mentagrophytes, Microsporum canis* **Tinea cruris (jock itch)** – *Epidermophyton floccosum, Trichophyton rubrum, Trichophyton mentagrophytes* **Tinea pedis (athlete's foot)** – *Trichophyton rubrum, Trichophyton interdigitale, Epidermophyton floccosum*	
› Oral griseofulvin. › Topical antifungal (tolnaftate, clotrimazole). › Apply wet compresses or take sitz bath.	› Wear light-colored socks, well-ventilated shoes. › Treat infected pets (Tinea corporis).

- Client Teaching
  - Reinforce teaching to client and family how to avoid the spread of infections.
    - Use appropriate hand hygiene.
    - Avoid sharing clothing, hats, combs, brushes, and/or towels.
    - Keep the child from touching the affected area by using distraction.
    - Do not squeeze vesicles.
    - Apply topical medications as prescribed.
    - Administer oral medications as prescribed.

ARTHROPOD BITES AND STINGS

Overview

- Scorpions, black widow, and brown recluse spiders inject venom that requires immediate attention.

Data Collection

- Risk Factors
  - Geographic area
- Assessment Data
  - Subjective Data
    - History of causative agent/exposure

○ Objective Data

CAUSATIVE AGENT	CLINICAL MANIFESTATIONS
Mosquitoes, fleas, flies	› Variable, from no reaction to hypersensitivity reaction › Papular urticaria › Firm papules
Bees, wasps, hornets, fire ants, yellow jackets	› Local reaction: small red itchy wheal that is warm to the touch › Systemic reaction: mild to severe – generalized edema, pain, nausea and vomiting, confusion, respiratory problems, and shock
Chiggers	› Bites on warm parts of the body › Variable, from no reaction to hypersensitivity reaction › Papular urticaria › Firm papules
Ticks	› Attaches to the skin with head embedded › Firm, discrete, pruritic nodule at site › Possible urticaria or persistent localized edema
Brown recluse spiders	› Mild sting leads to transient erythema and to blister › Pain 2 to 8 hr following bite › Star-shaped purple area in 3 to 4 days › Necrotic ulceration in 7 to 14 days
Black widow spiders	› Mild sting leads to swollen, painful, and erythematous site › Dizziness, weakness, and abdominal pain › Possible delirium, paralysis, seizures, and death
Scorpions	› Intense pain › Erythema, burning, numbness › Restlessness and vomiting › Ascending paralysis: seizures, weakness, increase in pulse, thirst, salivation, dysuria, pulmonary edema leading to coma and death › Death for children less than age 4 in the first 24 hr

Lyme disease (tick infected with *Borrelia burgdorferi*)	› May appear in any of these stages
	» Stage 1
	  › 3 to 31 days following bite – erythema migrans at site
	  › Chills, fever, itching, headache, fainting, stiff neck, muscle weakness; bulleye rash at the site of the bite
	» Stage 2: systematic involvement begins (neurologic, cardiac, and musculoskeletal); occurs several weeks following bite
	  › Paralysis or weakness in the face, muscle pain, swelling in large joints (knees), heart problems
	» Stage 3: systemic involvement is advanced (musculoskeletal pain that includes the muscles, tendons, bursae and synovia); possible arthritis, deafness and encephalopathy.
	  › Abnormal muscle movement and weakness, numbness and tingling, speech problems

- Patient-Centered Care
  - Nursing Care

CAUSATIVE AGENT	MANAGEMENT
Mosquitoes, fleas, flies	› Use antipruritic agent › Administer oral and topical antihistamines › Baths
Bees, wasps, hornets, fire ants, yellow jackets	› Remove the stinger › Cleanse with soap and water › Apply cool compresses › Apply home products (baking soda, lemon juice) › Administer topical and oral antihistamines › Epinephrine and corticosteroids for severe cases
Chiggers	› Systemic steroids for severe cases
Ticks	› Remove by pulling straight up with steady, even pressure with tweezers to remove the tick › Remove any remaining parts using a sterile needle › Cleanse site with soap and disinfectant
Brown recluse spiders	› Apply cool compresses › Administer antibiotic, corticosteroids › Analgesic for pain › Possible skin graft
Black widow spiders	› Cleanse bite with antiseptic › Apply cool compresses › Administer antivenom › Administer muscle relaxant
Scorpions	› Position site in dependant position › Keep child calm › Administer antivenom › Analgesic for pain › Admit to intensive care unit
Lyme disease (tick infected with *Borrelia burgdorferi*)	› Observe clients bitten by a tick for 30 days › Antibiotic (single dose) for clients who meet criteria › Antibiotic (2- to 3-week course) for clients who have confirmed disease › Doxycycline for children older than 8 years and amoxicillin for children under 8 years; cefuroxime or erythromycin for children who have an allergy to penicillin

Q
PCC

- Client Teaching
  - Prevent secondary infections.
  - Wear medical alert bracelet for severe reactions.
  - Inspect skin after possible exposure.
  - Prevent bites.
    - Avoid areas of tall grass.
    - Use insect repellent.
    - Avoid contact with insects.
    - Avoid wood piles.
    - Inspect and treat pets, carpets, and furniture.
    - Avoid flowery prints and bright clothing.
    - Avoid perfumes and colognes.

SKIN INFESTATIONS

Overview

- Scabies mite, *Sarcoptes scabiei*, is spread by direct contact with an infected person. The mite burrows into the skin and lays eggs. The eggs mature in 21 days.
- Pediculosis capitis (head lice), *Pediculus humanus capitis*, is spread by direct contact with an infected person, bedding, and clothing. The life span of the adult louse is 1 month, and it can live up to 48 hr without a human host. The female lays eggs at night, close to the skin surface and at the junction of the hair shaft. The nits hatch in 7 to 10 days.
- Pediculosis corporis (body lice), *Pediculus humanus corporis*, is spread by direct contact with an infected person, bedding, and clothing. The adult louse feeds on human blood and can live in folds of clothing for 1 month. They die at room temperature in 5 to 7 days.

Data Collection

- Risk Factors
  - Scabies: nursing homes, nursing facilities, and day care settings
  - Head lice: day care and schools; overcrowded conditions; sharing of combs, brushes, or hats
  - Body lice: overcrowded conditions and poor hygiene
  - Pubic lice: multiple sex partners

- Data Collection
  - Subjective Data
    - Itching
  - Objective Data

CAUSATIVE AGENT	CLINICAL MANIFESTATIONS

Scabies mite – *Sarcoptes scabiei*	› Itchy, especially at night
	› Rash, especially between fingers
	› Thin, pencil marks lines on the skin
	› Infants
	  » Widespread on the body
	  » Pimples on the trunk
	  » Blisters on the palms of the hands and soles of the feet
	› Young children: Most common on head, neck, shoulders, palms, and soles
	› Older Children: Most common on hands, wrists, genitals, and abdomen

Pediculosis capitis (head lice) – *Pediculus humanus capitis*	› Intense itching › Small, red bumps on the scalp › Nits (white specks) on the hair shaft
Pediculosis corporis (body lice) – *Pediculus humanus corporis*	› Intense itching, worse around the waist, under the arms and anywhere clothing is tight › Red bumps on the skin › Changes in skin if lice have been present for extended period
Pediculosis pubis (pubic lice) – *Pediculus humanus pubis*	› Intense itching › Bluish-gray skin › Sores

- Diagnostic tests
  - Scabies: examination under a microscope or skin biopsy
- Patient-Centered Care
  - Nursing Care
    - Collect data for infestation.
      - Scabies: Pencil-like mark on skin
      - Head Lice: Adult lice are hard to see. They're small, greyish-tan, and have no wings. Nits look like dandruff on the hair shaft and are firmly attached.
      - Body Lice: Adult lice are larger than other lice. They are the size of a sesame seed, tan to greyish-white, and have six legs. Nits are small grey-white ovals seen on clothing, and around the waist or armpits.
      - Pubic Lice: Adult lice have a crablike appearance. Nits are small grey-white ovals attached to the hair shaft

▪ Collect data for secondary skin infection.

CAUSATIVE AGENT	NURSING INTERVENTIONS
Scabies mite – *Sarcoptes scabiei*	› Apply 5% permethrin cream (Elimite) over the entire body as a one-time treatment; may need to repeat in 1 week › Treat entire family and persons that have been in contact with infected person during and 60 days after infection › Wash underwear, towels, clothing, and sleepwear in hot water › Vacuum carpets and furniture › Apply calamine lotion or cool compresses until itching subsides following treatment › Difficult cases: use oral ivermectin
Pediculosis capitis (head lice) – *Pediculus humanus capitis*	› Shampoos containing 1% permethrin as prescribed › Remove nits with a nit comb, repeat in 7 days after shampoo treatment › Wash clothing, bedding in hot water with detergent › Difficult cases: use malathion 0.5% in isopropanol
Pediculosis corporis (body lice) – *Pediculus humanus corporis*	› Lotions containing 1% permethrin as prescribed › Wash clothing, bedding, and towels in hot water (130° or more) then machine dry in hot cycle › Proper hygiene practices
Pediculosis pubis (pubic lice) – *Pediculus humanus pubis*	› Shampoos containing 1% permethrin as prescribed › Remove nits with a nit comb, repeat in 7 days after shampoo treatment › Wash clothing, bedding in hot water with detergent › Collect data related to other STIs › Difficult cases: repeat shampoo in 4 to 7 days

● Client Teaching
  ○ Reinforce teaching to the child and parents about medications.
  ○ Reinforce teaching to the child and parents to avoid home remedies, as they can worsen infection.
  ○ Reinforce teaching to the parent about correct laundering of potentially infected clothing, bedding.
  ○ Reinforce teaching to the parent to bag items that cannot be laundered into tightly sealed bag for 14 days.
  ○ Reinforce teaching to the parents to boil combs, brushes, and hair accessories in lice-killing products for 1 hr.
  ○ Discourage sharing of personal items.
● Complications
  ○ Secondary infections
    ▪ Examples include *staphylococcus, streptococcus,* and *Haemophilus influenzae.*
    ▪ Nursing Actions
      ▢ Ensure the family understands prescribed plan of care to prevent secondary infections.
      ▢ Monitor for secondary infections.
      ▢ Administer medications as prescribed for secondary infection.
      ▢ Reinforce teaching about clinical manifestations of secondary infections.

APPLICATION EXERCISES

1. A nurse is collecting data on an infant who has scabies. Which of the following are expected findings? (Select all that apply.)

_____ A. Presence of nits on the hair shaft

_____ B. Pencil-like marks on hands

_____ C. Blisters on the soles of the feet

_____ D. Bluish-gray skin color

_____ E. Pimples on the trunk

2. A nurse is reinforcing teaching with a group of parents about preventing insect bites. Which of the following should the nurse include when she reinforces the teaching? (Select all that apply.)

_____ A. Wear perfumes when outside.

_____ B. Avoid areas of tall grass.

_____ C. Wear bright-colored clothing.

_____ D. Wear insect repellent.

_____ E. Check house pets frequently.

3. A nurse is reinforcing teaching with the parent of a child who has pediculosis capitis. Which of the following should the nurse include when she reinforces the teaching?

A. Apply mayonnaise to the affected area at night.

B. Treat all household pets.

C. Use an over-the-counter medication containing 1% permethrin.

D. Discard the child's stuffed animals.

4. A nurse is caring for a child who has cellulitis on the hand. Which of the following is an appropriate action for the nurse to take?

A. Apply hot compresses.

B. Cleanse area using Burow's solution.

C. Prepare for cryotherapy.

D. Administer antifungal medication.

5. A nurse is contributing to the plan of care for a child who has tinea capitis. Which of the following should the nurse contribute to the plan of care? (Select all that apply.)

_____ A. Instruct parents to treat infected house pets.

_____ B. Use selenium sulfide shampoo.

_____ C. Cleanse area with Burow's solution.

_____ D. Administer antiviral medication.

_____ E. Use moist, warm compresses.

6. A nurse is reinforcing teaching with a group of parents about preventing skin infections. Use the ATI Active Learning Template: Systems Disorder to complete this item to include Client Education: Describe five teaching points to reinforce with the group.

APPLICATION EXERCISES KEY

1. A. INCORRECT: Presence of nits on the hair shaft is a clinical manifestation of pediculosis capitis.

    B. **CORRECT:** Pencil-like marks on hands is a clinical manifestation of scabies.

    C. **CORRECT:** Blisters on the soles of the feet is a clinical manifestation of scabies.

    D. INCORRECT: Bluish-gray skin color is a clinical manifestation of pediculosis pubis.

    E. **CORRECT:** Pimples on the trunk is a clinical manifestation of scabies.

    Ⓝ NCLEX® Connection: Physiological Adaptations, Basic Pathophysiology

2. A. INCORRECT: Parents should have their children avoid perfumes because they attract insects.

    B. **CORRECT:** Parents should have their children avoid places where insects live, such as tall grasses.

    C. INCORRECT: Parents should have their children avoid bright clothing because it attracts insects.

    D. **CORRECT:** Parents should apply insect repellent to their children to prevent insect bites.

    E. **CORRECT:** Parents should inspect and treat house pets frequently to prevent exposing family members.

    Ⓝ NCLEX® Connection: Physiological Adaptations, Alterations in Body Systems

3. A. INCORRECT: Home remedies such as mayonnaise increase the risk of infection.

    B. INCORRECT: Pediculosis capitis is transmitted person-to-person and does not host on household pets.

    C. **CORRECT:** The parent can purchase 1% permethrin to treat the child.

    D. INCORRECT: The parent can place unwashable items in a sealed bag for 14 days to kill the lice.

    Ⓝ NCLEX® Connection: Physiological Adaptations, Alterations in Body Systems

4. A. **CORRECT:** Hot compresses increase circulation, promote healing, and are an appropriate action for the nurse to take.

    B. INCORRECT: The nurse should use Burow's solution to clean lesions from impetigo contagiosa or herpes simplex virus.

    C. INCORRECT: Cryotherapy is recommended for human papillomavirus.

    D. INCORRECT: Cellulitis is a bacterial infection and requires antibiotic therapy.

    (N) NCLEX® Connection: Physiological Adaptations, Basic Pathophysiology

5. A. **CORRECT:** Parents should treat infected house pets because tinea capitis is transmitted from pets to persons.

    B. **CORRECT:** Selenium sulfide shampoo is recommended for use for children who have tinea capitis.

    C. INCORRECT: A topical antifungal medication is recommended for children who have tinea capitis.

    D. INCORRECT: Tinea capitis is a fungal infection. Therefore, the nurse should administer antifungal medications.

    E. INCORRECT: The nurse should apply moist, warm compresses to bacterial skin infections.

    (N) NCLEX® Connection: Physiological Adaptations, Basic Pathophysiology

6. *Using the ATI Active Learning Template: Systems Disorder*
    - Client Education
        - Use good hand hygiene.
        - Avoid sharing clothing, hats, combs, brushes, and towels.
        - Use distraction to keep the child from touching the affected area.
        - Do not squeeze vesicles.
        - Apply topical medications.
        - Administer oral medications.

    (N) NCLEX® Connection: Physiological Adaptations, Alterations in Body Systems

chapter 29

Overview

- Common skin conditions of the pediatric population include the following.
  - Contact dermatitis
  - Atopic dermatitis
  - Acne

CONTACT DERMATITIS

Overview

- Contact dermatitis is an inflammatory reaction of the skin. It is caused when the skin comes into contact with chemicals or other irritants (feces, urine, soaps, poison ivy, animals, metals, dyes, medications).
  - Diaper dermatitis can be caused by detergents, soaps, and/or chemicals that come in contact with the genital area. It also can be a result of *Candida albicans*.
  - Seborrheic dermatitis (cradle cap, blepharitis, otitis externa) has an unknown etiology but is most common in infancy and then again at puberty.

Data Collection

- Risk Factors
  - Use of diapers
  - Exposure to an irritant
- Subjective Data
  - Pruritus
- Objective Data
  - Physical Assessment Findings (depends on the cause of the irritation and the client)
    - Contact dermatitis
      - Red bumps that can form moist, weeping blisters
      - Skin warm and tender to the touch
      - Presence of oozing, drainage, or crusts
      - Skin becomes scaly, raw, or thickened

- Diaper dermatitis
  - □ Bright-red rash that extends gradually
  - □ Fiery-red and scaly areas on the scrotum and penis
  - □ Red or scaly areas on the labia
  - □ Blisters, ulcers, large bumps, or pus-filled sores
  - □ Smaller red patches that blend together

Patient-Centered Care

- Nursing Care
  - ○ Diaper dermatitis
    - Promptly remove the wet diaper.
    - Clean urine off the perineal area with a nonirritating cleanser. Cleanse the perineal area of feces with warm water and mild soap.
    - Wash skin folds and the genital area frequently with water.
    - Expose the affected area to air.
    - Use superabsorbent disposable diapers to reduce skin exposure.
    - Apply a skin barrier, such as zinc oxide. Do not wash it off with each diaper change.
    - Use cornstarch to reduce friction between the diaper and the skin. Shake a small amount into the hand and then apply to the diaper area.
  - ○ Contact dermatitis
    - Remove irritant, and limit further exposure.
    - Poisonous plant exposure

 View Image: Poison Ivy Rash and Poison Ivy Plant

      - □ Rinse area with cold running water immediately after exposure.
      - □ Cleanse exposed area as soon as possible with isopropyl alcohol followed by water, then soap and water shower.
      - □ Clothes, shoes should be cleansed with alcohol and then hot water and detergent.
      - □ Apply calamine lotion, Burow's solution compresses, or Aveeno baths.
      - □ Use topical corticosteroid gel.
      - □ Oral corticosteroids for severe reactions.
  - ○ Seborrheic dermatitis
    - Treat by gently scrubbing the scalp with mild pressure, and shampoo daily with mild soap or antiseborrheic shampoo.
    - Use a fine-tooth comb to remove the loosened crusts from the hair.

- Medications
  - Antihistamines – hydroxyzine (Atarax) or diphenhydramine
    - Administer in cases of allergic/medication reactions.
    - Client Education
      - Reinforce teaching to the family on the importance of the medication and administering on schedule.
      - Reinforce the sedating effect of some antihistamines and the need for parents to monitor the child and provide for safety during use.

  - Antibiotics
    - Use to treat secondary infections.
    - Client Education
      - Reinforce teaching to the family about the importance of continuing the medication as prescribed.
  - Antifungal ointments – clotrimazole (Lotrimin)
    - Used to treat *Candida albicans*.
    - Client Education
      - Reinforce teaching to the family on the importance of the medication and administration schedule.
- Care After Discharge
  - Client Education
    - Encourage frequent diaper changes.
    - Advise parents that their child should avoid bubble baths and harsh soaps.
    - Encourage children to wear long sleeves and pants when there is risk of possible exposure to irritants.
    - Reinforce teaching to the parents about removing an offending agent as soon as exposure takes place.

Complications

- Bacterial Infections
  - Caused by breaks in the skin from scratching
  - Nursing Actions
    - Monitor the area for signs of infection.
    - Keep fingernails trimmed short.
    - Cleanse the area with mild soap and water.
    - Administer antipruritics and antibiotics as prescribed.
  - Client Education
    - Reinforce teaching to the family and child about avoiding offending agents.

ATOPIC DERMATITIS (AD)

Overview

- Atopic dermatitis (AD) is a type of eczema (eczema describes a category of integumentary disorders, not a specific disorder with a determined etiology) that is characterized by pruritus and associated with a history of allergies that are of an inherited tendency (atopy).

- Lesions disappear if the scratching is stopped.

- Classifications of atopic dermatitis are based on the child's age, how the lesions are distributed, and the appearance of the lesions.

- AD cannot be cured but can be well controlled.

Data Collection

- Risk Factors
  - Presence of allergic condition and family history of atopy
  - Previous skin disorder and exacerbation of present skin disorder
  - Exposure to irritating and/or causative agents

- Subjective Data
  - Recent exposure to any irritant (medication, food, soap, contact with animals)
  - Intense pruritus

- Objective Data
  - Physical Assessment Findings

CLASSIFICATION	DISTRIBUTION	LESIONS
› Infants – Onset at 2 to 6 months of age with spontaneous remission by 3 years of age	› Generalized distribution of lesions on cheeks, scalp, trunk, hands and feet, as well as extensor surfaces of extremities	› Erythema › Vesicles, papules › Weeping, oozing, crusting, scaling
› Children – Onset at 2 to 3 years of age with 90% of children having manifestations by 5 years of age; can follow infantile eczema	› Lesions in the flexural areas (antecubital and popliteal fossae, neck), wrists, ankles, and feet with symmetric involvement	› Clusters › Erythematous or flesh-colored papules › Dry › Lichenification › Keratosis pilaris
› Adolescents – Onset at age 12 and can continue into adulthood	› Similar distribution to children	› Same as for children › Dry, thick › Confluent papules

- Unaffected skin can appear dry and rough.
- Hypopigmentation of skin can occur in small, diffuse areas.
- Pallor surrounds the nose, mouth, and ears.

- A bluish discoloration is present underneath the eyes.

- Numerous infections of the nails are present.

- Lymphadenopathy occurs, especially around affected areas.

- Signs of a wound infection are present (swelling, purulent drainage, pain, increased temperature, redness extending beyond the wound margin).

Patient-Centered Care

- Nursing Care

  ○ Keep skin hydrated with tepid baths (with/without mild soap or emulsifying oil), then apply an emollient within 3 min of bathing. Two or three baths can be given daily, with one prior to bedtime.

  ○ Dress the child in cotton clothing. Avoid wool and synthetic fabrics.

  ○ Avoid excessive heat and perspiration, which increases itching.

  ○ Avoid irritants (bubble baths, soaps, perfumes, fabric softeners).

  ○ Provide support to the child and family.

  ○ Wash skin folds and genital area frequently with water.

    - Assist in identifying causative agent.

- Medications

  ○ Antihistamines – hydroxyzine (Atarax) or diphenhydramine

    - Client Education

      □ Reinforce the sedating effect of some antihistamines and the need for parents to monitor the child during use.

      □ Reinforce safety of the child when using sedating antihistamines.

  ○ Antihistamines – loratadine (Claritin) or fexofenadine (Allegra)

    - Oral antihistamine for antipruritic effect

    - Client Education

      □ Inform the parents that it is preferred for use during the daytime.

  ○ Antibiotics

    - Antibiotics should be used to treat secondary infections.

  ○ Topical corticosteroids

    - Topical corticosteroids can be used intermittently to reduce or control flare-ups. They can be low-, moderate-, or high potency-and are prescribed based on the degree of skin involvement (extremity vs. eyelids), age of the child, and consequences from side effects.

  ○ Nonsteroidal agents

    - Used to decrease inflammation during flare-ups

    - Nursing Considerations

      □ Use for children older than 2 years of age.

      □ Use at the start of an exacerbation of AD when skin turns red and starts to itch.

○ Client Education

- Signs of infection.

- Advise the family to do the following.

    □ Change diapers when wet or soiled.

    □ Keep nails short and trimmed.

    □ Place gloves or cotton socks over hands for sleeping.

    □ Dress young children in soft, cotton, one-piece, long-sleeve, long-pant outfits.

    □ Remove items that can promote itching (woolen blankets, scratchy fabrics). Use cotton items whenever possible.

    □ Use mild detergents to wash clothing and linens. The wash cycle can be repeated without soap.

    □ Avoid latex products, second-hand smoke, furry pets, dust, and molds.

    □ Provide tepid baths without the use of soap. Avoid oils and powders.

    □ Follow specific directions regarding topical medications, soaks, and baths. Emphasize the importance of understanding the sequence of treatments to maximize the benefit of therapy and prevent complications.

    □ Avoid overheating the bedroom during winter months. Use a room humidifier.

    □ Maintain treatment to prevent flare-up.

    □ Follow up with the provider as directed.

    □ Participate in support groups.

Complications

- Infection

    ○ Caused by breaks in the skin from scratching

    ○ Nursing Actions

    - Keep nails trimmed.

    - Administer antipruritics as prescribed.

    - Monitor the area for signs of infection.

    - Cleanse the area with mild soap and water.

    ○ Client Education

    - Reinforce teaching to the family and child about avoiding offending agents.

ACNE

Overview

- Acne is the most common skin condition during adolescence.

- Acne is self-limiting and non-life-threatening. However, it poses a threat to self-image for adolescents.

- Acne involves the pilosebaceous follicles (hair follicle and sebaceous gland complex) of the face, neck, chest, and upper back.

- *Propionibacterium acnes* (*P. acnes*) is the bacteria associated with inflammation in acne.

Data Collection

- Risk Factors

  ○ Acne can be genetic.

  ○ Acne is more common in males than in females.

  ○ Hormonal fluctuations can result in acne flares in females.

  ○ The use of cosmetic products containing ingredients such as petrolatum and lanolin can increase acne outbreaks.

  ○ Although there is no dietary intake link with acne, adolescents working at fast food restaurants can have an increased incidence of acne due to exposure to cooking grease.

- Subjective and Objective Data

  ○ Report of exacerbations and remissions

  ○ Physical Assessment Findings

    ▪ Lesions (comedones) are either open (blackheads) or closed (whiteheads). Both are most often found on the face, neck, back, and chest.

    ▪ *P. acnes* can lead to inflammation manifesting as papules, pustules, nodules, or cysts.

Patient-Centered Care

- Nursing Care

  ○ Discuss the process of acne with the child and family.

  ○ Discuss the importance of adherence with the prescribed plan of care.

  ○ Provide written instructions to accompany verbal instructions.

  ○ Reinforce teaching to the child about gently washing the face and other affected areas, avoiding scrubbing and abrasive cleaners.

  ○ Reinforce teaching to the child and family about medications prescribed, especially side effects.

  ○ Monitor for and report signs of mood changes or suicidal ideation in adolescents who are taking isotretinoin 13-cis-retinoic acid (Accutane).

  ○ Provide support and encouragement to the child and family.

MEDICATION	ACTION	NURSING CONSIDERATIONS
Tretinoin (Retin-A)	› Interrupts abnormal keratinization that causes microcomedones	› Inform the client that tretinoin can irritate the skin. Instruct the client to apply within 20 to 30 min after washing the face. › Tell the client to: » Use a pea-size amount of medication and apply at night. » Avoid sun exposure. » Use sunscreen (SPF 15 or greater) to avoid sunburn.
Benzoyl peroxide	› Antibacterial agent › Inhibits growth of *P. acnes*	› Benzoyl peroxide can bleach bed linens, towels, and clothing, but not skin.
Topical antibacterial agents	› Inhibits growth of *P. acnes*	› Various topical or oral antibacterial agents can be used. However, be alert to allergic reactions. › Avoid overexposure to the sun. › Use sunscreen with an SPF of 15 or greater when exposure to sun is unavoidable.
isotretinoin 13-cis-retinoic acid (Accutane)	› Affects factors involved in the development of acne	› Isotretinoin 13-cis-retinoic acid is prescribed only by dermatologists. › Side effects include dry skin and mucous membranes, dry eyes, decreased night vision, headaches, photosensitivity, elevated cholesterol and triglycerides, depression, suicidal ideation, and/or violent behaviors. › Monitor for behavioral changes. › Isotretinoin 13-cis-retinoic acid is teratogenic. Therefore, it is contraindicated in women of childbearing age who are not taking oral contraceptives.

- Care After Discharge
  - Client Education
    - Reinforce that adherence to the therapeutic plan is essential to preventing acne flares.
    - Encourage the child to eat a balanced, healthy diet.
    - Encourage sleep, rest, and daily exercise.
    - Reinforce teaching to the child about washing the affected area gently with a mild cleanser once or twice daily, and not to pick or squeeze comedones.
    - Encourage frequent shampooing.
    - Encourage family support of the child and family members to assist the child in coping with body-image changes.
    - Instruct the child to wear protective clothing and sunscreen when outside.
    - Reinforce teaching to the child about avoiding the use of tanning beds.
    - Reinforce the need for follow-up and monitoring of cholesterol and triglycerides, especially in adolescents who are taking isotretinoin 13-cis-retinoic acid.
    - Reinforce the importance of using oral contraceptives while taking isotretinoin 13-cis-retinoic acid.

Complications

- Infection and cellulitis
  - ○ Caused by lesions of dermatitis and/or acne or breaks in the skin from scratching
  - ○ Nursing Actions
    - Monitor the area for signs of infection.
    - Cleanse the area with mild soap and water.
    - Monitor for signs of redness, swelling, and pain, which can indicate cellulitis.
    - Check for fever.
  - ○ Client Education
    - Reinforce teaching to the family and child about offending agents.
    - Encourage the child and family to keep fingernails trimmed and short.
    - Use antipruritics as prescribed.
    - Reinforce teaching about the manifestations of cellulitis and to notify the provider if they occur.

APPLICATION EXERCISES

1. A nurse is reinforcing teaching with the parent of an infant who has seborrheic dermatitis. Which of the following should be included in the teaching?

    A. "The patches are from not washing the infant's head regularly."

    B. "The cause is unknown and not contagious."

    C. "The patches are due to an infection the infant has."

    D. "The cause is due to the infant acquiring it from another child at day care."

2. A nurse is caring for a child who has contact dermatitis due to poison ivy. Which of the following actions should the nurse take? (Select all that apply.)

    _____ A. Remove the clothing over the rash.

    _____ B. Initiate contact isolation precautions.

    _____ C. Expose the rash to a heat lamp for 15 min.

    _____ D. Cleanse the affected skin with hydrogen peroxide solution.

    _____ E. Apply calamine lotion to the skin.

3. A nurse is caring for an adolescent who has acne and is prescribed isotretinoin 13-cis-retinoic acid (Accutane). Which of the following laboratory findings should be monitored?

    A. Cholesterol and triglycerides

    B. BUN and creatinine

    C. Serum potassium

    D. Serum sodium

4. A nurse is caring for an infant who has diaper dermatitis. Which of the following actions should the nurse take? (Select all that apply.)

    _____ A. Apply talcum powder with every diaper change.

    _____ B. Allow the buttocks to air dry.

    _____ C. Use commercial baby wipes to cleanse the area.

    _____ D. Use cloth diapers until the rash is gone.

    _____ E. Apply zinc oxide ointment to the affected area.

5. A nurse is collecting data from an infant who has eczema. Which of the following are clinical manifestations of eczema in an infant? (Select all that apply.)

_____ A. Generalized distribution

_____ B. Papules

_____ C. Clusters

_____ D. Crusting lesions

_____ E. Lichenification

6. A nurse is reinforcing teaching with a parent of a child who has eczema. Use the ATI Active Learning Template: Systems Disorder to complete this item to include the following sections:

A. Description of the Disorder/Disease Process

B. Client Education

APPLICATION EXERCISES KEY

1. A. INCORRECT: The cause of seborrheic dermatitis is unknown. Not washing the infant's head is not the cause of seborrheic dermatitis.

    B. **CORRECT:** The cause of seborrheic dermatitis is unknown. The condition is not contagious. This should be included in the teaching.

    C. INCORRECT: Seborrheic dermatitis is not caused by an infection. This should not be included in the teaching.

    D. INCORRECT: Seborrheic dermatitis is not contagious and not acquired from another child. This should not be included in the teaching.

    Ⓝ NCLEX® Connection: Physiological Adaptations, Alterations in Body Systems

2. A. **CORRECT:** Removing the irritant from the skin will decrease the exposure. The nurse should remove the clothing over the rash.

    B. INCORRECT: The irritant in poison ivy is not spread by contact or scratching. Contact isolation precautions are not necessary.

    C. INCORRECT: Using a heat lamp can cause skin burns and should be avoided.

    D. INCORRECT: The affected area should be cleansed with isopropyl alcohol followed by water.

    E. **CORRECT:** Calamine lotion will assist in relieving discomfort and should be included in the plan of care.

    Ⓝ NCLEX® Connection: Physiological Adaptations, Basic Pathophysiology

3. A. **CORRECT:** Adverse effects of 13-cis-retinoic acid include elevated cholesterol and triglycerides. These laboratory findings should be monitored.

    B. INCORRECT: Medications such as cephalosporins and furosemide can alter serum BUN and creatinine levels. However, they do not to be monitored in clients taking 13-cis-retinoic acid.

    C. INCORRECT: Medications such as diuretics and corticosteroids can alter serum potassium levels. However, it does not need to be monitored in clients taking 13-cis-retinoic acid.

    D. INCORRECT: Medications such as IV fluids and corticosteroids can alter the serum sodium level. However, it does not need to be monitored in clients taking 13-cis-retinoic acid.

    Ⓝ NCLEX® Connection: Reduction of Risk Potential, Laboratory Values

4.   A. INCORRECT: Talcum powder can cake and cause inhalation injury. It should not be used for infants who have diaper dermatitis.

   B. **CORRECT:** Allowing the buttocks to air-dry facilitates thorough drying of the skin and should be included in the plan of care.

   C. INCORRECT: Commercial baby wipes contain chemicals that can irritate the skin. They should not be used for infants who have diaper dermatitis.

   D. INCORRECT: Superabsorbent diapers should be used for infants who have diaper dermatitis to assist in keeping the skin dry.

   E. **CORRECT:** Zinc oxide ointment protects the skin from moisture and irritation and should be included in the plan of care.

   Ⓝ NCLEX® Connection: Physiological Adaptations, Alterations in Body Systems

5.   A. **CORRECT:** Generalized distribution is a clinical manifestation found in infants who have eczema.

   B. **CORRECT:** Papules are a clinical manifestation found in infants who have eczema.

   C. INCORRECT: Clusters are a clinical manifestation found in children who have eczema.

   D. **CORRECT:** Crusting lesions are a clinical manifestation found in infants who have eczema.

   E. INCORRECT: Lichenification is a clinical manifestation found in children who have eczema.

   Ⓝ NCLEX® Connection: Physiological Adaptations, Basic Pathophysiology

6. *Using ATI Active Learning Template: Systems Disorder*

   A. Description of the Disorder/Disease Process

     • Eczema describes a category of integumentary disorders, not a specific disorder with a determined etiology, that is characterized by pruritus and associated with a history of allergies that are of an inherited tendency (atopy).

   B. Client Education

     • Clinical signs of infection.

     • Change diapers when wet or soiled.

     • Keep nails short and trimmed.

     • Place gloves or cotton socks over hands for sleeping.

     • Dress young children in soft, cotton, one-piece, long-sleeve, long-pant outfits.

     • Remove items that can promote itching (woolen blankets, scratchy fabrics). Use cotton items whenever possible.

     • Use mild detergent to wash clothing and linens. The wash cycle can be repeated without soap.

     • Avoid latex products, secondhand smoke, furry pets, dust, and molds.

     • Encourage tepid baths without the use of soap. Avoid oils and powders.

     • Follow specific directions regarding topical medications, soaks, and baths.

     • Emphasize the importance of understanding the sequence of treatments to maximize the benefit of therapy and prevent complications.

     • Avoid overheating the bedroom during winter months. Use a room humidifier.

     • Maintain treatment to prevent flare-up.

     • Follow up with the provider as directed.

     • Participate in support groups.

Ⓝ NCLEX® Connection: Physiological Adaptations, Alterations in Body Systems

chapter 30

Overview

- Thermal, chemical, electrical, and radioactive agents can cause burns, which result in cellular destruction of the skin layers and underlying tissue. The type and severity of the burn affect the treatment plan.

  - Thermal burns occur when there is exposure to flames, steam, or hot liquids.

  - Chemical burns occur when there is exposure to a caustic agent. Cleaning agents used in the home (drain cleaner, bleach) and agents used in the industrial setting (caustic soda, sulfuric acid) cause chemical burns.

  - Electrical burns occur when an electrical current passes through the body. This type of burn can result in severe damage, including loss of organ function, tissue destruction with the subsequent need for amputation of a limb, and cardiac and/or respiratory arrest.

 View Image: Percentage of Burns

Data Collection

- Risk Factors
  - Lack of supervision, abuse, or neglect
  - Developmental stage of the child
- Subjective Data
  - Type of burning agent (dry heat, moist heat, chemical, electrical, ionizing radiation)
  - Duration of contact
  - Area of the body in which the burn occurred
- Objective Data
  - Physical Findings

DEPTH	APPEARANCE	SENSATION/HEALING
› Superficial (first-degree) » Damage to epidermis	› Pink to red in color with no blisters, mild edema, and no eschar › Blanches with pressure	› Painful. › Heals within 5 to 10 days. › No scarring.
› Superficial partial thickness (second-degree) » Damage to the entire epidermis » Dermal elements are intact	› Pink to red in color with blisters, mild to moderate edema, and no eschar › Blanches with pressure	› Pain is present. › Heals within 14 to 21 days. › Variable amounts of scarring. › Sensitive to temperature changes and light touch.

DEPTH	APPEARANCE	SENSATION/HEALING
› Deep partial thickness (second-degree) » Damage to the entire epidermis and some parts of the dermis » Sweat glands and hair follicles remain intact	› Red to white in color with blisters and moderate edema › Blanches with pressure	› Pain is present. › Sensitive to temperature changes and light touch. › Healing time can extend beyond 21 days. › Scarring is likely.
› Full thickness (third-degree) » Damage to the entire epidermis and dermis, and possible damage to the subcutaneous tissue » Nerve endings, hair follicles, and sweat glands are destroyed	› Red to tan, black, brown, or white in color › Dry, leathery appearance › No blanching	› As burn heals, painful sensations return and severity of pain increases. › Heals within weeks to months. › Scarring is present. › Grafting is required.
› Deep full thickness (fourth-degree) » Damage to all layers of the skin that extends to muscle, tendons, and bones	› Color variable › Dull and dry › Charring › Possible visible ligaments, bone or tendons	› No pain is present. › Heals within weeks to months. › Scarring is present. › Grafting is required. › Amputation possible.

 View Image: Stages of Burns

- ○ Extent of Injury
  - ■ Total Body Surface Area (TBSA)
    - □ Age-related charts determine the extent of injury to body surface, which is expressed in percentages.
    - □ Infant's skin is thin. Therefore, injury is likely to be deeper
  - ■ Burns are classified as minor, moderate, or major.
    - □ Minor: treated in a clinic setting
    - □ Moderate: treated in a hospital with expertise in burn care
    - □ Major: require medical services of a burn center
- ○ Laboratory Tests (for injury greater than 30% TBSA)
  - ■ CBC, serum electrolytes, BUN, ABGs, fasting blood glucose, random blood glucose, liver enzymes, urinalysis, and clotting studies

Patient-Centered Care

- Nursing Care
  - Minor burns
    - Stop the burning process.
      - Remove clothing or jewelry that can conduct heat.
      - Apply cool water soaks or run cool water over the injury. Do not use ice.
      - Flush chemical burns with large amounts of water.
    - Cover the burn with a clean cloth to prevent contamination.
    - Cleanse with mild soap and tepid water. (Avoid excess friction.)
    - Removing blisters is controversial.
    - Use antimicrobial ointment.
    - Apply dressing (nonadherent, hydrocolloid).
    - Provide warmth.
    - If necessary, child is seen in a health care facility.
    - Provide analgesia.
    - Check immunization status and determine the need for immunization. Administer tetanus vaccine if it has been more than 5 years since last immunization.
    - Reinforce teaching to the family about avoiding use of greasy lotions or butter on burns.
    - Reinforce teaching to the family about monitoring for signs of infection.
  - Moderate and major burns
    - Maintain airway and ventilation.
    - Provide humidified 100% supplemental oxygen as prescribed.
    - Monitor vital signs.
    - Maintain cardiac output.
      - Fluid replacement is important during the first 24 hr.
        - Isotonic crystalloid solutions, such as 0.9% sodium chloride or lactated Ringer's, are used during the early stage of burn recovery.
        - Colloid solutions, such as albumin or synthetic plasma expanders (Hespan), can be used after the first 24 hr of burn recovery.
        - Urine output should be 1 to 2 mL/kg/hr if the child weighs less than 30 kg (66 lb).
        - Urine output should be 30 mL/hr if the child weighs more than 30 kg (66 lb).
        - Monitor administration of blood products, if prescribed.
      - Monitor for manifestations of septic shock.
        - Alterations in sensorium (confusion)
        - Increased capillary refill
        - Spiking fever
        - Decreased bowel sounds
        - Decreased urine output
      - Notify the provider of findings.

- Manage pain.
  - Establish ongoing monitoring of pain and effectiveness of pain management.
  - Avoid IM or subcutaneous injections.
  - Monitor effectiveness of intravenous opioid analgesics, such as morphine sulfate, hydromorphone (Dilaudid), and fentanyl (Sublimaze).
  - Monitor for respiratory depression when using opioid analgesics.
  - Administer pain medications prior to dressing changes or procedures.
  - Use nonpharmacologic methods for pain control (guided imagery, music therapy, therapeutic touch) to enhance the effects of analgesics and promote improved pain management.
- Prevent infection.
  - Follow standard precautions when performing wound care.
  - Restrict plants and flowers due to the risk of contact with pseudomonas.
  - Change position frequently to prevent contractures and prolonged pressure.
  - Limit visitors.
  - Use reverse isolation if prescribed.
  - Monitor for manifestations of infection and report to the provider.
  - Use client-designated equipment, such as blood pressure cuffs and thermometers.
  - Administer tetanus toxoid if indicated.
  - Administer antibiotics if infection is present.
- Provide nutritional support.
  - Increase caloric intake to meet increased metabolic demands and prevent hypoglycemia.
  - Increase protein intake to prevent tissue breakdown and promote healing.
  - Provide enteral therapy and monitor total parenteral nutrition (TPN) if necessary due to decreased gastrointestinal motility and increased caloric needs.
  - Administer vitamins A and C to facilitate cell growth, and zinc for wound healing.
- Restore mobility.
  - Maintain correct body alignment, splint extremities, and facilitate position changes to prevent contractures.
  - Encourage and assist with active and passive range of motion.
  - Assist with ambulation as soon as the child is stable.
  - Assist with application of pressure dressings to prevent contractures and scarring.
  - Closely monitor areas at high risk for pressure sores (heels, sacrum, back of head).
- Provide psychological support.
  - Provide developmentally appropriate support for the child.
  - Assist with coping.
  - Use family-centered approach.
  - Assist with referrals as needed.

- Medications
  - Topical agents
    - Silver sulfadiazine (Silvadene)
      - Use with second- and third-degree burns.
      - Apply to cleansed, debrided area.
      - Wear sterile gloves for application.
      - Apply thickness of 1/16th inch.
    - Mafenide acetate (Sulfamylon)
      - Use with second- and third-degree burns.
      - Apply to cleansed, debrided area.
      - Wear sterile gloves for application.
      - Apply thickness of 16 mm.
    - Bacitracin
      - Use for prevention of secondary infection.
      - Apply thin film two to four times per day.
  - Morphine sulfate
    - Analgesia
    - Nursing Considerations
      - Care for the client receiving medication via continuous IV infusion and ensure boluses are administered prior to procedures.
      - Monitor for respiratory depression.
      - Monitor pain relief.
    - Client Education
      - Reinforce teaching to the child and family on the safety precautions needed with opioid administration.
  - Midazolam (Versed), fentanyl (Sublimaze), propofol (Diprivan), and nitrous oxide
    - Sedation and analgesia
    - Nursing Considerations
      - Ensure medication is administered IV just prior to the start of a procedure.
      - Monitor the need for sedation.
      - Monitor pain relief.
    - Client Education
      - Reinforce teaching to the child and the family about the safety precautions needed with opioid administration.
- Teamwork and Collaboration – Assist with referrals to services such as nutrition, child life, social support, respiratory therapy, occupational/physical therapy, and individual and family counseling.

- Therapeutic Procedures
  - ○ Wound care
    - ▪ Nursing Actions
      - ▢ Premedicate prior to wound care.
        - ▸ Administer analgesics.
        - ▸ Administer hydroxyzine (Vistaril) or diphenhydramine for pruritus.
      - ▢ Remove previous dressings.
      - ▢ Check for odors, drainage, and discharge.
      - ▢ Cleanse the wound as prescribed.
      - ▢ Assist with debridement.
        - ▸ Provide hydrotherapy (place client or affected extremity in a warm tub of water or use warm running water, as if to shower) to cleanse the wound. Use once or twice a day for up to 20 min.
          - ▹ Use mild soap or detergent to gently wash burns and then rinse with room-temperature water.
          - ▹ Encourage active range of motion during hydrotherapy.
          - ▹ Monitor for cold stress and hypothermia.
  - ○ Skin coverings
    - ▪ Biologic skin coverings can be used to promote healing of large burns. Requires repeated surgical application.
      - ▢ Allograft (homograft) – Skin from human cadavers that is used for partial- and full-thickness burn wounds
      - ▢ Xenograft – Obtained from animals, such as pigs, for partial thickness burn wounds
      - ▢ Synthetic skin coverings – Used for partial thickness burn wounds
    - ▪ Permanent skin coverings can be the treatment of choice for burns covering large areas of the body.
      - ▢ Autografts (client's skin)
        - ▸ Sheet graft – Sheet of skin used to cover the wound
        - ▸ Mesh graft – Sheet of skin placed in a mesher so skin graft has small slits in it; allows graft to cover larger areas of burn wound
        - ▸ Cultured epithelium – Epithelial cells cultured for use when grafting sites are limited
      - ▢ Artificial skin – Synthetic product that is used for partial and full thickness burn wounds (healing is faster)
    - ▪ Nursing Actions
      - ▢ Maintain immobilization of the graft site.
      - ▢ Elevate the extremity.
      - ▢ Provide wound care to the donor site.
      - ▢ Administer analgesics.

□ Monitor for infection before and after skin coverings or grafts are applied.

  ▸ Discoloration of unburned skin surrounding burn wound

  ▸ Green color to subcutaneous fat

  ▸ Degeneration of granulation tissue

  ▸ Development of subeschar hemorrhage

  ▸ Hyperventilation indicating systemic involvement of infection

  ▸ Unstable body temperature

- Client Education

  □ Reinforce teaching to the child about keeping the extremity elevated.

  □ Reinforce teaching to the family about reporting evidence of infection.

- Care After Discharge

  ○ Assist with a referral for home health services.

  ○ Assist with a referral to occupational therapy for evaluation of the home environment and assistance relearning how to perform ADLs.

  ○ Assist with a referral to social services for community support services.

  ○ Client Education

    - Reinforce teaching to the child about continuing to perform range-of-motion exercises and to work with a physical therapist to prevent contractures.

    - Reinforce teaching about how to check the wound for infection and how to perform wound care.

    - Reinforce teaching about age-appropriate safety measures for the home (covering electrical outlets, supervising children when in the bath, keeping irons out of reach of children, teaching the dangers of playing with matches).

    - Reinforce teaching to the family about avoiding sun exposure between 1000 and 1600, wearing protective clothing, and applying sunscreen to prevent sunburn.

Complications

- Inhalation injury

  ○ Direct thermal injury

    - Occurs with burns to the face and lips.

    - Manifestations can be delayed 24 to 48 hr.

    - Findings include wheezing, increased secretions, hoarseness, wet crackles in the lungs, singed nasal hairs, laryngeal edema, and carbonaceous secretions.

  ○ Carbon monoxide injury

    - Occurs when incident took place in an enclosed area.

    - Findings include mucosal erythema and edema followed by sloughing of the mucosa.

  ○ Nursing Actions

    - Maintain airway and ventilation, and provide 100% oxygen as prescribed.

- Shock/Systemic Sepsis
  - Nursing Actions
    - Care for the client receiving IV crystalloid solutions for the first 24 hr followed by colloid solutions.
    - Meticulous monitoring of intake and output.
    - Monitor laboratory findings, noting indications of anemia and infection.
    - Monitor vital signs.
    - Determine sensorium.
    - Check capillary refill in extremities.
- Pulmonary problems include edema, infections, aspiration, embolus, and posttraumatic pulmonary insufficiency.
  - Nursing Actions
    - Administer oxygen as prescribed.
- Wound infections
  - Nursing Actions
    - Check for discoloration, edema, odor, and drainage.
    - Identify fluctuations in temperature and heart rate.
    - Obtain a wound culture.
    - Administer antibiotics as prescribed.
    - Monitor laboratory findings, noting indications of anemia and infection.
    - Maintain surgical aseptic technique with dressing changes.

APPLICATION EXERCISES

1. A nurse is caring for a client who has a superficial partial thickness burn. Which of the following is an appropriate action for the nurse to take?

    A. Place the client in a cool area.

    B. Apply cool, wet compresses to affected area.

    C. Clean the affected area using a soft-bristle brush.

    D. Apply a hydrocolloid dressing.

2. A nurse is caring for a client who has major burns and suspected septic shock. Which of the following findings are consistent with septic shock? (Select all that apply.)

    _____ A. Increased body temperature

    _____ B. Altered sensorium

    _____ C. Decreased capillary refill

    _____ D. Decreased urine output

    _____ E. Increased bowel sounds

3. A nurse is assisting with the care of a child who is being treated with skin grafts. Which of the following actions should the nurse take? (Select all that apply.)

    _____ A. Elevate the involved extremity.

    _____ B. Apply topical enzymes.

    _____ C. Provide wound care to the donor site.

    _____ D. Exercise the joints of the involved extremity.

    _____ E. Observe for hyperventilation.

4. A nurse is caring for a client who has a skin graft. Which of the following clinical manifestations indicate infection? (Select all that apply.)

    _____ A. Green color to subcutaneous fat

    _____ B. Unstable body temperature

    _____ C. Generation of granulation tissue

    _____ D. Subeschar hemorrhage

    _____ E. Change in skin color around the affected area

5. A nurse is caring for a client who has a moderate burn. Which of the following is an appropriate action for the nurse to take?

      A. Maintain immobilization of the affected area.

      B. Expose affected area to the air.

      C. Initiate a high-protein, high-calorie diet.

      D. Implement contact isolation.

6. A nurse is assisting with the development of an education program about clinical manifestations of burns. Use the ATI Active Learning Template: Basic Concept to complete this item to include Underlying Principles. List the depth, appearance, sensation, and healing of first-, second-, third-, and fourth-degree burns.

APPLICATION EXERCISES KEY

1. A. INCORRECT: The nurse should place the client in a warm area to prevent decrease in the core body temperature.

    B. INCORRECT: The nurse should apply cool, wet compresses to stop the burning process.

    C. INCORRECT: Gentle cleansing with tepid water, not a soft-bristle brush, is recommended for a superficial partial thickness burn.

    D. **CORRECT:** The nurse should apply a hydrocolloid dressing to the burn to promote healing and prevent infection.

    (N) NCLEX® Connection: Physiological Adaptations, Basic Pathophysiology

2. A. **CORRECT:** Increased body temperature is a clinical manifestation of septic shock.

    B. **CORRECT:** Altered sensorium is a clinical manifestation of septic shock.

    C. INCORRECT: Increased capillary refill is a clinical manifestation of septic shock.

    D. **CORRECT:** Decreased urine output is a clinical manifestation of septic shock.

    E. INCORRECT: Decreased bowel sounds is a clinical manifestation of septic shock.

    (N) NCLEX® Connection: Physiological Adaptations, Basic Pathophysiology

3. A. **CORRECT:** The nurse should elevate the involved extremity to reduce the risk of edema.

    B. INCORRECT: The nurse should apply topical enzymes during debridement of a wound, not to a skin graft.

    C. **CORRECT:** The nurse should provide wound care to the donor site to prevent infection.

    D. INCORRECT: The nurse should immobilize the joints of the involved extremity to promote adherence of the grafts.

    E. **CORRECT:** The nurse should observe for hyperventilation, which indicates systemic involvement of infection.

    (N) NCLEX® Connection: Physiological Adaptations, Basic Pathophysiology

4.   A. **CORRECT:** Green color to subcutaneous fat is a clinical manifestation of infection.

   B. **CORRECT:** Unstable body temperature is a clinical manifestation of infection.

   C. INCORRECT: Degeneration of granulation tissues is a clinical manifestation of infection.

   D. **CORRECT:** Subeschar hemorrhage is a clinical manifestation of infection.

   E. **CORRECT:** A discoloration of the skin around the burn is a clinical manifestation of infection.

    NCLEX® Connection: Physiological Adaptations, Alterations in Body Systems

5.   A. INCORRECT: Active and passive range of motion of the affected area is recommended to prevent contractures.

   B. INCORRECT: Dressings should be applied to the burned area to prevent infection.

   C. **CORRECT:** A high-protein, high-calorie diet is initiated to meet increased metabolic demands and promote healing.

   D. INCORRECT: Reverse isolation precautions are recommended to prevent wound infections.

    NCLEX® Connection: Physiological Adaptations, Basic Pathophysiology

6. *Using the ATI Active Learning Template: Basic Concept*
   - Underlying Principles
     - Superficial (first-degree)
       - Damage to the epidermis.
       - Pink to red in color with no blisters.
       - Blanches with pressure.
       - Mild edema.
       - No eschar.
       - Painful.
       - Heals within 5 to 10 days with no scarring.
     - Superficial partial thickness (second-degree)
       - Damage to the entire epidermis with intact dermal elements.
       - Pink to red in color with blisters.
       - Blanches with pressure.
       - Mild to moderate edema.
       - No eschar.
       - Painful, sensitive to temperature changes and light touch.
       - Heals within 14 to 21 days with variable scarring.
     - Deep partial thickness (second-degree)
       - Damage to the entire epidermis and some parts of the dermis. Sweat glands and hair follicles remain intact.
       - Red to white in color with blisters.
       - Blanches with pressure.
       - Moderate edema.
       - Painful, sensitive to temperature changes and light touch.
       - Healing can go beyond 21 days with scarring.
     - Full thickness (third degree)
       - Damage to the entire epidermis and dermis with possible damage to the subcutaneous tissue. Nerve endings, hair follicles, and sweat glands are destroyed.
       - Red to tan, black, brown, or white in color.
       - Dry, leathery appearance.
       - No blanching.
       - As burn heals, painful sensations return and severity of pain increases.
       - It heals within weeks to months. Scarring is present. Grafting is required.
     - Deep full thickness (fourth-degree)
       - Damage to all layers of the skin that extends to the muscle, tendons, and bones.
       - Color variable, dull, and dry with charring. Possible visible ligaments, bone, or tendons.
       - No pain is present.
       - Heals within weeks to months. Scarring is present and grafting is required. Amputation possible.

Ⓝ NCLEX® Connection: Physiological Adaptations, Basic Pathophysiology

UNIT 2   Nursing Care of Children with System Disorders

SECTION: ENDOCRINE DISORDERS

› Diabetes Mellitus
› Growth Hormone Deficiency

NCLEX® CONNECTIONS

When reviewing the chapters in this section, keep in mind the relevant sections of the NCLEX® outline, in particular:

Client Needs: Pharmacological and Parenteral Therapies	Client Needs: Reduction of Risk Potential	Client Needs: Physiological Adaptations

› Relevant topics/tasks include:
  » Dosage Calculations
  › Perform calculations needed for medication administration.
  » Expected Actions/Outcomes
  › Apply knowledge of pathophysiology when addressing pharmacological agents.
	› Relevant topics/tasks include:
	  » Diagnostic Tests
	  › Perform diagnostic testing.
	  » Therapeutic Procedures
	  › Assist with the performance of a diagnostic or invasive procedure.
		› Relevant topics/tasks include:
		  » Alterations in Body Systems
		  › Reinforce education to client regarding care and condition.
		  » Basic Pathophysiology
		  › Identify signs and symptoms related to an acute or chronic illness.
		  › Apply knowledge of pathophysiology to monitoring client for alterations in body systems.

chapter 31

Overview

- Diabetes mellitus is characterized by a partial or complete metabolic deficiency of insulin.

- Diabetes mellitus is a contributing factor for the development of cardiovascular disease, hypertension, renal failure, blindness, and stroke as individuals age.

Data Collection

- Risk Factors

  - Genetics can predispose a person to the occurrence of type 1 and type 2 diabetes mellitus.

  - Toxins and viruses can predispose an individual to diabetes by destroying the beta cells, leading to type 1 diabetes mellitus.

  - Obesity, physical inactivity, high triglycerides (greater than 250 mg/dL), and hypertension can lead to the development of insulin resistance and type 2 diabetes mellitus.

- Subjective and Objective Data

  - Blood glucose alterations

    - Hypoglycemia – blood glucose level less than 60 mg/dL

AUTONOMIC NERVOUS SYSTEM RESPONSES RAPID ONSET	IMPAIRED CEREBRAL FUNCTION GRADUAL ONSET
› Hunger, lightheadedness, and shakiness	› Strange or unusual feelings
› Headache	› Decreasing level of consciousness
› Anxiety and irritability	› Difficulty in thinking and inability to concentrate
› Pale, cool skin	› Change in emotional behavior
› Diaphoresis	› Slurred speech
› Irritability	› Headache and blurred vision
› Normal or shallow respirations	› Seizures leading to coma
› Tachycardia and palpitations	

    - Hyperglycemia – blood glucose levels usually greater than 250 mg/dL

      - Thirst

      - Polyuria (early), oliguria (late)

      - Nausea, vomiting, abdominal pain

      - Skin that is warm, dry, and flushed with poor turgor

      - Dry mucous membranes

- ▫ Confusion
- ▫ Weakness
- ▫ Lethargy
- ▫ Weak pulse
- ▫ Diminished reflexes
- ▫ Rapid, deep respirations with acetone/fruity odor due to ketones (Kussmaul respirations)
- ○ Laboratory Tests
    - ▪ Diagnostic criteria for diabetes
        - ▫ An 8-hr fasting blood glucose level of 126 mg/dL or more
        - ▫ A random blood glucose of 200 mg/dL or more with classic signs of diabetes
        - ▫ An oral glucose tolerance test of 200 mg/dL or more in the 2-hr sample
    - ▪ Fasting blood glucose
        - ▫ Client Education
            - ‣ Ensure that the child has fasted (no food or drink other than water) for 8 hr prior to the blood draw. Antidiabetic medications should be postponed until after the level is drawn.
    - ▪ Oral glucose tolerance test
        - ▫ Client Education
            - ‣ Reinforce teaching to the child to consume a balanced diet for the 3 days prior to the test. Then instruct the child to fast for 8 hr prior to the test. A fasting blood glucose level is drawn at the start of the test. Reinforce teaching as to when the child is instructed to consume a specified amount of glucose. Blood glucose levels are drawn every 30 min for 2 hr. The child must be monitored for hypoglycemia throughout the procedure.
    - ▪ Glycosylated hemoglobin (HbA1c)
        - ▫ The expected reference range is 4% to 6%, but an acceptable target for children who have diabetes may be 6.5% to 8% with a total target goal of less than 7%.
- ○ Diagnostic Procedures
    - ▪ Self-monitored blood glucose (SMBG)
        - ▫ Blood glucose monitoring is essential to management of diabetes. Measurements should be checked at a minimum before meals and at bedtime.
        - ▫ Reinforce importance of teaching to ensure that the child follows the proper procedure for blood sample collection and use of a glucose meter.
        - ▫ Client Education
            - ‣ Reinforce the importance of teaching to the child to check the accuracy of the strips with the control solution provided.
            - ‣ Advise the child to keep a record of the SMBG that includes time, date, serum glucose level, insulin dose, food intake, and other events that may alter glucose metabolism, such as activity level or illness.

Patient-Centered Care

Q
TC

- Nursing Care
  - ○ Monitor the following.
    - ▪ Vital signs
    - ▪ Blood glucose levels and factors affecting levels (other medications, diet, and/or activity)
    - ▪ Intake and output, and weight
    - ▪ Skin integrity and healing status of any wounds, paying close attention to the feet and folds of the skin
    - ▪ Sensory alterations (tingling, numbness)
    - ▪ Visual alterations
    - ▪ Presence of recurrent infections
    - ▪ Dietary practices
    - ▪ Exercise patterns
    - ▪ The child's proficiency at self-monitoring blood glucose
    - ▪ The child's proficiency at self-administering medication
  - ○ Follow agency policy for nail care. Some protocols allow for trimming toenails straight across with clippers and filing edges with a nail file. If clippers or scissors are contraindicated, the child should file the nails straight across.
  - ○ Reinforce teaching on proper foot care.
    - ▪ Inspect feet daily. Wash feet daily with mild soap and warm water.
    - ▪ Pat feet dry gently, especially between the toes.
    - ▪ Use mild foot powder (powder with cornstarch) on sweaty feet.
    - ▪ Do not use commercial remedies for the removal of calluses or corns.
    - ▪ Perform nail care after a bath/shower if possible.
    - ▪ Separate overlapping toes with cotton or lambs' wool.
    - ▪ Avoid open-toe, open-heel shoes. Leather shoes are preferred to plastic ones. Wear slippers with soles. Do not go barefoot. Shake out shoes before putting them on.
    - ▪ Wear clean, absorbent socks or stockings that are made of cotton or wool and have not been mended.
    - ▪ Do not use hot water bottles or heating pads to warm feet. Wear socks for warmth.
    - ▪ Avoid prolonged sitting, standing, and crossing of legs.
  - ○ Reinforce teaching to the caregiver and the child to cleanse cuts with warm water and mild soap, gently dry, and apply a dry dressing. Reinforce teaching to the child and parents to monitor healing and to seek intervention promptly.
  - ○ Have the child's eyes examined yearly.
  - ○ Emphasize the importance of regular dental and health care visits.

○ Provide nutritional guidelines.

- Read labels for nutritional value.

- Meal planning is based on the requirements of growth and development of the child.

- Plan meals to achieve appropriate timing of food intake, activity, onset, and peak of insulin. Calories and food composition should be similar each day.

- Eat at regular intervals and do not skip meals.

- Count grams of carbohydrates consumed.

- Recognize that 15 g of carbohydrates are equal to 1 carbohydrate exchange.

- Avoid high-fat and high-sugar/high-carbohydrate food items.

- Use artificial sweeteners in moderation.

○ Reinforce teaching related to appropriate techniques for SMBG, including obtaining blood samples, recording and responding to results, and correctly handling supplies and equipment.

○ Assist with an exercise plan.

- Children active with team sports will require a snack 30 min prior to activity.

- Adjustment in diet and insulin may be required with changes in activities.

○ Reinforce teaching to caregiver and the child regarding guidelines to follow when sick.

- Monitor blood glucose levels every 3 hr.

- Continue to take insulin or oral antidiabetic agents.

- Encourage sugar-free, non-caffeinated liquids to prevent dehydration.

- Meet carbohydrate needs by eating soft foods if possible. If not, consume liquids that are equal to the usual carbohydrate content.

- Test urine for ketones every 3 hr.

- Rest.

- Call the health care provider if:

  □ Blood glucose is higher than 240 mg/dL.

  □ Fever higher than 38.9° C (102° F), fever does not respond to acetaminophen (Tylenol), or fever lasts more than 12 hr.

  □ Positive ketones in the urine.

  □ Disorientation or confusion occurs.

  □ Rapid breathing is experienced.

  □ Vomiting occurs more than once.

  □ Diarrhea occurs more than five times or for longer than 24 hr.

  □ Liquids cannot be tolerated.

  □ Illness lasts longer than 2 days.

- ○ Reinforce teaching related to signs and symptoms of hypoglycemia (e.g., shakiness, diaphoresis, anxiety, nervousness, chills, headache, confusion, labile, difficulty focusing, hunger, dizziness, pallor, palpations).
  - ▪ Check blood glucose levels.
  - ▪ Follow guidelines outlined by the provider or diabetes educator. Guidelines may include the following.
    - □ Treat with 10 to 15 g simple carbohydrate (1 tbsp sugar).
      - ‣ Examples of 15 g of carbohydrate are 4 oz orange juice, 8 oz milk, 3 to 4 glucose tablets, 4 oz regular soft drink.
    - □ For mild reactions, use milk or fruit juice.
    - □ Monitor blood glucose frequently.
    - □ Follow with complex carbohydrate.
    - □ If the child is unconscious or unable to swallow, administer glucagon SC or IM and notify the health care provider. Administer simple carbohydrate as soon as tolerated. Watch for vomiting and take precaution against aspiration.
- ○ Reinforce teaching related to signs and symptoms of hyperglycemia (lethargy, confusion, thirst, nausea, vomiting, abdominal pain, signs of dehydration, rapid respirations, fruity breath).
  - ▪ Encourage oral fluid intake.
  - ▪ Administer insulin as prescribed.
  - ▪ Test urine for ketones and report if findings are abnormal.
  - ▪ Consult the health care provider if symptoms progress.
- ○ Encourage the child to wear a medical identification wristband.
- • Medications
  - ○ Insulin is used to manage type 1 diabetes mellitus.
    - ▪ Insulin pumps
      - □ Regular insulin
      - □ Deliver a programmed amount of insulin on a consistent basis
    - ▪ Insulin injections
      - □ Self-administered injections 2 or more times per day
      - □ Mixing insulin: usually rapid-acting and intermediate-acting

○ The rate of onset, peak, and duration of action varies for each different type of insulin.

TYPE	TRADE NAME	ONSET	PEAK	DURATION
Rapid-acting	› Insulin lispro (Humalog)	Less than 15 min	0.5 to 1 hr	3 to 4 hr
Short-acting	› Regular insulin (Humulin R)	0.5 to 1 hr	2 to 4 hr	5 to 7 hr
Intermediate-acting	› NPH insulin (Humulin N)	1 to 2 hr	4 to 12 hr	18 to 24 hr
Long-acting	› Insulin glargine (Lantus)	3-4 hr	None	10.4 to 24 hr

- Nursing Considerations
  - □ Observe the child and/or parent drawing up and administering the insulin injection, and offer additional instruction as indicated.
  - □ Do not mix insulin glargine (Lantus) with other insulins due to incompatibility.
  - □ Observe the child and/or parent using the insulin pump and offer additional instruction as indicated.
- Client Education
  - □ Reinforce information regarding self-administration of insulin.
    - ▸ Rotate injection sites (to prevent lipohypertrophy) within one anatomic site (to prevent day-to-day changes in absorption rates).
    - ▸ Inject at a 90° angle (45° angle if thin). Aspiration for blood is not necessary.
    - ▸ When mixing a rapid- or short-acting insulin with a longer-acting insulin, draw up the shorter-acting insulin into the syringe first and then the longer-acting insulin. (This reduces the risk of introducing the longer-acting insulin into the vial of the shorter-acting insulin.)
- Teamwork and Collaboration
  - ○ Refer the child and family to a diabetes educator for comprehensive education in diabetes management.

Complications

- Diabetic ketoacidosis (DKA)
  - ○ DKA is an acute, life-threatening condition characterized by hyperglycemia (greater than 300 mg/dL), resulting in the breakdown of body fat for energy, and an accumulation of ketones in the blood and urine. The onset is rapid, and the mortality rate is high.
  - ○ Causes of DKA include insufficient insulin (usually failure to take the appropriate dose), acute stress (as from trauma or surgery), and poor management of acute illness.

- ○ Nursing Actions
  - ▪ Assist with the emergency management.
    - ▫ Assist with cardiac monitoring.
  - ▪ Collect subjective and objective data related to DKA.
    - ▫ Ketones in the blood and urine
    - ▫ Fruity scent to the breath
    - ▫ Mental confusion
    - ▫ Dyspnea
    - ▫ Nausea and vomiting
    - ▫ Dehydration
    - ▫ Weight loss
    - ▫ Electrolyte imbalances
    - ▫ Untreated: coma
  - ▪ Monitor IV site for infiltration and the child when rapid isotonic fluid (0.9% sodium chloride) replacement is administered to maintain perfusion to vital organs. Often, large quantities are required to replace losses. Monitor the child for evidence of fluid volume excess.
  - ▪ Monitor IV site for infiltration when a hypotonic fluid (0.45% sodium chloride) is administered to continue replacing losses to total body fluid.
  - ▪ Monitor glucose levels hourly.
  - ▪ Monitor serum potassium levels. Potassium levels initially will be elevated. With insulin therapy, potassium will shift into cells and the child will need to be monitored for hypokalemia. Provide potassium replacement therapy in all replacement IV fluids as indicated by lab values. Make sure urinary output is adequate before administering potassium.
  - ▪ Client should receive sodium bicarbonate by slow IV infusion for severe acidosis (pH less than 7.0). Monitor potassium levels because a correction of acidosis that occurs too quickly may lead to hypokalemia.
  - ▪ Administer oxygen to client whose arterial oxygen level is less than 90%.
- ○ Client Education
  - ▪ Reinforce instructions to manage diabetes.
- • Long-Term Complications
  - ○ Nephropathy
  - ○ Retinopathy
  - ○ Neuropathy
  - ○ Cardiovascular disease
  - ○ Altered thyroid function
  - ○ Limited mobility of the small joints

APPLICATION EXERCISES

1. A nurse is reviewing sick day management with a parent of a child who has type 1 diabetes mellitus. Which of the following should the nurse reinforce in the teaching? (Select all that apply.)

_____ A. Monitor blood glucose levels every 3 hr.

_____ B. Discontinue taking insulin until feeling better.

_____ C. Drink 8 oz of fruit juice every hour.

_____ D. Test urine for ketones.

_____ E. Call the provider if blood glucose is greater than 240 mg/dL.

2. A nurse is reinforcing teaching with a child who has type 1 diabetes mellitus about self care. Which of the following statements by the child indicates understanding of the information on self care?

A. "I should skip breakfast when I am not hungry."

B. "I should increase my insulin with exercise."

C. "I should drink a glass of milk when I am feeling irritable."

D. "I should draw up the NPH insulin into the syringe before the regular insulin."

3. A nurse is caring for a child who has type 1 diabetes mellitus. Which of the following are clinical manifestations of diabetic ketoacidosis? (Select all that apply.)

_____ A. Blood glucose 58 mg/dL

_____ B. Weight gain

_____ C. Dehydration

_____ D. Mental confusion

_____ E. Fruity breath

4. A nurse is reinforcing teaching about foot care with an adolescent who has diabetes mellitus. Which of the following should the nurse include when reinforcing the teaching?

A. "You should inspect your feet once a week."

B. "You should cut your toe nails in a rounded fashion."

C. "You can use cornstarch on your feet."

D. "You can use over-the-counter callus removers."

5. A nurse is reinforcing teaching about clinical manifestations of hypoglycemia with an adolescent who has diabetes mellitus. Which of the following should be included when the nurse reinforces the teaching? (Select all that apply.)

_____ A. Increased urination

_____ B. Hunger

_____ C. Signs of dehydration

_____ D. Irritability

_____ E. Sweating and pallor

_____ F. Kussmaul respirations

6. A nurse is reinforcing teaching with the parent of a child who has type 1 diabetes mellitus. Use the ATI Active Learning Template: Systems Disorder to complete this item to include the following:

A. Description of the Disorder/Disease Process

B. Collaborative Care: Medications: List the types of insulin used for children who have type 1 diabetes mellitus.

C. Nursing Care: Describe eight interventions.

APPLICATION EXERCISES KEY

1. A. **CORRECT:** A client who is experiencing illness can have waning blood glucose levels. Therefore, frequent monitoring of blood glucose levels is done to identify hyper- or hypoglycemic episodes.

   B. INCORRECT: A client who is experiencing illness should continue taking insulin during to prevent hyperglycemic episodes.

   C. INCORRECT: A client who is experiencing illness should drink fluids without sugars.

   D. **CORRECT:** A client who is experiencing an illness should test her urine for ketones to assist in early detection of ketoacidosis.

   E. **CORRECT:** A client who is experiencing illness should notify the provider of blood glucose levels greater than 240 mg/dL to obtain further instructions in caring for the hyperglycemia.

   Ⓝ NCLEX® Connection: Physiological Adaptations, Alterations in Body Systems

2. A. INCORRECT: A client who has diabetes should eat three meals a day with snacks and should avoid skipping meals to prevent hypoglycemic episodes.

   B. INCORRECT: The insulin requirements of a client who has type 1 diabetes will decrease with exercise, therefore increasing the amount of insulin with exercise could precipitate a hypoglycemic episode.

   C. **CORRECT:** An early clinical manifestation of hypoglycemia is irritability. Therefore, drinking a glass of milk, which is approximately 15 g of carbohydrates, indicates understanding of the teaching.

   D. INCORRECT: The client should draw up the regular insulin into the syringe prior to drawing up NPH to avoid altering the regular insulin.

   Ⓝ NCLEX® Connection: Physiological Adaptations, Alterations in Body Systems

3. A. INCORRECT: Diabetic ketoacidosis is classified as a blood glucose level greater than 300 mg/dL.

    B. INCORRECT: Clients who have diabetic ketoacidosis display weight loss.

    C. **CORRECT:** Clients who have diabetic ketoacidosis experience osmotic diuresis because of the electrolyte shift.

    D. **CORRECT:** Clients who have diabetic ketoacidosis experience mental confusion because of the electrolyte shift.

    E. **CORRECT:** Clients who have diabetic ketoacidosis experience fruity breath because of the body's attempt to eliminate ketones.

    (N) NCLEX® Connection: Physiological Adaptations, Alterations in Body Systems

4. A. INCORRECT: Clients who have diabetes should inspect their feet daily.

    B. INCORRECT: Clients who have diabetes should cut their toenails straight across.

    C. **CORRECT:** Clients who have diabetes can use cornstarch to aid in moisture absorption.

    D. INCORRECT: Clients who have diabetes should avoid commercial remedies for callus removal.

    (N) NCLEX® Connection: Physiological Adaptations, Alterations in Body Systems

5. A. INCORRECT: An increase in urination is a clinical manifestation of hyperglycemia.

    B. **CORRECT:** Hunger is a clinical manifestation of hypoglycemia because of the increased adrenergic nervous system activity.

    C. INCORRECT: Signs of dehydration is a clinical manifestation of hyperglycemia.

    D. **CORRECT:** Irritability is a clinical manifestation of hypoglycemia because of the depleted glucose in the CNS.

    E. **CORRECT:** Sweating and pallor is a clinical manifestation of hypoglycemia because of the increased adrenergic nervous system activity.

    F. INCORRECT: Kussmaul respirations is a clinical manifestation of hyperglycemia.

    (N) NCLEX® Connection: Physiological Adaptations, Alterations in Body Systems

6. *Using the ATI Active Learning Template: Systems Disorder*

   A. Description of the Disorder/Disease Process
      • Diabetes mellitus is characterized by a partial or complete metabolic deficiency of insulin.

   B. Collaborative Care: Medications
      • Insulin lispro (Humalog): Rapid-acting
      • Regular Insulin (Humulin R): Short-acting
      • NPH insulin (Humulin N): Intermediate-acting
      • Insulin glargine (Lantus): Long-acting

   C. Nursing Care
      • Monitor clinical manifestations of hyper- and hypoglycemia.
      • Provide nail care according to policy.
      • Reinforce teaching regarding proper foot care.
      • Reinforce teaching regarding wound care.
      • Provide nutritional guidelines.
      • Encourage yearly eye exams.
      • Encourage dental and medical follow-up.
      • Explain self-monitoring of blood glucose.
      • Recommend guidelines to follow when sick.
      • Reinforce teaching about hypo- and hyperglycemia.
      • Reinforce teaching about medications.

   Ⓝ NCLEX® Connection: Physiological Adaptations, Alterations in Body Systems

chapter **32**

Overview

- Human growth hormone (GH), somatotropin, is a naturally occurring substance that is secreted by the pituitary gland.
- GH is important for normal growth, development, and cellular metabolism.
- A deficiency in GH prevents somatic growth throughout the body.
- Other hormones that work with GH to control metabolic processes include adrenocorticotropic hormone (ACTH), thyroid-stimulating hormone (TSH), and the gonadotropins (follicle-stimulating hormone [FSH] and luteinizing hormone [LH]).
- Hypopituitarism is the diminished or deficient secretion of pituitary hormones (primarily GH). Consequences of the condition depend on the degree of the deficiency.

Data Collection

- Risk Factors
  - Structural factors (tumors, trauma, structural defects, surgery).
  - Heredity disorders.
  - Other pituitary hormone deficiencies (deficiencies of TSH or ACTH).
  - Most often, GH deficiencies are idiopathic.
- Objective Data
  - Data Collection Findings
    - Short stature but proportional height and weight
    - Delayed epiphyseal closure
    - Increased insulin sensitivity
    - Delayed dentition
    - Underdeveloped jaw
    - Delayed sexual development
  - Laboratory Tests
    - Plasma insulin-like growth factor-1 (IGF-1) and IGF binding protein-3 (IGFBP-3) levels
      - Further evaluation is indicated if the values are one standard deviation below the mean for age.
    - Nursing Actions
      - Assist with collecting the appropriate amount of blood for the test.
      - Explain the laboratory procedure to the family and child.
    - Client Education
      - The child should fast the night before the test.

○ Diagnostic Procedures

- GH stimulation

  □ GH stimulation testing is generally done for children who have a low level of IGF-1 and IGFBP-3, and short stature.

  □ Nursing Actions

    ‣ Assist with collecting baseline blood sample between 0600 and 0800.

    ‣ Administer medication that triggers the release of GH (arginine or GH-releasing hormone).

    ‣ Assist with collecting blood sample every 30 min for a 3-hr period following medication administration.

  □ Client Education

    ‣ Have nothing to eat or drink 10 to 12 hr before the test.

    ‣ Limit activity 10 to 12 hr before the test.

- Radiologic assessments

  □ Collect data related to the child's skeletal maturity by comparing epiphyseal centers on an x-ray to age-appropriate published standards.

  □ Collect data related to a general skeletal survey in children under 3 years of age, or survey the hands and wrists in older children. This will provide information about growth as well as epiphyseal function.

  □ Nursing Actions

    ‣ Assist in positioning the child.

- Computed tomographic (CT) scanning, magnetic resonance imaging (MRI), and skull x-rays

  □ Used to identify tumors or other structural defects

  □ Nursing Actions

    ‣ Monitor the child during the procedure.

    ‣ Sedate the child if prescribed medication is oral, rectal, or subcutaneous.

  □ Client Education

    ‣ Provide emotional support.

- Evaluation of the growth curve

  □ Nursing Actions

    ‣ Accurately obtain and plot height and weight measurements.

    ‣ Collect data related to height velocity or height over time.

    ‣ Determine height-to-weight relationship.

    ‣ Assist in projecting target height in context of genetic potential.

Patient-Centered Care

- Nursing Care
  - The child's height and weight are measured and marked on a growth chart as part of every visit to the primary care provider.
    - The height of a child is more affected than weight. Bone age usually matches height age.
    - Measure children who are younger than 3 years of age at least every 6 months and children older than 3 years of age every year.
  - Monitor effectiveness of GH replacement. GH is supplied by recombinant DNA technology.
  - Administer other hormone replacements (thyroid hormone) if prescribed medication is oral, rectal, or subcutaneous.
  - Provide support to the child and family regarding psychosocial concerns (altered body image, depression). Reassure the child and family that there are no cognitive delays or deficits.
  - Stress the importance of maintaining realistic expectations based on the child's age and abilities.
- Medications
  - Somatropin
    - Used as a human growth hormone that is a replacement for deficiency in growth hormones
    - Nursing Considerations
      - Administer the medication via subcutaneous injections.
      - Use cautiously in children who are receiving insulin.
- Teamwork and Collaboration
  - Communicate with an endocrinologist when questions or concerns are noted.
  - Psychological counseling may be indicated to help the child and family cope during this period of time.
- Care After Discharge
  - Nursing Actions
    - Inform the child and parents that there should not be any significant side effects when GH replacement therapy is used in appropriate doses for GH deficiency.
    - Inform the child and parents that GH will assist with muscle growth and help improve self-esteem.
  - Client Education
    - Reinforce teaching to the child and parents how to administer medication by subcutaneous injection for home use.
    - Explain to the child and parents that GH should be administered 6 to 7 days a week.
    - Inform the child and parents that GH usually is continued until bone maturation takes place. Radiologic evidence of epiphyseal closure is a criterion for ending therapy. This can be 16 years of age or older for boys and 14 years of age or older for girls.
    - Encourage the child and family to seek evaluation during early adulthood. Children who have GH deficiency in childhood should be evaluated in early adulthood to determine the need for continued replacement therapy.

Complications

- GH deficiency without hormone replacement can result in disruption of vertical growth, delayed epiphyseal closure, retarded bone age, delayed sexual development, and premature aging later in life.

APPLICATION EXERCISES

1. A nurse is caring for a child who has short stature. Which of the following diagnostic tests should the child undergo to confirm growth hormone (GH) deficiency? (Select all that apply.)

_____ A. CT scan of the head

_____ B. Bone age scan

_____ C. GH stimulation test

_____ D. Serum IGF-1

_____ E. DNA testing

2. A parent of a school-age child who has GH deficiency asks the nurse how long his son will need to take injections for his growth delay. Which of the following is an appropriate response by the nurse?

A. "Injections are usually continued until age 10 for girls and age 12 for boys."

B. "Injections continue until your child reaches the fifth percentile on the growth chart."

C. "Injections should be continued until there is evidence of epiphyseal closure."

D. "The injections will need to be administered throughout your child's entire life."

3. A nurse is collecting data on a child with short stature. Which of the following findings indicates a growth hormone deficiency?

A. Proportional height to weight

B. Height proportionally greater than weight

C. Weight proportionally greater than height

D. BMI greater than height/weight ratio

4. A nurse is reinforcing teaching with the parent of a child who has a growth hormone deficiency. Which of the following are complications of untreated growth hormone deficiency? (Select all that apply.)

_____ A. Delayed sexual development

_____ B. Premature aging

_____ C. Advanced bone age

_____ D. Short stature

_____ E. Increased epiphyseal closure

5. A nurse is preparing to administer somatropin (Genotropin) 0.2 mg/kg/week divided into six doses to a child who weighs 22 kg. Available is somatropin 5 mg/1.5 mL. How many mL should the nurse administer per dose? (Round the answer to the nearest tenth.)

6. A nurse is planning care for a child who is to undergo a growth hormone (GH) stimulation test. What interventions should the nurse contribute to the plan of care? Use the ATI Active Learning Template: Nursing Skill to complete this item to include two preprocedure nursing actions and three intraprocedure actions.

APPLICATION EXERCISES KEY

1. A. **CORRECT:** The child should undergo a CT scan of the head to determine whether there is a structural component to the short stature.

    B. **CORRECT:** The child should undergo a bone age scan to determine the development of the bones.

    C. **CORRECT:** The child should undergo a GH stimulation test to confirm diagnosis of GH deficiency.

    D. **CORRECT:** The child should undergo a serum IGF-1 as a preliminary test to determine GH deficiency.

    E. INCORRECT: DNA testing is not a diagnostic test to determine GH deficiency.

    (N) NCLEX® Connection: Reduction of Risk Potential, Diagnostic Tests

2. A. INCORRECT: The age for continuing injections is variable among clients.

    B. INCORRECT: The amount of growth necessary before discontinuing injections is variable among clients.

    C. **CORRECT:** Injections are continued until there is evidence of epiphyseal closure on radiographic tests.

    D. INCORRECT: Children do not need to receive injections throughout life.

    (N) NCLEX® Connection: Pharmacological Therapies, Expected Actions/Outcomes

3. A. **CORRECT:** Children who have growth hormone deficiency present with short stature with proportional height and weight.

    B. INCORRECT: Children who have growth hormone deficiency present with short stature with proportional height and weight.

    C. INCORRECT: Children who have growth hormone deficiency present with short stature with proportional height and weight.

    D. INCORRECT: Children who have growth hormone deficiency present with short stature with proportional height and weight.

    (N) NCLEX® Connection: Physiological Adaptations, Basic Pathophysiology

4. A. **CORRECT:** Complications of untreated growth hormone deficiency include delayed sexual development.

    B. **CORRECT:** Complications of untreated growth hormone deficiency include premature aging.

    C. INCORRECT: Complications of untreated growth hormone deficiency include retarded bone age.

    D. **CORRECT:** Complications of untreated growth hormone deficiency include short stature.

    E. INCORRECT: Complications of untreated growth hormone deficiency include delayed epiphyseal closure.

    (N) NCLEX® Connection: Physiological Adaptations, Alterations in Body Systems

5. **0.2** mL

Using Ratio and Proportion

STEP 1: *What is the unit of measurement to calculate?*
mg

STEP 2: *Set up an equation and solve for X.*
mg x kg/week = X
0.2 mg x 22 kg = 4.4 mg

STEP 3: *Round if necessary.*

STEP 4: *Reassess to determine whether the amount makes sense.*
If the prescribed amount is 0.2 mg/kg/week and the client weighs 22 kg, it makes sense to give 4.4 mg/week or 0.7333 mg per dose.

STEP 5: *What is the unit of measurement to calculate?*
mL

STEP 6: *What is the dose available? Dose available = Have.*
5 mg

STEP 7: *Should the nurse convert the units of measurement?*
No

STEP 8: *What is the quantity of the dose available?*
1.5 mL

STEP 9: *Set up an equation and solve for X.*

$$\frac{Have}{Quantity} = \frac{Desired}{X}$$

$$\frac{5 \text{ mg}}{1.5 \text{ mL}} = \frac{0.7333 \text{ mg}}{X \text{ mL}}$$

X = 0.2199

STEP 10: *Round if necessary.*
0.2199 = 0.2

STEP 11: *Reassess to determine whether the amount to give makes sense.*
If there are 5 mg/1.5 mL and the prescribed amount is 0.7333 mg, it makes sense to give 0.2 mL. The nurse should administer somatropin injection 0.2 mL subcutaneous per dose.

Using Desired over Have

STEP 1: *What is the unit of measurement to calculate?*
mg

STEP 2: *Set up an equation and solve for X.*
mg x kg/week = X
0.2 mg x 22 kg = 4.4 mg

STEP 3: *Round if necessary.*

STEP 4: *Reassess to determine whether the amount makes sense.*
If the prescribed amount is 0.2 mg/kg/week and the client weighs 22 kg, it makes sense to give 4.4 mg/week or 0.7333 mg per dose.

STEP 5: *What is the unit of measurement to calculate?*
mL

STEP 6: *What is the dose available? Dose available = Have.*
5 mg

STEP 7: *Should the nurse convert the units of measurement?*
No

STEP 8: *What is the quantity of the dose available?*
1.5 mL

STEP 9: *Set up an equation and solve for X.*

$$\frac{Desired \text{ x } Quantity}{Have} = X$$

$$\frac{0.7333 \text{ mg x } 1.5 \text{ mL}}{5 \text{ mg}} = X \text{ mL}$$

0.2199 = X

STEP 10: *Round if necessary.*
0.2199 = 0.2

STEP 11: *Reassess to determine whether the amount to give makes sense.*
If there are 5 mg/1.5 mL and the prescribed amount is 0.7333 mg, it makes sense to give 0.2 mL. The nurse should administer somatropin injection 0.2 mL subcutaneous per dose.

Using Dimensional Analysis

STEP 1: *What is the unit of measurement to calculate?*
mg

STEP 2: *Set up an equation and solve for X.*
mg x kg/week = X
0.2 mg x 22 kg = 4.4 mg

STEP 3: *Round if necessary.*

STEP 4: *Reassess to determine whether the amount makes sense.*
If the prescribed amount is 0.2 mg/kg/week and the client weighs 22 kg, it makes sense to give 4.4 mg/week or 0.7333 mg per dose.

STEP 5: *What is the unit of measurement to calculate?*
mL

STEP 6: *What is the dose available? Dose available = Have.*
5 mg

STEP 7: *Should the nurse convert the units of measurement?*
No

STEP 8: *What is the quantity of the dose available?*
1.5 mL

STEP 9: *Set up an equation and solve for X.*

$$X = \frac{Quantity}{Have} \times \frac{Conversion\ (Have)}{Conversion\ (Desired)} \times \frac{Desired}{}$$

$$X\ mL = \frac{1.5\ mL}{5\ mg} \times \frac{0.7333\ mg}{}$$

X = 0.2199

STEP 10: *Round if necessary.*
0.2199 = 0.2

STEP 11: *Reassess to determine whether the amount to give makes sense.*
If there are 5 mg/1.5 mL and the prescribed amount is 0.7333 mg, it makes sense to give 0.2 mL. The nurse should administer somatropin injection 0.2 mL subcutaneous per dose.

(N) NCLEX® Connection: Pharmacological Therapies, Dosage Calculation

6. *Using the ATI Active Learning Template: Nursing Skill*

- Preprocedure
  - Have nothing to eat or drink 10 to 12 hr prior to procedure.
  - Limit activity 10 to 12 hr prior to procedure.
- Intraprocedure
  - Assist with obtaining a baseline blood sample between 0600 and 0800.
  - Administer medication that triggers the release of GH (arginine or GH-releasing hormone).
  - Assist with obtaining a blood sample every 30 min during a 3-hr period following medication administration.

(N) NCLEX® Connection: Reduction of Risk Potential, Therapeutic Procedures

UNIT 2   Nursing Care of Children with System Disorders

SECTION: IMMUNE AND INFECTIOUS DISORDERS

› Immunizations
› Communicable Diseases
› Acute Otitis Media
› HIV/AIDS

NCLEX® CONNECTIONS

When reviewing the chapters in this section, keep in mind the relevant sections of the NCLEX® outline, in particular:

Client Needs: Safety and Infection Control

› Relevant topics/tasks include
  » Standard Precautions/ Transmission-Based Precautions/Surgical Asepsis
    › Identify communicable diseases and modes of transmission.
    › Identify client knowledge of infection control procedures.
    › Identify the need for and implement appropriate isolation technique.

Client Needs: Pharmacological Therapies

› Relevant topics/tasks include
  » Medication Administration
    › Administer a subcutaneous, intradermal or intramuscular medication.

Client Needs: Health Promotion and Maintenance

› Relevant topics/tasks include
  » Health Promotion/Disease Prevention
    › Identify clients in need of immunizations.
    › Identify precautions and contraindications to immunizations.

Client Needs: Reduction of Risk Potential

› Relevant topics/tasks include
  » Therapeutic Procedures
    › Reinforce client teaching on treatments and procedures.

Client Needs: Physiological Adaptations

› Relevant topics/tasks include
  » Alterations in Body Systems
    › Reinforce education to client regarding care and condition.
  » Basic Pathophysiology
    › Identify sign and symptoms related to an acute or chronic illness.
    › Consider general principles of client disease process when providing care.
    › Apply knowledge of pathophysiology to monitoring client for alterations in body systems.

chapter 33

Overview

- Administration of a vaccine stimulates the immune system to produce antibodies against that specific disease.
- Vaccines have the same antigen as the disease, but it is either killed or weakened, and therefore not strong enough to cause the disease.
- Antibodies will disappear after they have destroyed the infection/antigen. But memory cells are formed to protect from future exposures to that same infection. This is called immunity.
- The Advisory Committee on Immunization Practices (ACIP) makes recommendations and creates guidelines regarding immunizations.
- The most up-to-date information can be found at the Centers for Disease Control and Prevention website (www.cdc.gov).

Childhood Immunizations

MINIMUM AGE	NUMBER OF DOSES	SCHEDULE	CONSIDERATIONS
Hepatitis B (HepB)			
Birth	3	Birth 1 to 2 months 6 to 18 months	› Minimum of 4 weeks between doses 1 and 2. › Minimum of 8 weeks between doses 2 and 3. › Final dose no earlier than 24 weeks, and at least 16 weeks after first dose.
Rotavirus (RV)			
6 weeks	2	2 months 4 months	› Maximum age for the first dose is 14 weeks, 6 days. › Maximum age for the last dose is 8 months. › Series should not be initiated for children older than 15 weeks.
Diphtheria, tetanus, pertussis (DTaP)			
6 weeks	5	2 months 4 months 6 months 15 to 18 months 4 to 6 years 11 to 12 years Booster every 10 years	› Minimum of 6 months between doses 3 and 4. › Booster can be either Tdap or Td.

MINIMUM AGE	NUMBER OF DOSES	SCHEDULE	CONSIDERATIONS
Haemophilus influenzae type b (Hib)			
6 weeks	3	2 months 4 months 12 to 15 months	
Pneumococcal (PCV)			
6 weeks	4	2 months 4 months 6 months 12 to 15 months	
Inactivated poliovirus (IPV)			
6 weeks	4	2 months 4 months 6 to 18 months 4 to 6 years	› Final dose should be administered after 4 years and at least 6 months from the previous dose.
Influenza (TIV)			
6 weeks	Yearly	Yearly	› Must be 2 years or older to receive live vaccine (LAIV). › Children who have medical conditions that predispose them to influenza should not receive the live vaccine. › Administer starting with availability, usually October.
Measles, mumps, rubella (MMR)			
12 months	2	12 to 15 months 4 to 6 years	› MMR should be given to children ages 6 months through 11 months if traveling internationally. However, these children still need the scheduled MMR immunizations.
Varicella (VAR)			
12 months	2	12 to 15 months 4 to 6 years	
Hepatitis A (HepA)			
12 months	2	12 months to 2 years 6 to 18 months following	› Administer the final dose 6 to 18 months after the first.
Meningococcal (MCV4)			
9 months	1	11 to 12 years	› Can be given earlier for high-risk groups. › If vaccine given prior to 16 years, a booster is recommended.
Human papillomavirus			
9 years	3	11 to 12 years	› Administer second dose 1 to 2 months after first. › Administer third dose 6 months after first dose.

- For children who have missed scheduled immunizations, use the "catch-up" schedule.

Purpose

- Decrease or eliminate certain infectious diseases in society.
- Prevent infectious diseases and their complications.

Complications/Contraindications/Precautions

Q
EBP

- An anaphylactic reaction to a vaccine is a contraindication for receiving further doses of that vaccine.
- An anaphylactic reaction to a vaccine is a contraindication for using other vaccines containing that substance.
- Contraindications to all immunizations include severe allergies to any component of a vaccine.
- Moderate or severe illnesses with or without fever are contraindications to receiving immunizations. With acute febrile illness, immunization is deferred until symptoms resolve. The common cold and other minor illnesses are not contraindications.
- Contraindications to immunizations require health care providers to analyze data and weigh the risks that come with vaccinating or not vaccinating.

ADVERSE EFFECTS	CONTRAINDICATIONS
DTaP	
› Local reaction at the injection site › Fever and irritability › Crying that cannot be consoled and lasts up to 3 hr › Seizures › Rare – acute encephalopathy	› An occurrence of encephalopathy 7 days after the administration of the vaccine › An occurrence of seizures within 3 days of the immunization › A history of uncontrollable, inconsolable crying after a prior immunization (may have lasted more than 3 hr and occurred within 48 hr of immunization)
Hib	
› Mild local reactions and a low-grade fever › Rare – temperature greater than 38.5° C (101.3° F), vomiting, and crying	
RV	
› Irritability › Mild, temporary diarrhea or vomiting	› Intussusception › Immunocompromised
IPV	
› Local reaction at injection site	› Allergy to neomycin (Mycifradin) and/or streptomycin and polymyxin B › Pregnancy
MMR	
› Local reactions (rash; fever; swollen glands in cheeks, neck, and under the jaw) › Possibility of joint pain lasting for days to weeks › Risk for anaphylaxis and thrombocytopenia	› Pregnancy › Allergy to gelatin and neomycin › History of thrombocytopenia or thrombocytopenic purpura › Immunosuppression (with HIV infection or from medication administration) › Recent transfusion with blood products or immunoglobulins

ADVERSE EFFECTS	CONTRAINDICATIONS
Varicella vaccine	
› Varicella-like rash that is local or generalized (vesicles on the body) › Seizure	› Pregnancy › Cancers of blood and lymphatic system › Allergy to gelatin neomycin › Corticosteroids › Immunosuppression (with HIV or from medication administration)
PCV	
› Mild local reactions	
HepA	
› Local reaction at the injection site › Headache › Loss of appetite › Tiredness	
HepB	
› Local reaction at the injection site › Temperature of 37.7° C (99.9° F) or higher	› Allergy to baker's yeast
Influenza vaccine; TIV: Influenza (inactivated) vaccine; LAIV: Influenza (live) vaccine (nasal)	

› TIV – mild local reaction, and fever
› LAIV – headache, cough, and fever
› Rare – risk for Guillain-Barré syndrome
	› Hypersensitivity to eggs
	› LAIV
	  » Younger than 2 years old
	  » Immunosuppression
	  » Chronic disease

Meningococcal Conjugate vaccine (MCV4)	
› Mild local reaction › Rare – risk for allergic response	› History of Guillain-Barré syndrome
HPV2 and HPV4	
› Mild local reaction and fever › Fainting (shortly after receiving the immunization) › Headache	› Pregnancy › Hypersensitivity to yeast

Nursing Administration

- Infants and Children
  - Obtain parental consent for children.
  - Note the date, route, and site of immunization on the child's immunization record at the time of immunization.
  - Give intramuscular immunizations in the vastus lateralis or ventrogluteal muscle in infants and young children, and into the deltoid muscle for older children and adolescents.
  - Give subcutaneous injections in the outer aspect of the upper arm or anterolateral thigh.
  - Use an appropriately sized needle for the route, site, age, and amount of medication.
  - Use strategies to minimize discomfort.
  - Provide for distraction.
  - Encourage the parents to use comforting measures during the procedure (cuddling, pacifiers) and after the procedure (application of cool compresses to injection site, gentle movement of the involved extremity).
  - Provide praise afterward.
  - Apply a colorful bandage, if appropriate.
  - Have emergency medications and equipment on standby in case the child experiences an allergic response, such as anaphylaxis (rare).
  - Follow storage and reconstitution directions. If reconstituted, use within 30 min.
  - Provide written vaccine information sheets and review the content with parents or clients.
  - Reinforce teaching to the parents and child about observing for complications and to notify the provider if adverse effects occur.
  - Encourage the parents to maintain up-to-date immunizations for the child.
  - Document the administration of the vaccine, including the date, route, and site of immunization; type, manufacturer, lot number, and expiration date of the vaccine; and name, address, and signature of the child and/or parent.
  - Reinforce teaching to the parents about avoiding administration of aspirin to the child to treat fever or local reaction due to the risk of the development of Reye syndrome.
  - Give an infant concentrated oral sucrose solution on a pacifier 2 min prior to, during, and 3 min after injections.
  - Apply a topical anesthetic prior to the injection.
  - Observe for and report adverse reactions to the provider, who will provide updates to the Vaccine Adverse Event Reporting System.

Nursing Evaluation of Medication Effectiveness

- Depending on therapeutic intent, effectiveness may be evidenced by:
  - Improvement of local reaction to immunization with absence of pain, fever, and swelling at the site of injection
  - Development of immunity

APPLICATION EXERCISES

1. A nurse is preparing to administer immunizations to a 6-month-old infant. Which of the following is an appropriate action for the nurse to take in providing atraumatic care?

    A. Administer 81 mg of aspirin.

    B. Use the Z-track method when injecting.

    C. Ask the parents to leave the room during the injection.

    D. Provide sucrose solution on the pacifier.

2. A nurse is planning to administer immunizations to a 2-month-old infant. Which of the following should the nurse anticipate giving? (Select all that apply.)

    _____ A. Rotavirus (RV)

    _____ B. Diphtheria, tetanus, pertussis (DTaP)

    _____ C. Haemophilus influenzae type b (Hib)

    _____ D. Hepatitis A (HepA)

    _____ E. Pneumococcal (PCV)

    _____ F. Varicella (VAR)

3. A nurse is planning to administer immunizations to a 4-year-old child who has up-to-date immunizations. Which of the following should the nurse anticipate giving? (Select all that apply.)

    _____ A. Inactivated poliovirus (IPV)

    _____ B. Haemophilus influenzae type b (Hib)

    _____ C. Measles, mumps, rubella (MMR)

    _____ D. Varicella (VAR)

    _____ E. Hepatitis B (HepB)

    _____ F. Diphtheria, tetanus, pertussis (DTaP)

4. A nurse is preparing to administer varicella vaccine to an adolescent. Which of the following questions should the nurse ask to determine whether there is a contraindication to administering the vaccine?

    A. "Do you have an allergy to eggs?"

    B. "Have you ever had encephalopathy following immunizations?"

    C. "Are you currently taking a corticosteroid medication?"

    D. "Do you have a hypersensitivity to yeast?"

5. A nurse is preparing to administer an immunization intramuscularly to an infant. In which of the following sites should the nurse administer the injection?

    A. Deltoid

    B. Outer aspect of the upper arm

    C. Ventrogluteal

    D. Anterolateral thigh

6. A nurse is preparing to work in an immunization clinic. Use the ATI Active Learning Template: Basic Concept to complete this item to include the following:

    A. Related Concept: List all immunizations given during childhood.

    B. Underlying Principles: List the recommended ages of each immunization.

APPLICATION EXERCISES KEY

1.   A. INCORRECT: Aspirin is contraindicated in children due to the risk of Reye's syndrome. This is not an appropriate action for the nurse to take.

   B. INCORRECT: Using the Z-track method is not recommended with immunizations. This is not an appropriate action for the nurse to take.

   C. INCORRECT: Separating the parents from the infant can produce anxiety in the infant. This is not an appropriate action for the nurse to take.

   D. **CORRECT:** Allowing an infant to suck on a pacifier with sucrose solution can decrease pain with immunizations and is an appropriate action for the nurse to take in providing atraumatic care.

   Ⓝ NCLEX® Connection: Pharmacological Therapies, Medication Administration

2.   A. **CORRECT:** Two doses of rotavirus vaccine are given during childhood starting at 2 months of age.

   B. **CORRECT:** Six doses of diphtheria, tetanus, pertussis vaccine are given during childhood starting at 2 months of age.

   C. **CORRECT:** Three doses of haemophilus influenzae type b vaccine are given during childhood starting at 2 months of age.

   D. INCORRECT: Two doses of hepatitis A vaccine are given during childhood starting at 12 months of age.

   E. **CORRECT:** Four doses of pneumococcal vaccine are given during childhood starting at 2 months of age.

   F. INCORRECT: Two doses of varicella vaccine are given during childhood starting at 12 months of age.

   Ⓝ NCLEX® Connection: Health Promotion and Maintenance, Health Promotion/Disease Prevention

3.   A. **CORRECT:** Four doses of IPV are given during childhood with a dose given at 4 years of age.

   B. INCORRECT: Three doses of Hib vaccine are given during childhood scheduled at 2, 4, and 12 months of age.

   C. **CORRECT:** Two doses of MMR vaccine are given during childhood with a dose given at 4 years of age.

   D. **CORRECT:** Two doses of VAR are given during childhood with a dose given at 4 years of age.

   E. INCORRECT: Three doses of HepB vaccine are given during childhood scheduled at birth, 2, and 6 to 18 months of age.

   F. **CORRECT:** Five doses of DTaP vaccine are given during childhood with a dose given at 4 years of age.

   Ⓝ NCLEX® Connection: Health Promotion and Maintenance, Health Promotion/Disease Prevention

4.   A. INCORRECT: Influenza vaccine is contraindicated in clients who have an allergy to eggs.

    B. INCORRECT: DTaP vaccine is contraindicated in clients who have a history of encephalopathy following immunizations.

    C. **CORRECT:** Varicella vaccine is contraindicated in clients who are currently taking corticosteroid medications.

    D. INCORRECT: HepB vaccine is contraindicated in clients who have a hypersensitivity to yeast.

    (N) NCLEX® Connection: Health Promotion and Maintenance, Health Promotion/Disease Prevention

5.   A. INCORRECT: The deltoid muscle is an appropriate administration site for older children and adolescents, but is not appropriate for an infant.

    B. INCORRECT: The outer aspect of the upper arm is an appropriate administration site for subcutaneous injections, not intramuscular injections.

    C. **CORRECT:** The ventrogluteal or vastus lateralis muscle is the recommended administration site for intramuscular injections in infants.

    D. INCORRECT: The anterolateral thigh is an appropriate administration site for subcutaneous injections, not intramuscular injections.

    (N) NCLEX® Connection: Pharmacological Therapies, Medication Administration

6.   *Using the ATI Active Learning Template: Basic Concept*

    A. Related Concept/B. Underlying Principles

- Hepatitis B (HepB)
  - Birth
  - 1 to 2 months
  - 6 to 18 months
- Rotavirus (RV)
  - 2 months
  - 4 months
- Diphtheria, tetanus, pertussis (DTaP)
  - 2 months
  - 4 months
  - 6 months
  - 15 to 18 months
  - 4 to 6 years
  - 11 to 12 years
  - Booster every 10 years

- Haemophilus influenzae type b4 (Hib)
  - 2 months
  - 4 months
  - 12 to 15 months
- Pneumococcal (PCV)
  - 2 months
  - 4 months
  - 6 months
  - 12 to 15 months
- Inactivated poliovirus (IPV)
  - 2 months
  - 4 months
  - 6 to 18 months
  - 4 to 6 years

- Measles, mumps, rubella (MMR)
  - 12 to 15 months
  - 4 to 6 years
- Varicella (VAR)
  - 12 to 15 months
  - 4 to 6 years
- Hepatitis A (HepA)
  - 12 months to 2 years
  - 6 to 18 months following
- Meningococcal (MCV4)
  - 11 to 12 years
- Influenza (TIV)
  - Yearly
- Human papillomavirus
  - 11 to 12 years (3 doses)

    (N) NCLEX® Connection: Health Promotion and Maintenance, Health Promotion/Disease Prevention

chapter 34

Overview

- Communicable diseases are spread easily through airborne, droplet, or direct contact transmission.
- Most communicable diseases can be prevented with immunizations.

Health Promotion and Disease Prevention

SPREAD	INCUBATION	COMMUNICABILITY
Conjunctivitis		
› Direct contact (viral and bacterial)	› Depends on the infection	› Viral: Appears secondary to a viral infection; clears on own in 7 to 14 days.
		› Bacterial: Starts in one eye, spreads to the other; clears with antibiotics.
		› Allergic: Occurs in people who have other allergic conditions; clears with allergy medications.
Epstein-Barr virus (EBV)/mononucleosis		
› Saliva	› 4 to 6 weeks	› Healthy people can carry EBV in saliva, transmitting the virus for a lifetime.
		› People who have mononucleosis can transmit for weeks.
Erythema infectiosum (fifth disease)/parvovirus B19		
› Droplet › Blood	› 4 to 14 days, sometimes up to 20 days	› Onset of symptoms before rash appears.
Hand, foot, and mouth disease (HFMD)		
› Direct contact	› 4 to 6 days	› Most contagious during the first week of illness, contagious even when free from symptoms.
Mumps/paramyxovirus		
› Direct contact › Droplet › Surfaces, contaminated objects	› 12 to 25 days	› Immediately before and 5 days after swelling begins.

SPREAD	INCUBATION	COMMUNICABILITY
Pertussis (whooping cough)/Bordetella pertussis		
› Direct contact › Droplet	› 7 to 10 days	› Catarrhal stage through 2 weeks into the paroxysmal stage.
Rubella (German measles)/rubella virus		
› Direct contact › Droplet	› 12 to 23 days	› 7 days before to 5 to 7 days after the rash.
Rubeola (measles)/rubeola virus		
› Direct contact › Droplet › Can survive 2 hr on surfaces	› 7 to 18 days	› 4 days before to 4 days after rash.
Varicella (chickenpox)/varicella-zoster virus		
› Direct contact › Droplet › From person with shingles	› 10 to 21 days	› 1 to 2 days before lesions appear until all lesions have scabs.

M View Images
 › Chickenpox   › Rubella   › Mumps

Data Collection

- Risk Factors
  - Immunocompromised status
  - Crowded living conditions
  - Poor sanitation
  - Poor nutrition
  - Poor oxygenation and impaired circulation
  - Chronic illness
  - Recent exposure to a known case of a communicable disease
  - Not immunized or up to date on immunizations
- Subjective and Objective Data
  - Conjunctivitis
    - Pink or red color in the whites of the eyes
    - Swelling of the conjunctiva
    - Tearing
    - Yellow-green pus discharge from the eyes
    - Crusting of the eyelids in the morning

- ○ Fifth Disease
  - ▪ Before rash (several days)
    - ▫ Fever, runny nose, headache
  - ▪ Rash (7 to 10 days to several weeks)
    - ▫ Red rash on face (slapped cheek)
    - ▫ Secondary itchy rash can appear on rest of body, especially on the soles of the feet
- ○ Hand, Foot, and Mouth Disease
  - ▪ 1 to 2 days before rash and mouth sores
    - ▫ Fever and sore throat
    - ▫ Malaise and poor appetite
  - ▪ Rash and mouth sores
    - ▫ Painful sores in the mouth, blisters that become ulcers
    - ▫ Skin rash that is flat or raised red spots, usually on the hands and soles of the feet
- ○ Infectious Mononucleosis
  - ▪ Fever
  - ▪ Sore throat
  - ▪ Swollen lymph glands
  - ▪ Increased WBC
  - ▪ Atypical lymphocytes
  - ▪ Splenomegaly
  - ▪ Enlarged liver
- ○ Measles (rubeola)
  - ▪ 3 to 5 days prior to rash
    - ▫ Mild to moderate fever
    - ▫ Cough, runny nose, red eyes, sore throat
  - ▪ Rash
    - ▫ Koplik's spots (tiny white spots) appear in mouth
    - ▫ Red or reddish-brown rash beginning on the face spreading downward
    - ▫ Spike in fever with rash
- ○ Mumps
  - ▪ Painful swollen salivary glands
  - ▪ Fever and muscle aches
  - ▪ Abdominal pain
  - ▪ Fatigue and loss of appetite

- ○ Pertussis (whooping cough)
  - ▪ Common cold symptoms (runny nose/congestion, sneezing, mild fever, mild cough)
  - ▪ Severe coughing starts in 1 to 2 weeks
    - □ Coughing fits
    - □ Violent and rapid coughing
    - □ Loud "whooping" sound
- ○ Rubella (German measles)
  - ▪ Low-grade fever and sore throat
  - ▪ Red rash that starts on the face and spreads to the rest of the body, lasting 2 to 3 days
- ○ Varicella (chickenpox)
  - ▪ Symptoms 1 to 2 days prior to rash
    - □ High fever
    - □ Fatigue
    - □ Loss of appetite
    - □ Headache
  - ▪ Rash
    - □ Macules start in trunk and face, spreading to rest of the body, progressing to papules.
    - □ Vesicles follow, with crusts forming.
    - □ Scabs appear in approximately 1 week.
- • Laboratory Tests
  - ○ CBC
  - ○ Electrolyte panels
  - ○ Mono spot blood test for infectious mononucleosis

Patient-Centered Care

- • Nursing Care
  - ○ Symptomatic treatment
    - ▪ Isolation Precautions
      - □ Airborne/Contact
        - ▸ Varicella
      - □ Droplet
        - ▸ Rubella
        - ▸ Fifth disease
        - ▸ Pertussis
        - ▸ Mumps
      - □ Standard
        - ▸ Mononucleosis
        - ▸ Hand, foot, and mouth disease
        - ▸ Conjunctivitis

- Administer an antipyretic for fever. Do not administer aspirin, due to the risk of Reye syndrome.
- Administer analgesics for pain.
- Provide fluids and nutritious foods the child prefers.
- Skin care
  - Provide calamine lotion for topical relief.
  - Keep the child's skin clean and dry to prevent secondary infection.
  - Keep the child cool, but prevent chilling.
  - Dress the child in lightweight, loose clothing.
  - Give baths in tepid water, possibly with oatmeal.
  - Keep the child's fingernails clean and short.
  - Apply mittens if the child scratches.
  - Teach good oral hygiene. The child can gargle with warm water for a sore throat.
  - Change linens daily.
- Provide quiet diversional activities.
- Promote adequate rest with naps if necessary.
- Keep lights dim if the child develops photophobia.
- Keep the child out of the sun.
- Notify the child's school or day care center of the child's infection. Obtain a plan from the school so that the child can continue working on schoolwork at home.
- Notify the health department of communicable diseases.

- Medications
  - Antihistamine – diphenhydramine and hydroxyzine (Atarax)
    - Used to control pruritus
    - Nursing Considerations
      - Monitor the child's reaction to the medication because some children can become hyperalert with the administration of a medication from this group.
      - Monitor the child for drowsiness.
    - Client Education
      - Educate the family about safety precautions.
  - Antibiotic or antiviral therapy
    - Acyclovir (Zovirax) for high-risk clients who have varicella or mononucleosis
    - Antibiotics for pertussis
    - Antibiotic eye drops for bacterial conjunctivitis
  - NSAIDs or acetaminophen (Tylenol)
    - Decreases fever
    - Nursing Consideration – Be alert for allergies.
    - Client Education – Reinforce teaching to parents about the appropriate dosing for acetaminophen.

- Care After Discharge
  - Client Education
    - Good hand hygiene prevents spread of infection.
    - Encourage adherence with antibiotic or antiviral therapy.
    - Reinforce teaching to the parents about having the child cover her nose and mouth when coughing or sneezing.
    - Reinforce teaching to parents about washing the child's bed linens daily in mild detergent.
    - Reinforce teaching to parents of children who are immunocompromised to seek prompt medical care if symptoms develop.
    - Encourage adolescents to participate in decision-making.

Complications

- Fifth Disease
  - People who have a weakened immune system are at risk for serous complications, anemia, secondary infections
- Hand, Foot, and Mouth Disease
  - Viral or aseptic meningitis
- Mononucleosis
  - Ruptured spleen
- Mumps
  - Orchitis, encephalitis, meningitis, oophoritis, mastitis, deafness
- Pertussis
  - Infants and children: pneumonia, convulsions, apnea, encephalopathy, death
  - Teens and adults: weight loss, loss of bladder control, passing out, rib fractures
- Rubella
  - Birth defects (deafness; heart defects; mental, liver, and spleen damage) in fetus of women infected during pregnancy
- Rubeola
  - Ear infections, pneumonia, diarrhea, encephalitis, death
- Varicella
  - Dehydration, pneumonia, bleeding problems, bacterial infection of the skin, sepsis, toxic shock syndrome, bone or joint infections, death

APPLICATION EXERCISES

1. A nurse is reinforcing teaching to a group of parents about complications of communicable diseases. Which of the following communicable diseases can lead to pneumonia? (Select all that apply.)

_____ A. Rubella (German measles)

_____ B. Rubeola (measles)

_____ C. Pertussis (whooping cough)

_____ D. Varicella (chickenpox)

_____ E. Mumps

2. A nurse is collecting data from an adolescent client who has mononucleosis. The client exhibits fever, fatigue, swollen lymph nodes, sore throat, and a sore upper abdomen. The nurse should reinforce which of the following instructions with the adolescent and her parents? (Select all that apply.)

_____ A. Take antibiotics until symptoms subside.

_____ B. Drink plenty of liquids.

_____ C. Avoid participating in strenuous activities.

_____ D. Allow for periods of rest.

_____ E. Take aspirin as needed for fever and discomfort.

_____ F. Gargle with saltwater every 2 to 3 hr.

3. A nurse is reinforcing teaching to the parent of a child who has hand, foot, and mouth disease. Which of the following should be included in the teaching?

A. "Your child can be contagious when the symptoms are gone."

B. "The incubation period is 10 to 21 days."

C. "It is transmitted by droplet."

D. "Once infected, your child will be a lifetime carrier."

4. A nurse is collecting data from a client who has pertussis. Which of the following are clinical manifestations of pertussis? (Select all that apply.)

_____ A. Runny nose

_____ B. Mild fever

_____ C. Whooping sound cough

_____ D. Swollen salivary glands

_____ E. Red rash

5. A nurse is reinforcing teaching to a group of parents about communicable diseases. Which of the following is the most appropriate method to prevent a communicable disease?

A. Handwashing

B. Avoiding persons with active disease

C. Covering your cough

D. Obtaining immunizations

6. A nurse is planning care for a group of clients who have communicable diseases. Use the ATI Active Learning Template: Basic Concept to complete this item to include the following sections:

A. Related Content: List the communicable diseases that require more than standard isolation precautions during hospitalization.

B. Nursing Interventions: Identify the type of isolation precaution to be implemented with the communicable disease identified above.

APPLICATION EXERCISES KEY

1. A. INCORRECT: Complications of rubella include birth defects (deafness; heart defects; brain, liver, and spleen damage) in the fetus of a woman infected during pregnancy.

   B. **CORRECT:** Complications of rubeola include ear infections, pneumonia, diarrhea, encephalitis, and death.

   C. **CORRECT:** Complications of pertussis include pneumonia, convulsions, apnea, encephalopathy, and death in infants and children; and weight loss, loss of bladder control, passing out, and rib fractures in teens and adults.

   D. **CORRECT:** Complications of varicella include dehydration, pneumonia, bleeding problems, bacterial infection of the skin, sepsis, toxic shock syndrome, bone or joint infections, and death.

   E. INCORRECT: Complications of mumps include orchitis, encephalitis, meningitis, oophoritis, mastitis, and deafness.

   (N) NCLEX® Connection: Safety and Infection Control, Standard Precautions/Transmission-Based Precautions/Surgical Asepsis

2. A. INCORRECT: Antivirals are prescribed to clients who have mononucleosis.

   B. **CORRECT:** Fluids are encouraged to prevent dehydration with illness.

   C. **CORRECT:** The spleen could rupture as a result of injury. Therefore, strenuous activities should be avoided.

   D. **CORRECT:** Fatigue is common in clients who have mononucleosis. Therefore, allowing for periods of rest facilitates healing.

   E. INCORRECT: Acetaminophen (Tylenol) is used to control fever and discomfort.

   F. **CORRECT:** Gargling with saltwater can soothe discomfort associated with a sore throat.

   (N) NCLEX® Connection: Physiological Adaptations, Alterations in Body Systems

3. A. **CORRECT:** Children are most contagious the first week of illness. However, they can be contagious even when symptoms are gone.

   B. INCORRECT: The incubation period of varicella is 10 to 21 days.

   C. INCORRECT: Varicella, rubella, rubeola, and mumps are examples of communicable diseases transmitted by droplet.

   D. INCORRECT: Healthy people who have EBV can transmit infection for a lifetime.

   (N) NCLEX® Connection: Physiological Adaptations, Alterations in Body Systems

4.   A. **CORRECT:** A client who has pertussis has coldlike symptoms, including runny nose, congestion, and mild fever.

   B. **CORRECT:** A client who has pertussis has coldlike symptoms, including runny nose, congestion, and mild fever.

   C. **CORRECT:** A client who has pertussis will experience coughing fits and a whooping sound.

   D. INCORRECT: A client who has mumps will have enlarged lymph nodes.

   E. INCORRECT: A client who has measles will have a red rash.

   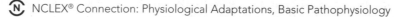 NCLEX® Connection: Physiological Adaptations, Basic Pathophysiology

5.   A. INCORRECT: Handwashing will decrease the spread of infection. However, this is not the best method to prevent communicable disease.

   B. INCORRECT: Avoiding people who have active disease will decrease the spread of infection. However, this is not the best method to prevent communicable disease.

   C. INCORRECT: Covering coughs will decrease the spread of infection. However, this is not the best method to prevent communicable disease.

   D. **CORRECT:** Obtaining immunizations has decreased the rate of communicable diseases and is the best method to prevent further spread of illness.

   N NCLEX® Connection: Safety and Infection Control, Standard Precautions/Transmission-Based Precautions/Surgical Asepsis

6.   *Using ATI Active Learning Template: Basic Concept*

   A. Related Content
   - Varicella
   - Rubella
   - Fifth disease
   - Pertussis
   - Mumps

   B. Nursing Interventions
   - Airborne/contact: varicella
   - Droplet: rubella, fifth disease, pertussis, mumps

   N NCLEX® Connection: Safety and Infection Control, Standard Precautions/Transmission-Based Precautions/Surgical Asepsis

chapter 35

Overview

- Acute otitis media (AOM) is an infection of the structures of the middle ear with rapid clinical symptoms of infection.

- Otitis media with effusion (OME) is a collection of fluid in the middle ear but with no symptoms of infection.

- Repeated infections can cause impaired hearing and speech delays.

- Many infections clear spontaneously in a few days.

- The majority of incidences are related to eustachian tube malfunction.

Data Collection

- Risk Factors

  - The eustachian tubes in children are shorter and more horizontal than those of adults. Otitis media is most common in the first 24 months of life and again when children enter school (ages 5 to 6). Otitis media occurs infrequently after age 7.

  - Otitis media usually is triggered by a bacterial infection (Streptococcus pneumoniae, Haemophilus influenzae, Moraxella catarrhalis), a viral infection (respiratory syncytial virus or influenza), allergies, or enlarged adenoids.

  - There is a lower incidence of otitis media in infants who are breastfed (possibly due to the presence of immunoglobulin A [IgA] in breast milk), which protects against infection.

  - Incidence is higher in the winter months.

  - Exposure to large numbers of children (day care).

  - Exposure to secondhand smoke.

  - Cleft lip and/or cleft palate.

  - Down syndrome.

- Subjective Data

  - Recent history of upper respiratory infection

  - Acute onset of changes in behavior

  - Frequent crying, irritability, and fussiness

  - Inconsolability

  - Tugging at ear

  - Reports of ear pain, loss of appetite, nausea, and vomiting

- Objective Data
  - Physical Assessment Findings
    - AOM
      - Rubbing or pulling on ear
      - Crying
      - Lethargy
      - Bulging yellow or red tympanic membrane

 View Image: Acute Otitis Media

      - Purulent material in middle ear or drainage from external canal
      - Decreased or no tympanic movement with pneumatic otoscopy
      - Lymphadenopathy of the neck and head
      - Temperature (can be as high as 40° C [104° F])
      - Hearing difficulties and speech delays if otitis media becomes a chronic condition
    - OME
      - Feeling of fullness in the ear
      - Orange discoloration of the tympanic membrane with decreased movement
      - Vague findings including rhinitis, cough, and diarrhea
      - Transient hearing loss and balance disturbances
  - Diagnostic Procedures
    - Pneumatic otoscope
      - A pneumatic otoscope is used to visualize the tympanic membrane and middle ear structures. The otoscope also assesses tympanic membrane movement.
      - Nursing Actions
        - Gently pull the pinna down and back to visualize the tympanic membrane of a child younger than 3 years old. For a child older than 3 years, gently pull the pinna up and back.

Patient-Centered Care

- Nursing Care
  - Provide comfort measures.
    - Administer pain medication as needed.
    - Provide diversional activities.
  - Place child in an upright position.
  - Management of fevers.
- Medications
  - Acetaminophen (Tylenol) or ibuprofen (Advil)
    - Used to provide analgesia and reduce fever
    - Nursing Considerations
      - Obtain a liquid preparation.
      - Use age-appropriate techniques to administer medication.
  - Antibiotics
    - Amoxicillin (Amoxil), amoxicillin-clavulanate (Augmentin), or azithromycin (Zithromax) PO (10 to 14 days)
    - Ceftriaxone (Rocephin) IM (once)
    - Nursing Considerations
      - Wait 72 hr for spontaneous resolution of otitis media before starting antibiotic.
      - Administer in high doses orally, usually 80 to 90 mg/kg/day in two divided doses.
      - The usual course of treatment orally is 10 to 14 days in children younger than 6 years of age. The course can be shorter for older children.
      - IM is used for resistant organisms or for client-specific reasons (difficulty taking oral medications, inability to complete the oral course).
    - Client Education
      - Reinforce teaching to the family that the child should complete the total course of treatment.
      - Observe for signs of allergy to the antibiotic, such as rash or difficulty breathing.
  - Benzocaine (Americaine Otic)
    - Ear drops for topical pain relief
    - Client Education
      - Reinforce teaching to the family on appropriately administering ear drops.
      - Discourage the use of decongestants or antihistamines.

- Therapeutic Procedures
  - Myringotomy and placement of tympanoplasty tubes may be indicated for a child who has multiple episodes of otitis media. This procedure can now be performed by laser treatment.
    - This procedure is performed in an outpatient setting with the administration of general anesthesia. It is usually completed in 15 min.
    - A small incision is made in the tympanic membrane, and tiny plastic or metal tubes are placed into the eardrum to equalize pressure and minimize effusion.
    - Recovery takes place in a PACU, and discharge usually occurs within 1 hr.
    - Postoperative pain is not common and, if present, will be mild.
    - The tubes come out spontaneously (usually in 6 to 12 months).
    - Client Education
      - Limit the child's activities for a few days following surgery.
      - Inform the parents to notify the provider when tubes come out. This usually does not require replacement of tubes.
- Surgical Interventions
  - Reinforce instruction to the family about not allowing water to enter the child's ears while the tubes are in place. The effectiveness of earplugs is not conclusive. Encourage the parents to follow the health care provider's instructions.
- Care After Discharge
  - Client Education
    - Inform the client/parents about comfort measures.
    - Encourage the parents to feed the child in an upright position when bottle or breastfeeding.
    - If drainage is present, clean the external ear with sterile cotton swabs. Apply antibiotic ointment.
    - Reinforce teaching to the parents about avoiding exposure of child to risk factors if possible (secondhand smoke, exposure to individuals with viral/bacterial respiratory infections).
    - Stress the importance of seeking medical care at initial signs and symptoms of infections (change in child's behavior, tugging on ear).
    - Encourage the parents to keep the child's immunizations up to date.

Complications

- Hearing loss and/or speech delays
  - Nursing Actions
    - Monitor for deficits.
    - Assist with referral for audiology testing if needed.
  - Client Education
    - Speech therapy may be necessary.

APPLICATION EXERCISES

1. A nurse is reinforcing instructions with the parent of a child who is postoperative following a myringotomy and placement of tympanostomy tubes. Which of the following statements by the parent indicates a need for further teaching?

    A. "The tubes should come out on their own in 2 to 3 years."

    B. "If my child has any pain after we get home, it should be minimal."

    C. "I have canceled my child's gymnastics lesson that is scheduled for tomorrow."

    D. "I will rinse my child's hair with water from the tap when she takes a bath."

2. A nurse is caring for a 2-year-old child who has had three ear infections in the past 5 months. The nurse should know that the child is at risk for developing which of the following as a long-term complication?

    A. Balance difficulties

    B. Lymphadenopathy

    C. Speech delays

    D. Mastoiditis

3. An infant who has clinical manifestations of acute otitis media (AOM) is brought to an outpatient facility by his parent. The nurse should recognize that which of the following factors place the infant at risk for otitis media? (Select all that apply.)

    _____ A. Breastfeeding without formula supplementation.

    _____ B. Attends day care 4 days per week.

    _____ C. Immunizations are up to date.

    _____ D. History of a cleft palate repair.

    _____ E. Parents smoke cigarettes outside.

4. A nurse is caring for a toddler who has rhinitis, cough, and diarrhea for 2 days. When collecting data, the nurse notes that the tympanic membrane has a orange discoloration and decreased movement. Which of the following is an appropriate statement for the nurse to make?

    A. "Your child has an ear infection that requires antibiotics."

    B. "Your child could experience transient hearing loss."

    C. "Your child will need to be on a decongestant until this clears."

    D. "Your child will need to have a myringotomy."

5. A nurse is collecting data from an infant. Which of the following findings are clinical manifestations of acute otitis media? (Select all that apply.)

    _____ A. Decreased pain in the supine position

    _____ B. Rolling head side to side

    _____ C. Loss of appetite

    _____ D. Increased sensitivity to sound

    _____ E. Crying

6. A nurse is caring for an infant who has acute otitis media for the first time. Use the ATI Active Learning Template: Systems Disorder to complete this item to include the following:

    A. Description of Disorder/Disease Process

    B. Nursing Care: Describe two interventions.

    C. Medications: List two.

    D. Care After Discharge: Describe two teaching points to reinforce.

    E. Potential Complication: Identify one.

APPLICATION EXERCISES KEY

1.   A. **CORRECT:** Tympanostomy tubes come out spontaneously in 6 to 12 months. Therefore, this statement indicates a need for further teaching.

   B. INCORRECT: Postoperative pain is not common, but will be mild if present.

   C. INCORRECT: The child's activities should be limited for a few days following surgery.

   D. INCORRECT: The parent should rinse the child's hair with water from the tap because bath water or shampoo water allows easier entry of water into the middle ear due to reduced surface tension.

   N NCLEX® Connection: Reduction of Risk Potential, Therapeutic Procedures

2.   A. INCORRECT: Balance difficulties can be present with otitis media. However, it is not a long-term complication.

   B. INCORRECT: Lymphadenopathy can be present with otitis media. However, it is not a long-term complication.

   C. **CORRECT:** Speech delay is a long-term complication of recurrent otitis media.

   D. INCORRECT: Mastoiditis can be a result of otitis media. However, it is not a long-term complication.

   N NCLEX® Connection: Physiological Adaptations, Basic Pathophysiology

3.   A. INCORRECT: Breastfeeding helps to protect against AOM because breast milk contains secretory immunoglobulin A.

   B. **CORRECT:** Infants who attend day care have an increased risk of AOM because of the exposure to multiple people.

   C. INCORRECT: The pneumococcal conjugate vaccine decreases the incidence of AOM.

   D. **CORRECT:** Infants born with cleft palate are more prone to AOM because micro-organisms can easily enter the eustachian tubes.

   E. **CORRECT:** Exposure to secondhand smoke increases an infant's risk for AOM.

   N NCLEX® Connection: Physiological Adaptations, Basic Pathophysiology

4.   A. INCORRECT: Rhinitis, cough, diarrhea, and an orange discoloration of the tympanic membrane are clinical findings of otitis media with effusion (OME). Therefore, antibiotics are not recommended.

B. **CORRECT:** Rhinitis, cough, diarrhea, and an orange discoloration of the tympanic membrane are clinical findings of OME. Transient hearing loss is a complication of OME.

C. INCORRECT: Rhinitis, cough, diarrhea, and an orange discoloration of the tympanic membrane are clinical findings of OME. Therefore, decongestants are not recommended.

D. INCORRECT: Myringotomy is recommended for clients with chronic OME.

 NCLEX® Connection: Physiological Adaptations, Basic Pathophysiology

5.   A. INCORRECT: Infants who have acute otitis media will have an increase in pain in the supine position from the fluid and pressure in the ear.

B. **CORRECT:** Infants who have acute otitis media will roll their head side to side because of the pain and pressure in the ear.

C. **CORRECT:** Infants who have acute otitis media will exhibit a loss of appetite due to the pain and pressure in the ear.

D. INCORRECT: Infants who have acute otitis media have a decreased sensitivity to sound from the fluid and pressure in the ear.

E. **CORRECT:** Infants who have acute otitis media will exhibit crying and irritability from the pain.

 NCLEX® Connection: Physiological Adaptations, Basic Pathophysiology

6. *Using the ATI Active Learning Template: Systems Disorder*

    A. Description of Disorder/Disease Process

       • Acute otitis media (AOM) is an infection of the structures of the middle ear with rapid clinical symptoms of infection.

    B. Nursing Care

       • Comfort care with pain medications and distraction

       • Management of fevers

       • Place child in an upright position

    C. Medications

       • Amoxicillin (Amoxil), amoxicillin-clavulanate (Augmentin), or azithromycin (Zithromax) PO, or ceftriaxone (Rocephin) IM

       • Acetaminophen (Tylenol) or ibuprofen (Advil) for pain and fever

       • Benzocaine (Americaine Otic)

    D. Care After Discharge

       • Inform the parents about comfort measures.

       • Encourage the parents to feed the child in an upright position when bottle or breastfeeding.

       • If drainage is present, clean the external ear with sterile cotton swabs. Apply antibiotic ointment.

       • Reinforce the need to avoid risk factors (secondhand smoke, exposure to individuals with viral/bacterial respiratory infections).

       • Stress the importance of seeking medical care at the onset of signs and symptoms of infections (change in child's behavior, tugging on ear).

       • Eliminate exposure to secondhand smoke.

       • Encourage the parents to keep the child's immunizations up to date.

    E. Potential Complication

       • Hearing loss and/or speech delays

    ⓝ NCLEX® Connection: Physiological Adaptations, Basic Pathophysiology

chapter 36

Overview

- HIV infection is a viral infection in which the virus infects the T-lymphocytes, causing immune dysfunction. This leads to organ dysfunction and a variety of opportunistic illnesses in a weakened host.

Data Collection

- Risk Factors

  - Infants of mothers who are infected with HIV/AIDS can transmit the virus perinatally or by breast milk.

  - Blood products that contain the HIV virus.

  - Sexual abuse.

  - Risky behaviors such as unprotected sexual activity and IV drug use.

  - Sexually transmitted infections.

  - Lack of awareness.

- Objective Data

  - Physical Assessment Findings and Laboratory Tests

    - HIV infection – Birth to 12 years

HIV INFECTION: BIRTH TO 12 YEARS						
	LESS THAN 12 MONTHS		1 TO 5 YEARS		6 TO 12 YEARS	
	Cells/mEq/L* %**		Cells/mEq/L %		Cells/mEq/L %	
No suppression	1,500 or more	25% or more	1,000 or more	25% or more	500 or more	25% or more
Moderate suppression	750 to 1,499	15% to 24%	500 to 999	15% to 24%	200 to 499	15% to 24%
Severe suppression	Less than 750	Less than 15%	Less than 500	Less than 15%	Less than 200	Less than 15%

*   CD4+ T-lymphocyte count = cells/mEq/L

** CD4+ T-lymphocyte percentage of total lymphocytes = %

NOT SYMPTOMATIC

› No signs or symptoms considered to be the result of HIV infection are present, or the child has only one of the conditions listed in the mildly symptomatic section.

MILDLY SYMPTOMATIC

› Two or more of the following conditions are present, but the child has none of the conditions listed in the moderately or severely symptomatic sections.

  » Lymphadenopathy

  » Hepatomegaly

» Splenomegaly

» Recurrent upper respiratory infections, sinusitis, or otitis media

» Dermatitis

» Parotitis

MODERATELY SYMPTOMATIC

› Children with the following conditions are considered moderately symptomatic.

  » Anemia

  » Bacterial meningitis, pneumonia, or sepsis (single episode)

  » Oropharyngeal candidiasis

  » Cardiomyopathy

  » Cytomegalovirus infection, with onset before 1 month of age

  » Recurrent or chronic diarrhea

  » Hepatitis

» Herpes simplex virus (HSV), stomatitis, bronchitis, pneumonitis, or esophagitis

» Herpes zoster

» Nephropathy

» Leiomyosarcoma

» Lymphoid interstitial pneumonia (LIP) or pulmonary lymphoid hyperplasia complex

» Persistent fever (lasting more than 1 month)

» Toxoplasmosis before 1 month of age

» Disseminated varicella

SEVERELY SYMPTOMATIC

› Children with the following conditions are considered severely symptomatic.

  » Multiple serious bacterial infections (meningitis, bone or joint, abscesses of internal organ or body cavity, septicemia, pneumonia)

  » Esophageal or pulmonary candidiasis, (bronchi, trachea, lungs)

  » Cytomegalovirus disease (greater than 1 month of age with site other than liver, spleen, or lymph nodes)

  » HSV stomatitis, bronchitis, pneumonitis, or esophagitis lasting longer than 1 month

  » Kaposi's sarcoma

  » Brain or Burkitt's lymphoma

» Disseminated or extrapulmonary mycobacterium tuberculosis

» Encephalopathy with developmental delays

» Disseminated coccidioidomycosis

» Extrapulmonary cryptococcosis

» Cryptosporidiosis or isosporiasis with diarrhea longer than 1 month

» Disseminated histoplasmosis

» Pneumocystis carinii pneumonia

» Multifocal leukoencephalopathy

» Salmonella septicemia

» Toxoplasmosis of the brain

» Wasting syndrome

* Human Immunodeficiency Virus Infection (HIV) (retrieved from www.cdc.gov). To read more about HIV, go to the website of the Centers for Disease Control and Prevention (www.cdc.gov).

  ▪ HIV infection – 13 to 20 years (See the chapter on *HIV/AIDS* in the *Adult Medical Surgical Nursing Review Module*.)

○ Diagnostic Procedures

■ Laboratory criteria for diagnosis – 18 months or older

☐ Positive result from HIV enzyme-linked immunosorbent assay (ELISA) and Western blot immunoassay.

■ Laboratory criteria for diagnosis of infants who are less than 18 months of age and were born to infected mothers

☐ Positive result from polymerase chain reaction (PCR) and virus culture.

■ Classification

☐ Children less than 13 are classified by the following criteria.

▸ N: No signs or symptoms

▹ N1 = no evidence of suppression

▹ N2 = evidence of moderate suppression

▹ N3 = severe suppression

▸ A: Mild signs of symptoms

▹ A1 = no evidence of suppression

▹ A2 = evidence of moderate suppression

▹ A3 = severe suppression

▸ B: Moderate signs or symptoms

▹ B1 = no evidence of suppression

▹ B2 = evidence of moderate suppression

▹ B3 = severe suppression

▸ C: Severe signs or symptoms

▹ C1 = no evidence of suppression

▹ C2 = evidence of moderate suppression

▹ C3 = severe suppression

Patient-Centered Care

• Nursing Care

○ Encourage a balanced diet that is high in calories and protein. Obtain the child's preferred food and beverages. Give nutritional supplements.

○ Monitor total parental nutrition (TPN) if prescribed.

○ Provide good oral care and report abnormalities for treatment.

○ Keep the child's skin clean and dry.

○ Provide nonpharmacological methods of pain relief.

○ Determine the child's pain level and provide adequate pain management. Use of medications may include nonsteroidal anti-inflammatory drugs (NSAIDs), acetaminophen (Tylenol), opioids, muscle relaxants, and/or a eutectic mixture of local anesthetics (EMLA cream) for numerous diagnostic procedures.

Q
S

- ○ Protect/prevent infection using standard precautions.
  - ▪ Encourage deep breathing and coughing.
  - ▪ Maintain good hand hygiene.
  - ▪ Reinforce teaching to the child and parents about avoiding individuals who have colds/infections/viruses.
  - ▪ Encourage immunizations, such as pneumococcal vaccine (PCV) and yearly seasonal influenza vaccine.
  - ▪ Monitor for signs of opportunistic infections.
- ○ Administer medications as prescribed for opportunistic infections.
- • Medications
  - ○ Antiretroviral medications are given at various stages of the HIV cycle to inhibit reproduction of the virus.
    - ▪ Nucleoside reverse transcriptase inhibitors (NRTIs) – zidovudine, didanosine, lamivudine, abacavir
      - □ Suppress the synthesis of viral DNA
    - ▪ Non-nucleoside reverse transcriptase inhibitors (NNRTIs) – delavirdine, efavirenz, nevirapine
      - □ Bind to the viral DNA causing direct inhibition
    - ▪ Nucleotide reverse transcriptase inhibitors such as adefovir.
      - □ Inhibit viral DNA synthesis
    - ▪ Protease inhibitors – indinavir, ritonavir, nelfinavir, amprenavir
      - □ Inhibit an enzyme needed for the virus to replicate
    - ▪ Adjunctive antiretrovirals such as hydroxyurea
      - □ Suppress DNA replication
    - ▪ Nursing considerations
      - □ Monitor laboratory results (CBC, WBC, liver function tests). Antiretroviral medications can increase alanine aminotransferase (ALT), aspartate aminotransferase (AST), bilirubin, mean corpuscular volume (MCV), high-density lipoproteins (HDLs), total cholesterol, and triglycerides.
    - ▪ Client education
      - □ Reinforce teaching about the side effects of the medications and ways to decrease the severity of the side effects.
      - □ Reinforce teaching about the need to take the medication on a regular schedule and to not miss doses.
  - ○ Antibiotics
    - ▪ Trimethoprim-sulfamethoxazole (TMZ-SMZ)
      - □ Administer to all infants who are born to mothers who are infected until HIV infection is excluded.
  - ○ IV gamma globulin
    - ▪ To prevent recurrent or serious bacterial infections
- • Teamwork and Collaboration
  - ○ Social services can help with access to health care and medication acquisition.
  - ○ Dietitian can assist with nutritional support and promote good nutrition.

- Care After Discharge
  - Client Education
    - Reinforce teaching to the child and parents about the chronicity of the illness and the need for lifelong medication administration.
    - Reinforce teaching to the parents about when to notify the provider. Signs and symptoms requiring medical care include headache, fever, lethargy, warmth, tenderness, redness at joints, and neck stiffness.
    - Reinforce teaching to the child and parents about transmission of the virus (high-risk behaviors).
    - Identify stressors that may be affecting the family and assist with making needed referrals (school/community response to child, finances, access to health care).
    - Reinforce teaching to the child and parents about safe practice when using needles/syringes and administering medications.

Complications

- Failure to thrive
  - Nursing Actions
    - Obtain a baseline height and weight, and monitor.
    - Promote optimal nutrition.
    - Monitor growth and development.
    - Provide opportunities for normal development (age-appropriate toys, play with children of the same age).
  - Client Education
    - Reinforce teaching to the child and parents about appropriate nutrition and how to meet nutritional needs.
- *Pneumocystis carinii* pneumonia (PCP)
  - Nursing Actions
    - Monitor respiratory status, which includes respiratory rate and effort, oxygen saturation, and breath sounds.
    - Administer appropriate antibiotics.
    - Administer an antipyretic and/or analgesics.
    - Provide adequate hydration and monitor fluid and electrolyte balance as directed.
    - Use postural drainage and chest physiotherapy to mobilize and remove fluid from the lungs.
    - Promote adequate rest.
  - Client Education
    - Reinforce teaching to the child and parents about the infectious process and how to prevent infection.
    - Reinforce teaching to the child and parents about the importance of medication and the need to maintain the medication regimen.

APPLICATION EXERCISES

1. A nurse is reinforcing teaching to the parent of a child who has HIV. Which of the following should be included? (Select all that apply.)

_____ A. Avoid influenza immunizations.

_____ B. Protease inhibitors inhibit viral DNA replication.

_____ C. Avoid individuals who have colds.

_____ D. Provide nutritional supplements.

_____ E. Administer aspirin for fever.

2. A nurse is caring for a child who has AIDS. Which of the following isolation precautions should the nurse implement?

A. Contact

B. Airborne

C. Droplet

D. Standard

3. A nurse is admitting a child who has HIV. Which of the following are clinical manifestations of a child who is mildly symptomatic? (Select all that apply.)

_____ A. Herpes zoster

_____ B. Anemia

_____ C. Dermatitis

_____ D. Hepatomegaly

_____ E. Lymphadenopathy

4. A nurse is reinforcing teaching to a group of adolescents about HIV/AIDS. Which of the following should be included in the teaching?

A. "You can contract HIV through casual kissing."

B. "You can contract HIV by sharing eating utensils."

C. "The incubation period can be months to years."

D. "Medications inhibit transmission of the virus."

5. A nurse is collecting data from a child who has HIV. Which of the following are clinical manifestations of a child who is severely symptomatic? (Select all that apply.)

_____ A. Kaposi's sarcoma

_____ B. Hepatitis

_____ C. Wasting syndrome

_____ D. Pulmonary candidiasis

_____ E. Cardiomyopathy

6. A nurse is reinforcing teaching to the parent of a child who has AIDS. Use the ATI Active Learning Template: Systems Disorder to complete this item. List two complications of AIDS and include four nursing actions for each.

APPLICATION EXERCISES KEY

1. A. INCORRECT: Obtaining a yearly influenza vaccination is recommended to protect the child from opportunistic infections.

    B. **CORRECT:** Protease inhibitors are antiretroviral medications that suppress DNA replication.

    C. **CORRECT:** Avoiding individuals who have colds will assist in protecting the child from opportunistic infections.

    D. **CORRECT:** Nutritional supplements are recommended to promote improved nutrition of the child who has HIV.

    E. INCORRECT: Acetaminophen should be administered to a child who has a fever.

     NCLEX® Connection: Physiological Adaptations, Alterations in Body Systems

2. A. INCORRECT: Contact isolation precautions are used to protect transmission of disease that is skin-to-skin or direct contact.

    B. INCORRECT: Airborne isolation precautions are used to protect transmission of disease that is small-particle droplets.

    C. INCORRECT: Droplet isolation precautions are used to protect transmission of disease that is large-particle droplets.

    D. **CORRECT:** Standard isolation precautions are used to protect transmission of disease that is bloodborne or present in a body substance.

     NCLEX® Connection: Safety and Infection Control, Standard Precautions/Transmission-Based Precautions/Surgical Asepsis

3. A. INCORRECT: Herpes zoster is a clinical manifestation of a child who is moderately symptomatic.

    B. INCORRECT: Anemia is a clinical manifestation of a child who is moderately symptomatic.

    C. **CORRECT:** Dermatitis is a clinical manifestation of a child who is mildly symptomatic.

    D. **CORRECT:** Hepatomegaly is a clinical manifestation of a child who is mildly symptomatic.

    E. **CORRECT:** Lymphadenopathy is a clinical manifestation of a child who is mildly symptomatic.

     NCLEX® Connection: Physiological Adaptations, Basic Pathophysiology

4. A. INCORRECT: HIV is transmitted via blood, semen, vaginal secretions, and breast milk. There is no evidence that casual contact spreads the virus.

   B. INCORRECT: HIV is transmitted via blood, semen, vaginal secretions, and breast milk. There is no evidence that casual contact spreads the virus.

   C. **CORRECT:** The incubation period can be months to years depending on the individual, how HIV was acquired, and interventions.

   D. INCORRECT: Medications suppress the progression of the virus.

   Ⓝ NCLEX® Connection: Physiological Adaptations, Alterations in Body Systems

5. A. **CORRECT:** Kaposi's sarcoma is a clinical manifestation of a child who is severely symptomatic.

   B. INCORRECT: Hepatitis is a clinical manifestation of a child who is moderately symptomatic.

   C. **CORRECT:** Wasting syndrome is a clinical manifestation of a child who is severely symptomatic.

   D. **CORRECT:** Pulmonary candidiasis is a clinical manifestation of a child who is severely symptomatic.

   E. INCORRECT: Cardiomyopathy is a clinical manifestation of a child who is moderately symptomatic.

   Ⓝ NCLEX® Connection: Physiological Adaptations, Basic Pathophysiology

6. *Using the ATI Active Learning Template: Systems Disorder*
   - Failure to thrive
     - Nursing Actions
       - Obtain a baseline height and weight, and monitor.
       - Promote optimal nutrition.
       - Monitor growth and development.
       - Provide opportunities for normal development (age-appropriate toys, play with children of the same age).
       - Reinforce teaching to the child and parents about appropriate nutrition and how to meet nutritional needs.

   - *Pneumocystis carinii* pneumonia (PCP)
     - Nursing Actions
       - Monitor respiratory status, which includes respiratory rate and effort, oxygen saturation, and breath sounds.
       - Administer appropriate antibiotics.
       - Administer an antipyretic and/ or analgesics.
       - Provide adequate hydration and monitor fluid and electrolyte balance as directed.
       - Use postural drainage and chest physiotherapy to mobilize and remove fluid from the lungs.
       - Promote adequate rest.
       - Reinforce teaching to the child and parents about the infectious process and how to prevent infection.
       - Reinforce teaching to the child and parents about the importance of medication and the need to maintain the medication regimen.

   Ⓝ NCLEX® Connection: Physiological Adaptations, Alterations in Body Systems

UNIT 2   Nursing Care of Children with System Disorders

SECTION: NEOPLASTIC DISORDERS

› Pediatric Cancers

NCLEX® CONNECTIONS

When reviewing the chapter in this section, keep in mind the relevant sections of the NCLEX® outline, in particular:

Client Needs: Physiological Adaptations

› Relevant topics/tasks include:

» Alterations in Body Systems

› Reinforce education to client regarding care and condition.

» Basic Pathophysiology

› Identify signs and symptoms related to an acute or chronic illness.

› Consider general principles of client disease process when providing care.

chapter 37

Overview

- There are many organ neoplasms that both children and adults can acquire, such as lymphoma, brain tumor, and liver and testicular cancer. For information on these neoplasms, see the chapter on *General Principles of Cancer* in the *Adult Medical Surgical Review Module*.

- Certain neoplasms occur predominantly in children. Examples of these are Wilms' tumor (nephroblastoma) and neuroblastoma. Additional neoplasms that occur frequently in children include the following.

  ○ Wilms' tumor is a malignancy that occurs in the kidneys or abdomen.

    ▪ The tumor is usually unilateral, with 10% of cases affecting both kidneys.

    ▪ Diagnosis typically occurs at an age younger than 5, with the majority of cases being diagnosed at about age 3.

    ▪ Metastasis is rare.

  ○ Neuroblastoma is a malignancy that occurs in the adrenal gland, sympathetic chain of the retroperitoneal area, head, neck, pelvis, or chest.

    ▪ Diagnosis typically occurs during the toddler years, with 95% of cases prior to age 10.

    ▪ Half of all cases have metastasized before diagnosis.

  ○ Treatment varies with each child and can be any combination of surgery, chemotherapy, and radiation.

- Leukemia is the term for a group of malignancies that affect the bone marrow and lymphatic system.

  ○ Leukemia is classified by the type of WBCs that becomes neoplastic and is commonly divided into two groups: acute lymphoid leukemia (ALL) and acute myelogenous or nonlymphoid leukemia (AML/ANLL).

  ○ Leukemia causes an increase in the production of immature WBCs, which leads to infiltration of organs and tissues.

    ▪ Bone marrow infiltration causes crowding of cells that would normally produce RBCs, platelets, and mature WBCs.

      □ Deficient RBCs cause anemia.

      □ Deficient mature WBCs (neutropenia) increase the risk for infection.

      □ Deficient platelets (thrombocytopenia) cause bleeding and bruising.

    ▪ Infiltration of spleen, liver, and lymph nodes leads to tissue fibrosis.

    ▪ Infiltration of the CNS causes increased intracranial pressure.

    ▪ Other tissues can also be infiltrated (testes, prostate, ovaries, gastrointestinal tract).

- Malignant tumors in bone may originate from all tissues involved in bone growth, including osteoid matrix, blood vessels, and cartilage.

  ○ Osteosarcoma usually occurs in the metaphysis of long bones, most often in the femur. Treatment frequently includes amputation or limb salvage procedure of the affected extremity as well as chemotherapy.

  ○ Ewing's sarcoma (a primitive neuroectodermal tumor [PNET]) occurs in the shafts of long bones and of trunk bones. Treatment includes surgical biopsy, intensive radiation therapy to tumor site, and chemotherapy, but not amputation.

  ○ Prognosis depends on how quickly the disease is diagnosed and whether metastasis has occurred.

- Soft tissue malignancies arise from undifferentiated cells in the soft tissues (muscles, tendons), in connective or fibrous tissue, or in blood or lymph vessels. These malignancies can begin in any area of the body.

  ○ Rhabdomyosarcoma originates in skeletal muscle in any part of the body, but it most commonly occurs in the head and neck, with the orbit of the eye frequently affected. Treatment consists of surgical biopsy, local radiation therapy, and chemotherapy, rather than radical surgical procedures.

- Children who undergo irradiation for malignancies in or near the pelvic area can experience sterilization and/or secondary cancers.

Data Collection

- Wilms' Tumor

  ○ Risk Factors

    ■ There are no known risk factors for Wilms' tumor or neuroblastoma.

  ○ Subjective and Objective Data

    ■ Wilms' Tumor

      □ Firm, nontender abdominal swelling or mass

      □ Fatigue, malaise, weight loss

      □ Fever

      □ Hematuria

      □ Hypertension

      □ Signs and symptoms of metastasis include dyspnea, cough, and shortness of breath.

    ■ Neuroblastoma

      □ Symptoms depend upon the location and stage of disease.

      □ Half of children who have neuroblastoma have few symptoms.

      □ Signs and symptoms of metastasis include an ill appearance, periorbital ecchymoses, exophthalmos, bone pain, and irritability.

- Leukemia
  - Risk Factors
    - Leukemia is the most common cancer of childhood, with peak onset between 2 and 5 years of age.
    - There is a family history of leukemia.
  - Subjective Data
    - History and physical assessment findings may reveal vague reports (anorexia, headache, fatigue).
  - Objective Data
    - Physical Assessment Findings
      - Early manifestations
        - Low-grade fever
        - Pallor
        - Increased bruising and petechiae

 View Image: Petechiae

        - Listlessness
        - Enlarged liver, lymph nodes, and joints
        - Abdominal, leg, and joint pain
        - Constipation
        - Headache
        - Vomiting and anorexia
        - Unsteady gait
      - Late manifestations
        - Pain
        - Hematuria
        - Ulcerations in the mouth
        - Enlarged kidneys and testicles
        - Signs of increased intracranial pressure
- Bone and Soft Tissue Cancers
  - Risk Factors
    - Osteosarcoma peaks at age 15 during growth spurts and is more common in boys.
    - Ewing's sarcoma occurs prior to 30 years of age and is more common in Caucasians.
    - Rhabdomyosarcoma occurs in children of all ages (but more commonly in children younger than 5 years of age) and is more common in Caucasians.

○ Subjective and Objective Data

BONE CANCERS	
Subjective Data	› Nonspecific bone pain that is often mistaken for an injury or growing pains › Temporary relief of pain when extremity is flexed
Objective Data	› Weakness, swelling, or decreased movement of the extremity › Palpable lymph nodes near the tumor › Anemia, generalized infection, or unexplained weight loss › Limpness or inability to hold a heavy object
RHABDOMYOSARCOMA	
Subjective Data	› May cause pain in local areas related to compression by the tumor (sore throat may occur with tumor of the nasopharynx) › Possible absence of pain in some parts of the body, such as in the retroperitoneal area, until the tumor begins to obstruct organs
Objective Data	› Based on affected area » CNS – headaches, diplopia, vomiting » Orbit – unilateral proptosis, ecchymosis of conjunctiva, strabismus » Nasopharynx – stuffy nose, pain, nasal obstruction, epistaxis, palpable neck nodes, visible mass (late) » Paranasal sinuses – nasal obstruction, pain, discharge, sinusitis, swelling » Middle ear – chronic otitis media, pain, sanguinopurulent discharge, facial paralysis » Retroperitoneal area – usually no symptoms, abdominal mass, pain, intestinal or genitourinary obstruction » Perineum – visible superficial mass, bowel or bladder obstruction » Extremity – pain, palpable fixed mass, lymph node enlargement

Q
EBP

- Laboratory Tests
  - □ Complete Blood Counts
    - ▸ Anemia (low blood counts)
    - ▸ Thrombocytopenia (low platelets)
    - ▸ Neutropenia (low neutrophils)
    - ▸ Leukemic blasts (immature WBCs)
  - □ Coagulation studies
  - □ BUN, creatinine
  - □ Urine catecholamines (vanillylmandelic acid, homovanillic acid, dopamine, and norepinephrine)
  - □ Urinalysis
  - □ 24-hr urine specimen for protein and creatinine clearance

- Diagnostic Procedures
  - Wilms' Tumor
    - Abdominal ultrasonography
    - Abdominal and chest computed tomography (CT) scan
    - Inferior venacavogram (rule out involvement with the vena cava)
    - Bone marrow aspiration (rule out metastasis)
  - Neuroblastoma
    - Skeletal survey
    - Skull, neck, chest, abdominal, and bone CT scans
    - Bone marrow aspiration (rule out metastasis)
    - Metaiodobenzylguanidine (MIBG) scan (determine bone, bone marrow and soft tissue involvement)
    - Biopsy of tumor
  - Leukemia
    - Bone marrow aspiration or biopsy analysis is the most definitive diagnostic procedure. If leukemia is present, the specimen will show prolific quantities of immature leukemic blast cells and protein markers indicating a specific type of leukemia.
    - Cerebrospinal fluid (CSF) analysis to determine CNS involvement (increased intracranial pressure)
    - Liver and kidney function studies (provide baseline data prior to chemotherapy)
  - Bone Cancers
    - X-rays, CT scans, or magnetic resonance imaging (MRI) of the primary site
    - Bone marrow biopsy
    - CT of the chest and bone scans to evaluate metastasis.
  - Rhabdomyosarcoma
    - CT scans or MRI of the primary site
    - Biopsy of tumor if possible
    - CT of the chest, bone scans, bone marrow biopsy, and lumbar puncture to evaluate metastasis
  - Nursing Actions
    - Chest x-ray and CT, MRI, positron emission tomography (PET), and single photon emission computed tomography (SPECT) scans.
      - ▷ Check the child for allergies to contrast dye or shellfish.
      - ▷ Assist the child to remain still during the procedure.
      - ▷ Sedate the child if prescribed.

- ▶ Bone marrow aspiration or biopsy

  - ▷ Assist the provider with the procedure.

  - ▷ Topical anesthetic, such as a eutectic mixture of local anesthetics (EMLA), can be applied over the biopsy area 45 min to 1 hr prior to the procedure.

  - ▷ Unconscious sedation is induced using a general anesthetic, such as propofol (Diprivan).

  - ▷ Positioning depends on the access site to be used (posterior or anterior iliac crest is most common; tibia can be used in infants because it is easier to access and hold the infant).

  - ▷ The provider obtains a specimen by the provider.

  - ▷ Postprocedure

    - ◆ Apply pressure to the site for 5 to 10 min, then apply a pressure dressing.

    - ◆ Check vital signs frequently.

    - ◆ Monitor for signs of bleeding and infection for 24 hr.

    - ◆ Provide pain relief.

- ▶ Cerebrospinal fluid (CSF) analysis – obtained by lumbar puncture

  - ▷ Have the child empty his bladder.

  - ▷ Assist the provider with the procedure.

  - ▷ A topical anesthetic (EMLA cream) can be applied over the biopsy area 45 min to 1 hr prior to the procedure.

  - ▷ Place the child in the side-lying position with the head flexed and knees drawn up toward the chest, and assist in maintaining the position. Distraction may need to be used.

  - ▷ The child may be sedated with fentanyl (Sublimaze) and midazolam (Versed).

  - ▷ The provider will clean the skin and inject a local anesthetic.

  - ▷ The provider will take pressure readings and collect three to five test tubes of CSF.

  - ▷ Pressure and an elastic bandage will be applied to the puncture site after the needle is removed.

  - ▷ Label specimens appropriately, and deliver them to the laboratory.

  - ▷ Monitor the site for bleeding and infection for 24 hr.

- ▫ Client Education

  - ▶ Provide emotional support.

  - ▶ Educate the child and parents about the procedure and postprocedure care.

  - ▶ Assist the child to remain flat in bed for 4 to 8 hr to prevent leakage and spinal headache after lumbar puncture.

Patient-Centered Care

- Nursing Care
  - If Wilms' tumor is suspected, do not palpate the abdomen.
  - Assess pain using an age-appropriate pain scale.
  - Use pharmacological and nonpharmacological interventions to provide around the clock pain management.
  - Check for developmental delays related to illness.
  - Monitor physical growth (height and weight).
  - Monitor for signs of infection and administer antibiotics.
  - Keep the child's skin clean, dry, and lubricated.
  - Provide oral hygiene and keep the child's lips lubricated.
  - Provide age-appropriate diversional activities.
  - Provide support to the child and family.
    - Observe the child and family's ability to cope and available support.
    - Reinforce education regarding diagnostic testing, treatment plan, ongoing therapy, and prognosis.
    - Avoid false reassurance. Give honest answers and information.
    - Avoid overwhelming the child and family with information.
    - Listen to the child's concerns.
    - Encourage peer contact if appropriate.
    - Allow time for the child and family to discuss feelings regarding loss and to grieve.
- Teamwork and Collaboration
  - Request referral for social services to assist with access to medications and durable medical equipment if needed.
  - Request a referral for a nutritionist for development of a diet plan.
  - Suggest support group of older children and adolescents.
  - Request referral for mental health counseling to assist the child to resume normal activities.
  - Request referral for physical and occupational therapy referrals to start while in the hospital and to continue after discharge.
- Therapeutic Procedures
  - Treatment for Wilms' tumor
    - Surgical removal of the tumor and kidney soon after diagnosis
    - Preoperative chemotherapy or radiation if both kidneys are involved to decrease the size of the tumors and potentially preserve one kidney.
    - Postoperative radiation and/or chemotherapy for children with large tumors, metastasis, reoccurrence, and residual disease
  - Treatment for neuroblastoma
    - Surgical removal of the tumor
    - Chemotherapy and/or radiation used for metastasis and residual disease

○ Treatment for leukemias

- Chemotherapy in four phases (induction therapy, CNS prophylactic therapy, intensification therapy (consolidation), maintenance therapy)

- Radiation

- Hematopoietic stem cell transplant (HSCT)

○ Treatment for bone and soft tissue malignancies

- Chemotherapy

- Localized radiation therapy

- Limb salvage or amputation procedures

○ Nursing Actions

- Chemotherapy

  □ Assist with care of the child's long-term central venous access device or a peripherally inserted central catheter (PICC).

  □ Medicate the child with an antiemetic prior to administration.

  □ Assist the child to manage side effects.

- Client Education

  □ Reinforce education to the child and family about the side effects of chemotherapy (mouth sores, loss of appetite, nausea and vomiting, hair loss, diarrhea or constipation, increased risk of infection, easy bruising or bleeding, and fatigue).

  □ Instruct the parents that the use of steroid treatment can cause moon face.

  □ Instruct the parents that the child might experience mood changes.

  □ Instruct the parents to recognize signs of infection, skin breakdown, and nutritional deficiency.

  □ Encourage the child and parents to maintain good hygiene.

  □ Instruct the child and parents to avoid individuals who have infectious diseases.

  □ Instruct the child and parents how to administer medications and provide nutritional support at home.

  □ Instruct the parents in the proper use of vascular access devices.

  □ Instruct the child and parents about bleeding precautions and the management of active bleeding.

○ Radiation

- Radiation is dose-calculated and usually delivered in divided treatments over several weeks.

- Radiation affects rapidly growing cells in the body. Therefore, cells that normally have a fast turnover can be affected in addition to cancer cells.

- Nursing Actions

  □ Take care when radiation is in use. Wear lead aprons.

- Client Education

  □ Educate the child and family about the procedure and provide support.

  □ Instruct the child and family not to wash off marks on skin that outline the targeted areas.

  □ Teach the child and family to wash the marked areas with lukewarm water, use hands instead of a washcloth, pat dry, and take care not to remove the markings. Avoid using hot or cold water.

□ Teach the child and family to avoid the use of soaps, creams, lotions, and/or powders unless they are prescribed.

□ Encourage wearing loose cotton clothing.

□ Remind the child and family to keep the areas protected from the sun by wearing a hat and long-sleeved shirts.

□ Instruct the family to seek medical care for blisters, weeping, and red/tender skin.

- Surgical Interventions
  ○ Tumor debulking
    ▪ Nursing Actions
      □ Preoperative
        ▸ Avoid palpation of Wilms' tumor.
      □ Postoperative
        ▸ Monitor gastrointestinal activity (bowel sounds, bowel movements, distention, nausea, vomiting).
        ▸ Provide pain relief.
        ▸ Monitor vital signs and any manifestations of infection.
        ▸ Encourage pulmonary hygiene.
    ▪ Client Education
      □ Reinforce preoperative teaching to the child and family that includes length of surgery, where the child will recover, and what equipment will be in place (nasogastric tube, IV line, indwelling urinary catheter).
  ○ Surgical biopsy for any of the bone or soft tissue cancers
    ▪ Tumor is biopsied under anesthesia to determine presence and/or tissue type of cancer.
    ▪ Nursing Actions
      □ Provide routine pre- and postoperative care.
        ▸ Provide for adequate pain relief.
        ▸ Monitor wound for signs of infection.
    ▪ Client Education
      □ Educate the child and family regarding postoperative care.
  ○ Limb salvage procedure for bone cancers
    ▪ It involves a preoperative course of chemotherapy to shrink the tumor and then total bone and joint replacement after the tumor and affected bone are removed.
    ▪ Nursing Actions
      □ Assist with managing side effects.
      □ Provide routine postoperative care.
      □ Provide adequate pain relief.
    ▪ Client Education
      □ Educate the child and family regarding postoperative care.
      □ Teach the child and family about any expected effects of preoperative chemotherapy, such as hair loss.

- ○ Limb amputation for bone cancer
  - ▪ The child may receive chemotherapy both preoperatively and postoperatively.
  - ▪ Nursing Actions
    - □ Provide routine pre- and postoperative care.
    - □ Provide emotional support.
    - □ Provide stump care.
    - □ Monitor for the presence of phantom limb pain postoperatively, and medicate appropriately.
  - ▪ Client Education
    - □ Prepare the child for fitting of a temporary prosthesis, which can occur immediately after surgery.
    - □ Encourage cooperation with postoperative physical therapy.
    - □ Work with the child and family to plan for issues such as appropriate clothing to wear with a prosthesis.
    - □ Assist the family to recognize that the child's emotions, such as anger, are normal grief reactions after amputation, chemotherapy, and other treatments.
- ○ Hematopoietic stem cell transplant (HSCT)
  - ▪ Nursing Actions
    - □ Implement protective isolation.
      - ▸ A private, positive-pressure room
      - ▸ At least 12 air exchanges/hr
      - ▸ HEPA filtration for incoming air
      - ▸ Respirator mask, gloves, and gowns
      - ▸ No dried or fresh flowers, and no potted plants
  - ▪ Client Education
    - □ Instruct the child and parents to avoid individuals who have infectious diseases.
    - □ Instruct the child and parents how to administer medications and provide nutritional support at home.
    - □ Instruct the parents in the proper use of vascular access devices.
    - □ Instruct the child and parents about bleeding precautions and the management of active bleeding.

Complications

CHEMOTHERAPY AND RADIATION SIDE EFFECTS AND NURSING INTERVENTIONS	
SIDE EFFECT	**NURSING INTERVENTIONS**
Mucosal ulceration	› Provide frequent oral care.
	› Inspect the child's mouth for ulceration and hemorrhage.
	› Use a soft-bristled toothbrush or a soft, disposable toothbrush for oral care.
	› Lubricate lips with lip balm to prevent cracking.
	› Offer foods that are soft and bland (nonacidic), cool fluids. Can require a pureed or liquid diet.
	› Assist the child to use mouthwashes (such as 1 tsp salt mixed with 1 pint of water or 1 tsp baking soda mixed with 1 quart of water) frequently.
	› Apply local anesthetics (hydrocortisone dental paste [Orabase], antiseptic mouth rinse [UlcerEase]), aluminum and magnesium hydroxide (Maalox) to mucosa to minimize pain.
	› Use agents (mouthwashes, lozenges) that are effective against fungal and bacterial infections (chlorhexidine gluconate [Peridex]).
	› Avoid viscous lidocaine (causes risk of aspiration from depressed gag reflex), hydrogen peroxide (delays healing), milk of magnesia (dries mucous membranes), and lemon glycerin swabs (causes tooth decay and erosion of tissue).
Skin breakdown	› Inspect skin daily.
	› Check rectal mucosa for fissures.
	› Avoid rectal temperatures.
	› Provide sitz baths as needed.
	› Reposition frequently.
	› Use a pressure reduction system.
Neuropathy	› Foot drop
	» Use a footboard in bed.
	» Weakness and numbness of extremities
	» Assist with ambulation.
	› Jaw pain
	» Provide a soft diet.
Alteration in bowel elimination	› Constipation
	» Encourage a diet high in fiber.
	» Administer stool softeners and laxatives as needed.
	» Encourage fluids.
	› Diarrhea
	» Provide meticulous skin care.
	» Provide a nutritious diet.
	» Determine if certain foods or drinks (high-fiber, lactose-rich) worsen the child's condition.
	» Monitor intake and output and daily weight.

CHEMOTHERAPY AND RADIATION SIDE EFFECTS AND NURSING INTERVENTIONS	
SIDE EFFECT	**NURSING INTERVENTIONS**
Anorexia, nausea, and vomiting	› Monitor fluid intake and hydration status. › Administer antiemetics before meals. › Provide small, frequent, well-balanced meals. › Avoid strong odors. Provide a pleasant atmosphere for meals. › Involve the child in meal planning and the child to choose favorite foods. › Administer enteral nutrition if needed. › Weigh the child daily. › Monitor electrolyte values.
Hemorrhage cystitis	› Encourage fluid intake to 1½ times usual amount. › Encourage frequent voiding. › Administer mesna (Mesnex) to provide protection to the bladder.
Alopecia	› Prepare the child and parents in advance for hair loss. › Discuss cutting long hair. › Use gentle shampoos. Gently brush the child's hair. › Avoid blow dryers and curling irons. › Encourage the use of a cotton hat or scarf, or a wig if the child is self conscious about hair loss.

- Pancytopenia
  - Bone marrow depression resulting in anemia, neutropenia, and/or thrombocytopenia
  - Nursing Actions
    - Monitor vital signs and report them to the provider. Report a temperature greater than 37.8° C (100° F).
    - Monitor for signs of infection (lung congestion; redness, swelling, and pain around IV sites) and lesions in the mouth, and monitor the client's wound site and immunization status.
    - Administer antimicrobial, antiviral, and antifungal medications as prescribed.
    - Protect the child from sources of possible infection.
      - Use good hand hygiene.
      - Encourage the child and family to use good hand hygiene.
    - Encourage the child to avoid crowds while undergoing chemotherapy.
    - Instruct the child to avoid fresh fruits and vegetables.
    - Avoid invasive procedures (injections, rectal temperatures, catheters). Apply pressure to puncture sites for 5 min.
    - Monitor for signs of bleeding.
    - Avoid aspirin/NSAIDs.
    - Administer filgrastim (Neupogen) subcutaneously daily to stimulate WBC production.
    - Administer epoetin alfa (Procrit) subcutaneously two to three times per week to stimulate RBC formation.

- Administer oprelvekin (Interleukin-11, Neumega) subcutaneously daily to stimulate platelet formation.

- Encourage the use of a soft toothbrush.

- Use gentle handling and positioning to protect from injury.

- Organize care to provide for rest. Schedule rest periods.

- Infection

  - Infection can be a complication of myelosuppression.

  - Nursing Actions

    - Monitor for elevated WBC and fever.

    - Monitor for potential sites of infections (oral ulcer, open cut), and monitor temperature.

    - Provide the child with a private room. The room should be designed to allow for adequate air flow to reduce airborne pathogens.

    - Restrict visitors and health care personnel who have active illnesses.

    - Adhere to strict hand hygiene.

    - Administer antibiotics as prescribed.

    - Encourage adequate protein and caloric intake.

    - Avoid live vaccines during periods of immunosuppression.

    - Ensure that siblings are up to date on vaccinations.

    - Provide a diet adequate in proteins and calories.

- Hemorrhage

  - Bleeding (thrombocytopenia) can be a complication of myelosuppression.

  - Nursing Actions

    - Monitor for signs of bleeding (petechiae, ecchymoses, hematuria, bleeding gums, hematemesis, tarry stools).

    - Avoid unnecessary skin punctures, and use surgical aseptic technique when performed. Apply pressure for 5 min to stop bleeding.

    - Assist with platelet administration.

    - Treat a nosebleed with cold and pressure.

      - Use a strict aseptic technique for all invasive procedures.

      - Use gentle technique when providing mouth care.

      - Clean the perineal area carefully to prevent trauma, and avoid obtaining temperatures rectally.

- Anemia
  - Anemia can be a complication of myelosuppression.
  - Nursing Actions
    - Monitor for fatigue and decreased hemoglobin/hematocrit.
    - Assist with blood transfusions.
    - Allow for frequent rest periods.
    - Administer oxygen therapy.
    - Administer IV fluid replacement.
- Care After Discharge
  - Client Education
    - Educate the child and family regarding the importance of follow-up care.
    - Reinforce education the child and family about infection control procedures at home.
    - Reinforce education to the child and family about the importance of immunizations.
    - Encourage the parents and child to visit a dentist before therapy.
    - Encourage the use of mouth washes, such as 1 tsp salt mixed with 1 pint water or 1 tsp baking soda mixed with 1 quart water.
    - Discuss the use of a wig, turbans, or hats.
    - Instruct the child and family to avoid blow dryers and curling irons.
    - Encourage/provide meticulous oral care to prevent gingival bleeding. Use a soft toothbrush, and avoid astringent mouthwashes.
    - Instruct the parents about measures for controlling epistaxis.
    - Instruct the parents and child to avoid activities that may lead to injury or bleeding.
    - Educate the child and parents about foods high in iron.
  - Community Services
    - Request appropriate referrals to assist the child to resume normal activities (school attendance, physical activities).
    - Encourage attendance at support groups.

APPLICATION EXERCISES

1. A nurse is contributing to the plan of care for a toddler who has a Wilms' tumor. Which of the following should the nurse include?

    A. Palpate the abdomen to identify the size of the tumor.

    B. Prepare the toddler for surgery.

    C. Reinforce teaching to the parents about dialysis.

    D. Obtain 24-hr urine specimen.

2. A nurse is collecting data from a child who has Wilms' tumor. Which of the following findings should the nurse expect? (Select all that apply.)

    _____ A. Weight gain

    _____ B. Hematuria

    _____ C. Hypotension

    _____ D. Bone pain

    _____ E. Fatigue

3. A nurse is collecting data from a child who has leukemia. Which of the following are early clinical manifestations of leukemia? (Select all that apply.)

    _____ A. Hematuria

    _____ B. Anorexia

    _____ C. Petechiae

    _____ D. Ulcerations in the mouth

    _____ E. Unsteady gait

4. A nurse is caring for a child who is receiving chemotherapy. Which of the following are clinical manifestations of neuropathy? (Select all that apply.)

    _____ A. Constipation

    _____ B. Skin breakdown

    _____ C. Foot drop

    _____ D. Jaw pain

    _____ E. Hemorrhagic cystitis

5. A nurse is contributing to the plan of care for a child who has oral mucositis. Which of the following actions should the nurse include? (Select all that apply.)

_____ A. Swab the mucosa with lemon glycerine swabs.

_____ B. Apply viscous lidocaine.

_____ C. Offer soft foods.

_____ D. Use a soft, disposable toothbrush for oral care.

_____ E. Encourage gargling with a warm saline mouthwash.

6. A nurse is reviewing teaching with an adolescent client who is receiving epoetin alfa (Procrit) for side effects from chemotherapy. Which of the following statements indicates understanding of the teaching?

A. "I have to take Procrit so I will manufacture white blood cells."

B. "My platelet count is low, which is why I need Procrit."

C. "This medication is an iron supplement for anemia."

D. "Procrit helps build up my bone marrow so I make more red blood cells."

7. A nurse is reinforcing teaching to a parent of a child who has bone cancer and is receiving chemotherapy about myelosuppression. Use the ATI Active Learning Template: Systems Disorder to complete this item to include the following:

A. Nursing Actions: Describe two actions related to each of the following areas.
- Evaluate laboratory data for complications.
- Prevent infection.
- Prevent hemorrhage or injury from bleeding.
- Prevent anemia or injury from anemia.

APPLICATION EXERCISES KEY

1. A. INCORRECT: The nurse should not plan to palpate the abdomen because this can lead to rupture of the of encapsulated tumor.

    B. **CORRECT:** The nurse should plan to prepare the toddler for surgery because surgical removal of the tumor should take place within 24 to 48 hr of admission.

    C. INCORRECT: Wilms' tumor is usually unilateral. Therefore, it is unlikely the toddler will undergo dialysis.

    D. INCORRECT: The nurse should not plan to obtain a 24-hr urine specimen because the provider most likely used this specimen when diagnosing Wilms' tumor.

    Ⓝ NCLEX® Connection: Physiological Adaptations, Basic Pathophysiology

2. A. INCORRECT: The nurse should expect a child who has Wilms' tumor to have weight loss rather than weight gain.

    B. **CORRECT:** The nurse should expect a child who has Wilms' tumor to have hematuria.

    C. INCORRECT: The nurse should expect a child who has Wilms' tumor to have hypertension.

    D. INCORRECT: The nurse should expect a child who has metastatic neuroblastoma to have bone pain.

    E. **CORRECT:** The nurse should expect a child who has Wilms' tumor to have fatigue.

    Ⓝ NCLEX® Connection: Physiological Adaptations, Basic Pathophysiology

3. A. INCORRECT: Hematuria is a late clinical manifestation of leukemia.

    B. **CORRECT:** Anorexia is an early clinical manifestation of leukemia.

    C. **CORRECT:** Petechiae is an early clinical manifestation of leukemia.

    D. INCORRECT: Ulcerations in the mouth are a late clinical manifestation of leukemia.

    E. **CORRECT:** Unsteady gait is an early clinical manifestation of leukemia.

    Ⓝ NCLEX® Connection: Physiological Adaptations, Basic Pathophysiology

4. A. **CORRECT:** Constipation is a clinical manifestation of neuropathy.

    B. INCORRECT: Skin breakdown is an adverse effect of chemotherapy.

    C. **CORRECT:** Foot drop is a clinical manifestation of neuropathy.

    D. **CORRECT:** Jaw pain is a clinical manifestation of neuropathy.

    E. INCORRECT: Hemorrhagic cystitis is an adverse effect of chemotherapy.

     NCLEX® Connection: Physiological Adaptations, Basic Pathophysiology

5. A. INCORRECT: The nurse should not plan to use lemon glycerin swabs because they can cause tooth decay and erosion of the tissues.

    B. INCORRECT: The nurse should not plan to use viscous lidocaine because it can depress the gag reflex and cause aspiration.

    C. **CORRECT:** The nurse should plan to offer soft foods to decrease the amount of chewing needed and possible irritation.

    D. **CORRECT:** The nurse should plan to use a soft toothbrush to minimize irritation during oral care.

    E. **CORRECT:** The nurse should plan to offer warm saline mouthwash to provide pain relief.

     NCLEX® Connection: Physiological Adaptations, Basic Pathophysiology

6. A. INCORRECT: The client should take filgrastim (Neupogen) to stimulate WBC production.

    B. INCORRECT: The client should take oprelvekin (Interleukin-11) to simulate platelet production.

    C. INCORRECT: The client should take iron supplements for anemia.

    D. **CORRECT:** The client should take epoetin alfa to stimulate RBC formation.

     NCLEX® Connection: Physiological Adaptations, Alterations in Body Systems

7. *Using ATI Active Learning Template: Systems Disorder*
    A. Nursing Actions
        - Evaluate laboratory data for complications.
            ○ Infection – elevated WBC and fever
            ○ Hemorrhage – blood in urine or stool, bruising, and petechiae
            ○ Anemia – fatigue and decreased hemoglobin/hematocrit
        - Prevent infection.
            ○ Provide a private room when hospitalized.
            ○ Restrict staff/visitors who have infections.
            ○ Promote frequent hand hygiene by staff/visitors.
            ○ Avoid all live-virus vaccines during periods of immunosuppression.
            ○ Ensure that siblings are up to date on vaccinations.
            ○ Provide a diet adequate in proteins and calories.
        - Prevent hemorrhage or injury from bleeding.
            ○ Use a strict aseptic technique for all invasive procedures.
            ○ Use gentle technique when providing mouth care.
            ○ Clean the perineal area carefully to prevent trauma, and avoid obtaining temperatures rectally.
            ○ Assist with administering platelets.
        - Prevent anemia or injury from anemia.
            ○ Provide rest periods as needed.
            ○ Assist with administering packed red blood cells.

    N NCLEX® Connection: Physiological Adaptations, Basic Pathophysiology

UNIT 3   Nursing Care of Children with Special Needs

CHAPTERS

› Pediatric Emergencies
› Psychosocial Issues of Infants, Children, and Adolescents

NCLEX® CONNECTIONS

When reviewing the chapters in this section, keep in mind the relevant sections of the NCLEX® outline, in particular:

Client Needs: Psychosocial Integrity

› Relevant topics/tasks include:
  » Abuse or Neglect
    › Identify signs and symptoms of physical, psychological or financial abuse in client.

Client Needs: Physiological Adaptations

› Relevant topics/tasks include:
  » Alterations in Body Systems
    › Reinforce education to client regarding car and condition.
  » Basic Pathophysiology
    › Identify signs and symptoms related to an acute or chronic illness.
  » Medical Emergencies
    › Respond/intervene to a client life-threatening situation.

chapter 38

Overview

- In caring for children, nurses often deal with emergent care situations that require rapid assessment and intervention and offer opportunities for parent and community education.
  - Respiratory emergencies
  - Drowning
  - Apparent life-threatening event
  - Sudden infant death syndrome (SIDS)
  - Poisoning

RESPIRATORY EMERGENCIES

Overview

- Respiratory insufficiency
  - Increased work of breathing with mostly adequate gas exchange or hypoxia with acidosis
- Respiratory failure
  - Inability to maintain adequate oxygenation of the blood
- Apnea
  - The cessation of respirations for more than 20 seconds
  - May be associated with hypoxemia or bradycardia
  - Can be central or obstructive
- Respiratory arrest
  - The complete cessation of respirations
- Airway obstruction
  - May be due to aspiration of a foreign body

Data Collection

- Risk Factors
  - Toddlers
  - Primary inefficient gas exchange due to cerebral trauma, brain tumor, overdose, asphyxia, or CNS infection
  - Obstructive lung disease caused by aspiration, infection, tumor, anaphylaxis, laryngospasm, or asthma
  - Restrictive lung disease resulting from cystic fibrosis, pneumonia, or respiratory distress syndrome
- Subjective Data
  - History of illnesses (chronic or acute)
  - History of events leading to respiratory emergency
  - Allergies
- Objective Data
  - Early signs of respiratory distress
    - Restlessness
    - Tachypnea
    - Tachycardia
    - Diaphoresis
    - Nasal flaring
    - Retractions
    - Grunting
    - Dyspnea
    - Wheezing
  - Advanced hypoxia
    - Bradypnea
    - Bradycardia
    - Peripheral or central cyanosis
    - Stupor
    - Coma
  - Signs of choking
    - Universal choking sign (clutching neck with hands)
    - Inability to speak
    - Weak, ineffective cough
    - High-pitched sounds or no sound
    - Dyspnea
    - Cyanosis
- Laboratory Tests – arterial blood gases (ABGs)
- Diagnostic Procedures – chest x-rays

Patient-Centered Care

Q
EBP

- Nursing Care
  - Follow the American Heart Association (AHA) guidelines for CPR for respiratory and cardiac arrest.
  - Follow the facility's protocol for activating the rapid response team.
  - Use current basic life support (BLS) and advanced cardiac life support (ACLS) guidelines for neonates (NALS) and for pediatric clients (PALS).
  - Obstructed Airway
    - Follow the American Heart Association (AHA) guidelines for a choking child.
    - Infants – Use a combination of back blows and chest thrusts.
    - Children and adolescents – Use abdominal thrusts.
    - Remove any visual obstruction or large debris from the mouth, but do not perform blind finger sweep.
    - Place the recovered child (one who resumes breathing) into the recovery position (side-lying position with legs bent at knees for stability).
  - Position to maintain patent airway. Monitor respiratory status. Monitor vital signs.
  - Administer oxygen.
  - Suction as needed.
  - Assist with intubation if needed.
  - Use a calm approach with the child and family.
  - Assist with emergency medications.
  - Keep the family informed of the child's status.
  - Client Education
    - Teach the family clinical manifestations of respiratory distress.
    - Encourage the family to learn CPR.
    - Reinforce teaching with the family about strategies to prevent respiratory emergencies, such as recognizing choking hazards for toddlers.

DROWNING

Overview

- Asphyxiation while child is submerged in fluid may occur in any standing body of water that is at least 1 inch deep (bathtub, toilet, bucket, pool, pond, lake).
- Submersion injury (near-drowning) incidents are those in which children have survived for 24 hr after being submerged in fluid.

Data Collection

- Risk Factors
  - Children over 12 months of age
  - Swimming (may be overconfident or lack ability)
  - Inadequate supervision or unattended in bathtub, pools, or any source of water
  - Not wearing life jackets when in water
  - Diving
  - Child abuse
- Subjective Data
  - History of event including location and time of submersion
  - Type and temperature of the fluid
- Objective Data
  - Respiratory assessment (see the respiratory emergencies section)
  - Body temperature (hypothermia)
  - Bruising, spinal cord injury, or other physical injuries
- Laboratory Tests – ABGs
- Diagnostic Procedures – chest x-rays

Patient-Centered Care

- Nursing Care (based on degree of cerebral insult)
  - Administer oxygen; may need mechanical ventilation.
  - Monitor vital signs.
  - Assist with emergency medications.
  - Provide chest physiotherapy.
  - Monitor for complications that can occur 24 hr after incident (cerebral edema, respiratory distress).
  - Use a calm approach with the child and family.
  - Keep the family informed of the child's status.
  - Client Education
    - Instruct parents to provide supervision for children near any body of water, even if the child is able to swim.
    - Preventive measures include
      - Locking toilet seats if toddlers are in home.
      - Always attending children when in the bathtub or swimming pool.
      - Ensuring all private pools are surrounded by a fence and locked gate.
      - Securing life jackets when boating.

APPARENT LIFE-THREATENING EVENT

Overview

- Sudden event where the infant exhibits apnea, change in color, change in muscle tone, and choking

Data Collection

- Risk Factors
  - Gastroesophageal reflux
  - Respiratory infections
  - Seizure
  - Urinary tract infection (UTI)
- Subjective data
  - Description of the event by the observer
  - CPR efforts provided
  - Maternal history
  - Family history of seizures
- Objective data
  - Event
    - Apnea may or may not be present during event.
    - Change in color: pallor, redness, cyanosis.
    - Change in muscle tone: hypotonia.
    - Choking, gagging, coughing.
  - Head-to-toe assessment
- Laboratory Tests
  - Blood cultures – bacterial or viral infection
  - Urine culture – UTI
  - CBC
  - Serum glucose
  - Electrolytes
- Diagnostic Procedures
  - ECG (long QT syndrome or dysrhythmias)
  - EEG (epilepsy)
  - pH study (reflux)
  - MRI (hemorrhage or cerebral abnormalities/injuries)
  - Sleep study (sleep apnea)

Patient-Centered Care

- Nursing Care
  - Prepare infant and family for testing.
  - Monitor infant for recurrent events.
  - Encourage the family to learn CPR.
  - Reinforce teaching regarding use of an apnea monitor, if prescribed.

SUDDEN INFANT DEATH SYNDROME (SIDS)

Overview

- SIDS is the sudden, unpredictable death of an infant without an identified cause, even after investigation and autopsy.
- Preventive measures should be taught to families.

Data Collection

- Risk Factors
  - Maternal smoking during pregnancy
  - Secondhand smoke
  - Cosleeping with parent or adult
  - Nonstandard bed (sofa, soft bedding, water beds, pillows, or use of crib bumpers)
  - Prone or side-lying sleeping
  - Low birth weight
  - Prematurity
  - Twin or multiple birth
  - Low Apgar scores
  - Viral illness
  - Family history of SIDS
  - Poverty
- Subjective data
  - History of events prior to discovery of infant
  - History of illnesses
  - Pregnancy and birth history
  - Presence of risk factors

Patient-Centered Care

- Nursing Care
  - Teach the family how to reduce the risks of SIDS.
    - Place infant on back for sleep.
    - Avoid exposure to tobacco smoke.
    - Prevent overheating.
    - Use a firm, tight-fitting mattress in the infant's crib.
    - Remove all objects including blankets from the crib during sleep.
    - Ensure that the infant's head is kept uncovered during sleep.
    - Offer pacifier at naps and night.
    - Encourage breastfeeding.
    - Avoid cosleeping.
    - Maintain immunizations up to date.
  - Provide support.
  - Allow the infant's family an opportunity to express feelings.
  - Plan a home health visit to follow a death.
  - Refer to support groups, counseling, or community groups.

POISONING

Overview

- Ingestion of or exposure to toxic substances.
- Preventive measures should be taught to families.

Data Collection

- Risk Factors
  - Children younger than 6 years of age
  - Improperly stored medications, household chemicals, and hazardous substances
  - Exposure to plants, cosmetics, and heavy metals, which are potential sources of toxic substances
  - Lead ingestion from lead-based paint, soil contamination
- Subjective data
  - Information regarding poisonous agent
    - Name and location
    - Amount ingested
    - Time of ingestion

- Objective data
  - Physical response will depend on specific poison
    - Acetaminophen (Tylenol)
      - 2 to 4 hr after ingestion – nausea, vomiting, sweating, and pallor
      - 24 to 36 hr after ingestion – improvement in the child's condition
      - 36 hr to 7 days or longer (hepatic stage) – pain in upper right quadrant, confusion, stupor, jaundice, and coagulation disturbances
      - Final stage – death or gradual recovery
    - Acetylsalicylic acid (aspirin)
      - Acute poisoning – nausea, vomiting, disorientation, diaphoresis, tachypnea, tinnitus, oliguria, lightheadedness, and seizures
      - Chronic poisoning – subtle version of acute manifestations, bleeding tendencies, dehydration, and seizures more severe than acute poisoning
    - Supplemental iron
      - Initial period (30 min to 6 hr after ingestion) – vomiting, hematemesis, diarrhea, gastric pain, and bloody stools
      - Latency period (2 to 12 hr after ingestion) – improvement of condition
      - Systemic toxicity period (4 to 24 hr after ingestion) – metabolic acidosis, hyperglycemia, bleeding, fever, shock, and possible death
      - Hepatic injury period (48 to 96 hr after ingestion) – seizures or coma
    - Hydrocarbons (gasoline, kerosene, lighter fluid, paint thinner, turpentine)
      - Gagging, choking, coughing, nausea, and vomiting
      - Lethargy, weakness, tachypnea, cyanosis, grunting, and retractions
    - Corrosives (household cleaners, batteries, denture cleaners, bleach)
      - Pain and burning in mouth, throat, and stomach
      - Edematous lips, tongue, and pharynx with white mucous membranes
      - Violent vomiting with hemoptysis
      - Drooling
      - Anxiety
      - Shock
    - Lead
      - Low-dose exposure – easily distracted, impulsive, hyperactive, hearing impairment, and mild intellectual difficulty
      - High-dose exposure – cognitive delays varying in severity, blindness, paralysis, coma, seizures, and death
      - Other manifestations – kidney impairment, impaired calcium function, and anemia

- Laboratory Tests
  - Serum lead
  - CBC with differential
  - ABGs
  - Serum iron
  - Serum acetaminophen
  - Liver function tests
  - Blood alcohol and toxicology screening

Patient-Centered Care

- Nursing Care
  - Depends on the poison ingested. Monitor for ongoing changes.
  - Terminate exposure.
  - Provide cardiorespiratory support as needed.
  - Notify local or regional poison control center.
  - Administer IV fluids.
  - Provide for cardiac monitoring.
  - Monitor vital signs and oxygen saturation.
  - Monitor I&O.
  - Administer antidote if indicated.
  - Assist with gastric decontamination if indicated.
    - Activated charcoal.
    - Gastric lavage.
    - Increasing bowel motility.
    - Syrup of ipecac is contraindicated for routine poison control treatment.
  - Keep the family informed of the child's condition.

SUBSTANCE	INTERVENTION
Acetaminophen (Tylenol)	› N-acetylcysteine given orally
Acetylsalicylic acid (Aspirin)	› Activated charcoal › Gastric lavage › Sodium bicarbonate › Oxygen and ventilation › Vitamin K › Hemodialysis for severe cases

SUBSTANCE	INTERVENTION
Supplemental iron	› Emesis or lavage › Chelation therapy using deferoxamine mesylate (Desferal)
Hydrocarbons (gasoline, kerosene, lighter fluid, paint thinner, turpentine)	› Do not induce vomiting › Intubation with cuffed endotracheal tube prior to any gastric decontamination › Treatment of chemical pneumonia
Corrosives (household cleaners, batteries, denture cleaners, bleach)	› Airway maintenance › NPO › No attempt to neutralize acid (corrosive) › Do not induce vomiting › Analgesics for pain
Lead	› Chelation therapy using calcium EDTA (calcium disodium versenate)

- ○ Client Education
  - ▪ Poison prevention
    - ▫ Keep toxic agents out of reach of children.
    - ▫ Lock cabinets containing potentially harmful substances.
    - ▫ Do not take medication in front of children.
    - ▫ Discard unused medications.
    - ▫ When giving a child medication, do not tell them it is candy.
    - ▫ Use nonmercury thermometers.
    - ▫ Eliminate lead-based paint in the environment.
    - ▫ Encourage hand hygiene prior to eating.
    - ▫ Do not store food in lead-based containers.

Complications

- Cognitive Impairments
  - ○ Varies with degree of anoxic insult or lead levels in the blood.
  - ○ Provide prevention measures to families.
  - ○ Routine screening for lead levels at 1, 2, and 3 years of age.
  - ○ Provide case management for children who have elevated lead levels.
  - ○ Make appropriate referrals (community nurse, teacher, early intervention).

APPLICATION EXERCISES

1. A nurse is caring for a child who has respiratory distress. Which of the following are early clinical manifestations? (Select all that apply.)

_____ A. Bradypnea

_____ B. Peripheral cyanosis

_____ C. Tachycardia

_____ D. Diaphoresis

_____ E. Restlessness

2. A nurse is reinforcing teaching about SIDS prevention with a mother. Which of the following should the nurse include in the teaching? (Select all that apply.)

_____ A. Cover the infant's head when sleeping.

_____ B. Avoid exposure to smoke.

_____ C. Use a space heater in the infant's room.

_____ D. Use a firm, tight-fitting mattress for the crib.

_____ E. Place the newborn on her back for sleeping.

3. A nurse is reinforcing teaching to a parent about acetaminophen (Tylenol) poisoning. Which of the following statements by the nurse should be included in the teaching?

A. "Nausea begins 24 hours after ingestion."

B. "Pallor can appear as early as 2 hours after ingestion."

C. "Jaundice will appear in 12 hours if your child is toxic."

D. "Children can have 4 grams of acetaminophen per day."

4. A nurse is caring for a child who has swallowed paint thinner. The child is lethargic, gagging, and cyanotic. Which of the following is an appropriate action for the nurse to take?

A. Induce vomiting with syrup of ipecac.

B. Insert a nasogastric tube and administer activated charcoal.

C. Prepare for intubation with a cuffed endotracheal tube.

D. Administer chelation therapy using deferoxamine mesylate.

5. A nurse in the emergency department is assisting with the admission of a child who experienced an obstructed airway in which the parent performed CPR. Which of the following statements by the parent requires clarification?

    A. "I pushed on my son's abdomen."

    B. "I tilted my son's head back while lifting his chin."

    C. "I listened for sounds of breathing by my son."

    D. "I used my finger to check my son's mouth."

6. A nurse is reinforcing teaching with a group of parents about prevention of drowning. What should the nurse include? Use the ATI Active Learning Template: Basic Concept to identify methods to reduce the risk of drowning.

APPLICATION EXERCISES KEY

1. A. INCORRECT: Tachycardia is an early clinical manifestation of respiratory distress.

    B. INCORRECT: Cyanosis is an advanced clinical manifestation of hypoxia.

    C. **CORRECT:** Tachycardia is an early clinical manifestation of respiratory distress.

    D. **CORRECT:** Diaphoresis is an early clinical manifestation of respiratory distress.

    E. **CORRECT:** Restlessness is an early clinical manifestation of respiratory distress.

    Ⓝ NCLEX® Connection: Physiological Adaptations, Basic Pathophysiology

2. A. INCORRECT: The parent should keep the infant's head uncovered when sleeping to prevent overheating and increasing the risk of SIDS.

    B. **CORRECT:** The parent should avoid exposing the newborn to tobacco smoke to decrease the risk of SIDS.

    C. INCORRECT: Use of a space heater can cause the newborn to become overheated and increases the risk of SIDS.

    D. INCORRECT: Use of a firm, tight-fitting mattress in the crib decreases the risk for injury.

    E. **CORRECT:** Sleeping on the back decreases the risk of SIDS.

    Ⓝ NCLEX® Connection: Physiological Adaptations, Alterations in Body Systems

3. A. INCORRECT: Nausea is a clinical manifestation that begins 2 to 4 hr after ingestion.

    B. **CORRECT:** Sweating is a clinical manifestation that starts 2 to 4 hr after ingestion.

    C. INCORRECT: Jaundice will appear in 36 hr to 7 days.

    D. INCORRECT: The maximum dose of acetaminophen in children 2 to 5 years of age is 720 mg/day. In children 6 to 12 years of age, it is 2.6 g/day.

    Ⓝ NCLEX® Connection: Physiological Adaptations, Alterations in Body Systems

4. A. INCORRECT: Inducing vomiting with syrup of ipecac is contraindicated as a poison control measure.

    B. INCORRECT: Activated charcoal is indicated for acetylsalicylic acid poisoning.

    C. **CORRECT:** Treatment for poisoning with hydrocarbons includes intubation to protect the airway before proceeding with gastric decontamination.

    D. INCORRECT: Chelation therapy is indicated for lead poisoning.

    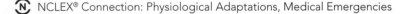 NCLEX® Connection: Physiological Adaptations, Medical Emergencies

5. A. INCORRECT: Abdominal thrusts are performed to open an obstructed airway in a child as part of CPR.

    B. INCORRECT: The head-tilt, chin-lift method during CPR is used to open an obstructed airway.

    C. INCORRECT: Checking for chest motion and listening for normal breath sounds are steps in evaluating airway clearance when performing CPR.

    D. **CORRECT:** Finger sweeps to check for an impaired airway are not performed as part of CPR.

    N NCLEX® Connection: Physiological Adaptations, Alterations in Body Systems

6. *Using the ATI Active Learning Template: Basic Concept*
    - Methods to reduce the risks of drowning
      - Provide supervision whenever children are near any body of water, even if the child is able to swim.
      - Lock toilet seats if toddlers are in home.
      - Attend to children when in the bathtub or swimming pool.
      - Ensure all private pools are surrounded by a fence and locked gate.
      - Have children wear life jackets when boating.
      - Encourage swimming lessons.

    N NCLEX® Connection: Physiological Adaptations, Alterations in Body Systems

chapter 39

Overview

- Depression
- Posttraumatic stress disorder (PTSD)
- Attention-deficit/hyperactivity disorder (ADHD)
- Autism spectrum disorder
- Cognitive impairment
- Failure to thrive (FTT)
- Maltreatment of infants and children

DEPRESSION

Overview

- Difficult to detect because children have limitations in expressing their feelings.
- Findings must be present for 1 year to diagnose major depressive disorder in children and adolescents.

Data Collection

- Risk Factors
  - Family history
  - Traumatic event
- Subjective and Objective Data
  - Sad facial expressions
  - Tendency to remain alone
  - Withdrawn from family, friends, and activities
  - Fatigue
  - Tearful/crying
  - Ill feeling
  - Weight loss or gain
  - Alterations in sleep
  - Lack of interest in school, drop in school performance
  - Statements regarding low self-esteem
  - Hopelessness
  - Suicidal ideations

Patient-Centered Care

- Nursing Care
  - Provide individualized care.
  - Obtain health history.
  - Determine substance use.
  - Identify actual or potential risk to self (including a suicide plan, the lethality of that plan, and the means to carry out the plan).
  - Assist with coping strategies.
  - Encourage peer group discussions, mentoring, and counseling.
- Medications
  - Tricyclic antidepressants (TCAs) or selective serotonin reuptake inhibitors (SSRIs)
    - Trazodone (Oleptro), sertraline (Zoloft), paroxetine (Paxil), bupropion (Wellbutrin)
    - Nursing Care
      - Monitor for adverse effects.
      - Monitor for suicidal ideations.
    - Client teaching
      - Reinforce teaching to the client and family about adverse effects.
      - Reinforce teaching to the client and family about when to expect therapeutic effectiveness.
      - Reinforce teaching to the client and family about not abruptly discontinuing the medication.

Complications

- Suicide

POSTTRAUMATIC STRESS DISORDER (PTSD)

Overview

- Develops following a traumatic event

Data Collection

- Risk Factors
  - Potential genetic predisposition
  - Traumatic incident
  - Repeated trauma
  - Psychiatric disorder

- Subjective and Objective Data
  - Initial response
    - Lasting a few minutes to 2 hr
    - Increased stress hormones (fight or flight)
  - Second phase
    - Lasting approximately 2 weeks
    - Period of calm (feeling of numbness, denial)
  - Third phase
    - Extends over 2 to 3 months
    - Client gets worse instead of better
    - Depression, phobias, anxiety, conversion reactions, repetitive movements, flashbacks

Patient-Centered Care

- Nursing Care
  - Assist with referral to psychotherapy services.
  - Monitor for behavior changes/behavior problems.
  - Monitor school work.
  - Assist the family and client with coping strategies.
  - Allow family and client to express their feelings.
- Medications
  - Selective norepinephrine reuptake inhibitor can be used on an individual basis.

ATTENTION-DEFICIT/HYPERACTIVITY DISORDER (ADHD)

Overview

- Inattentiveness, hyperactivity, and impulsiveness
- Diagnostic criteria for diagnosis
  - Symptoms typically are present between the ages of 4 and 18 years.
  - Manifestations are present in more than one setting.
  - Evidence of social or academic impairment.
  - Six or more findings from a category (inattention or hyperactivity-impulsive).

Data Collection

- Risk Factors
  - Can be a familial tendency
- Subjective and Objective Data
  - Inattention
    - Fails to pay close attention to detail or makes careless mistakes
    - Difficulty sustaining attention
    - Does not seem to listen
    - Fails to follow through on instructions
    - Difficulty organizing activities
    - Avoids or dislikes activities that require mental effort for a period of time
    - Loses things
    - Easily distracted
    - Forgetful
  - Hyperactivity
    - Fidgety
    - Fails to remain seated
    - Inappropriate running
    - Difficulty engaging in quiet play
    - Seems to be busy all the time
    - Talks excessively
  - Impulsivity
    - Blurts out response before question is asked
    - Difficulty waiting turns
    - Interrupts often

Patient-Centered Care

- Nursing Care/Client Teaching
  - Use a calm, firm, respectful approach with the child.
  - Use modeling to demonstrate acceptable behavior.
  - Obtain the child's attention before giving directions. Provide short and clear explanations.
  - Set clear limits on unacceptable behaviors and be consistent.
  - Provide physical activities through which the child can use energy and obtain success.
  - Focus on the family and child's strengths, not just the problems.
  - Support the parents' efforts to remain hopeful.

○ Provide a safe environment for the child and others.

○ Provide the child with specific positive feedback when expectations are met.

○ Identify issues that result in power struggles.

○ Assist the child in developing effective coping mechanisms.

○ Encourage the child to participate in a form of group, individual, or family therapy.

○ Assist the family with behavioral strategies.

  ▪ Positive reinforcement

  ▪ Rewards for good behavior

  ▪ Age-appropriate consequences

○ Assist family with modification of the environment to help the child become successful.

  ▪ Structured environment

  ▪ Charts to assist with organization

  ▪ Decreasing stimuli in the environment

  ▪ Consistent study area

  ▪ Model positive behaviors

○ Assist with appropriate classroom placement in the school.

  ▪ Allow more time for testing.

  ▪ Place in classroom that has order and consistent rules.

  ▪ Offer verbal instruction combined with visual cues.

  ▪ Plan academic subjects in the morning.

  ▪ Include regular breaks.

  ▪ Provide for small classroom settings or work groups.

● Medications

  ○ Methylphenidate (Ritalin) or dextroamphetamine (Dexedrine)

    ▪ Psychostimulant, which increases dopamine and norepinephrine levels

    ▪ Nursing Considerations/Client Education

      □ Gradually increase dose to reach therapeutic results.

      □ Give 30 min before meal.

      □ Give last dose of the day prior to 1800 to prevent insomnia.

      □ Monitor for adverse effects.

  ○ Atomoxetine (Strattera)

    ▪ Selective norepinephrine reuptake inhibitor

    ▪ Nursing Considerations/Client Education

      □ Gradual increase in dose to reach therapeutic results.

      □ Monitor for adverse effects (suicidal ideations).

AUTISM SPECTRUM DISORDER

Overview

- Complex neurodevelopmental disorders with spectrum of behaviors affecting an individual's ability to communicate and interact with others.

Data Collection

- Risk Factors
  - Possible genetic component
- Subjective and Objective Data
  - Delays in at least one of the following: social interaction, social communication, imaginative play prior to the age of 3 years
  - Distress when routines are changed
  - Unusual attachments to objects
  - Cannot start or continue conversation
  - Uses gestures instead of words
  - Delayed language development
  - Unable to adjust gaze to look at something else
  - Does not refer to self correctly
  - Withdrawn
  - Lack of empathy
  - Spends time alone rather than play with others
  - Avoids eye contact
  - Withdraw from physical contact
  - Heightened or lowered senses
  - Does not imitate actions of others
  - Minimal pretend play
  - Short attention span
  - Intense temper tantrums
  - Shows aggression
  - Exhibits repetitive movements

Patient-Centered Care

- Nursing Care/Client Education
  - Assist with screening assessment tools.
  - Assist with referrals to early intervention, physical therapy, occupational therapy, and speech and language therapy.
  - Assist with behavior modification program.
    - Promote positive reinforcement.
    - Increase social awareness.
    - Reinforce appropriate verbal communication.
    - Decrease unacceptable behaviors.
    - Set realistic goals.
    - Structure opportunities for small successes.
    - Set clear rules.
  - Decrease environmental stimulation.
  - Provide for nutritional needs.
  - Introduce the child to new situations slowly.
  - Monitor for behavior changes.
  - Encourage age appropriate play.
  - Communicate at an age-appropriate level.
  - Provide support to the family.
  - Encourage support groups.
- Medications
  - Used on an individual basis to control aggression, anxiety, hyperactivity, irritability, mood swings, compulsions, and attention problems.

COGNITIVE IMPAIRMENT

Overview

- Mental difficulty or deficiency

Data Collection

- Risk Factors
  - Infections (congenital rubella, syphilis)
  - Fetal alcohol syndrome
  - Chronic lead ingestion
  - Trauma to the brain
  - Preexisting disease (Down syndrome, psychiatric disorders, microcephaly, hydrocephaly, metabolic disorders)

- Subjective and Objective Data
  - Can range from mild to severe
  - Delayed developmental milestones
  - Early clinical manifestations
    - Abnormal eye contact
    - Feeding difficulties
    - Language difficulties
    - Gross motor delays
    - Decrease alertness
    - Unresponsive to contact

Patient-Centered Care

- Nursing Care/Client Education
  - Determine the child's deficiency.
  - Care and teaching should be individualized to the client's needs.
  - Assist with appropriate referrals such as early intervention program, social work, speech therapy, physical therapy, and occupational therapy.
  - Add visual cues with verbal instruction.
  - Give one-step instructions.
  - Assist the family in teaching the child self-care activities.
  - Assist the family in promoting development.
  - Encourage play.
  - Assist the family with appropriate activities and toys.
  - Assist with communication skills.
  - Encourage social activities.

FAILURE TO THRIVE (FTT)

Overview

- Inadequate growth resulting from the inability to obtain or use calories required for growth. It is usually described in an infant or child who falls below the fifth percentile for weight (and possibly for height) or who has persistent weight loss.
  - Inadequate caloric intake
  - Inadequate absorption
  - Increased metabolism
  - Defective utilization

Data Collection

- Risk Factor
  - Organic causes: cerebral palsy, chronic renal failure, congenital heart disease, hyperthyroidism, cystic fibrosis, celiac disease, hepatic disease, Down syndrome, prematurity, and gastroesophageal reflux
  - Parental neglect, lack of parental knowledge, or a disturbed maternal-child attachment
  - Poverty
  - Health or childrearing beliefs
  - Family stress
  - Feeding resistance
  - Insufficient breast milk
- Subjective and Objective Data
  - Less than the fifth percentile on the growth chart for weight
  - Malnourished appearance
  - No fear of strangers
  - Minimal smiling
  - Decreased activity level
  - Withdrawal behavior
  - Developmental delays
  - Feeding disorder
  - Wide-eyed gaze
  - Stiff or flaccid body

Patient-Centered Care

- Nursing Care
  - Assist with obtaining a nutritional history.
  - Observe parent-child interactions.
  - Collect baseline height and weight. Observe for low weight, malnourished appearance, and signs of dehydration.
  - Weigh the child daily without clothing or a diaper.
  - Maintain I&O and calorie counts as prescribed.
  - Reinforce teaching to the parents about recognizing and responding to the infant's cues of hunger.
  - Establish a routine for eating that encourages usual times, duration, and setting.
  - Reinforce proper positioning, latching on, and timing for mothers who are breastfeeding.
  - Provide 24 kcal/oz formula as prescribed.
  - Provide high-calorie milk supplements for children.

- ○ Administer multivitamin supplements including zinc and iron.
- ○ Reinforce teaching to parents regarding how to mix formula properly and provide step-by-step written instructions.
- ○ Limit juice to 4 oz/day.
- ○ Provide developmental stimulation.
- ○ Encourage parents to:
  - Maintain eye contact and face-to-face posture during feedings.
  - Talk to the infant while feeding.
  - Burp the infant frequently.
  - Keep the environment quiet and avoid distractions.
  - Be persistent, remaining calm during 10 to 15 min of food refusal.
  - Introduce new foods slowly.
  - Never force the infant to eat.

Complications

- Extreme malnourishment
  - ○ Nursing Care – Prepare the client and the parents for tube feedings or IV therapy.

MALTREATMENT OF INFANTS AND CHILDREN

Overview

- Maltreatment of infants and children is attributed to a variety of predisposing factors, which include parental, child, and environmental characteristics. Child maltreatment can occur across all economic and educational backgrounds and racial/ethnic/religious groups.
  - ○ Maltreatment of children is made up of several specific types of behaviors.
    - Physical – causing pain or harm to a child (shaken baby syndrome [due to violent shaking of infants], fractures, Munchausen syndrome by proxy)
    - Sexual – occurring when sexual contact takes place without consent, whether or not the victim is able to give consent (includes any sexual behavior toward a minor and dating violence among adolescents)
    - Emotional – humiliating, threatening, or intimidating a child (includes behavior that minimizes an individual's feelings of self-worth)
    - Neglect – includes failure to provide:
      - □ Physical care (feeding, clothing, shelter, medical or dental care, safety, education)
      - □ Emotional care and/or stimulation to foster normal development (nurturing, affection, attention)

Data Collection

- Warning signs of abuse
  - Physical evidence of abuse
  - History of injury incompatible with the findings
  - Vague explanation of injury
  - Other injuries are discovered that are not related to the original client concern
  - Delay in seeking care
  - Multiple fractures at different stages of healing
  - Bruising in a nonmobile client
  - Caregivers/client report conflicting histories
  - Statement of possible abuse from a caregiver or client
- Parental characteristics
  - Younger parents
  - Single parents
  - Social isolation
  - Low-income situation
  - Lack of education or lower education level
  - Low self-esteem
  - Lack of knowledge of parenting
  - Substance use disorder
  - History of having been abused
- Characteristics of the child
  - Child 1 year old or younger is at greater risk due to the need for constant attention and increased demands of caregiving.
  - Infants and children who are unwanted, hyperactive, or physically or mentally disabled are at risk due to their increased demands and need for constant attention.
  - Premature infants are at risk due to the possible failure of parent-child bonding at birth.
- Environmental characteristics
  - Chronic stress
  - Divorce, alcohol use disorder, drug addiction, poverty, unemployment, inadequate housing, and crowded living conditions
- Subjective and Objective Data
  - Inconsistencies between the parent/caregiver's report and the child's injuries
  - Inconsistency between nature of injury and developmental level of the child
  - Repeated injuries requiring emergency treatment
  - Inappropriate responses from the parents or child

- ○ Physical neglect
  - Failure to thrive, malnutrition
  - Lack of hygiene
  - Frequent injuries
  - Delay in seeking health care
  - Dull affect
  - School absences
  - Self-stimulating behaviors
- ○ Physical abuse
  - Bruises, welts in various stages of healing
  - Burns
  - Fractures
  - Lacerations
  - Fear of parents
  - Lack of emotional response/reaction
  - Superficial relationships
  - Withdrawal
  - Aggression
- ○ Emotional neglect and abuse
  - Failure to thrive
  - Eating disorder
  - Enuresis
  - Sleep disturbances
  - Self-stimulating behaviors
  - Withdrawal
  - Lack of social smile (infant)
  - Extreme behaviors
  - Delayed development
  - Attempts suicide
- ○ Sexual abuse
  - Bruises, lacerations
  - Bleeding of genitalia, anus, or mouth
  - Sexually transmitted infection
  - Difficulty walking or standing
  - UTI
  - Regressive behavior
  - Withdrawn
  - Personality changes

- ○ Shaken baby syndrome
  - ▪ Shaking can cause intracranial hemorrhage.
  - ▪ If bruising is present in an infant before 6 months of age, it should be deemed as suspicious by the nurse.
  - ▪ Manifestations
    - □ Vomiting, poor feeding and listlessness
    - □ Respiratory distress
    - □ Bulging fontanels
    - □ Retinal hemorrhages
    - □ Seizures
    - □ Posturing
    - □ Alterations in LOC
    - □ Apnea
    - □ Bradycardia
- ○ Laboratory Tests
  - ▪ CBC, urinalysis, and other tests that assess for sexually transmitted infections or bleeding
- ○ Diagnostic Procedures – depend upon the assessment findings and noted findings or injuries
  - ▪ Radiograph
  - ▪ CT scan or magnetic resonance imaging scan (MRI)

Patient-Centered Care

- Nursing Care
  - ○ Identify abuse as soon as possible.
  - ○ Determine presence of unusual bruising on the abdomen, back, and/or buttocks.
  - ○ Determine the mechanism of injury, which might not be congruent with the physical appearance of the injury. Many bruises at different stages of healing can indicate ongoing beatings.
  - ○ Observe for bruises or welts in the shape of a belt buckle or other objects.
  - ○ Observe for burns that appear glove- or stocking-like on hands or feet, which can indicate forced immersion into boiling water. Small, round burns can be caused by lit cigarettes.
  - ○ Note fractures with unusual features, such as forearm spiral fractures, which could be caused by twisting the extremity forcefully. The presence of multiple fractures is suspicious.
  - ○ Check the child for head injuries. Identify the child's level of consciousness, making sure to note equal and reactive pupils. Also, monitor the child for nausea/vomiting.
  - ○ The nursing priority is to have the child removed from the abusive situation.
  - ○ Mandatory reporting is required of all providers, including suspected or actual cases of child abuse. There are civil and criminal penalties for not reporting.

- ○ Clearly and objectively document information obtained in the interview and during the physical assessment.

- ○ Photograph and detail all visible injuries.

- ○ Conduct the interview with the child and parents individually.

- ○ Be direct, honest, and professional.

- ○ Use language the child understands.

- ○ Be understanding and attentive.

- ○ Inform the child and parents if a referral is made to child or adult protective services and explain the process.

- ○ Monitor safety and reduce danger for the victim.

- ○ Use open-ended questions that require a descriptive response. These questions are less threatening and elicit more relevant information.

- ○ Provide support for the child and parents.

- ○ Demonstrate behaviors for child-rearing with the parents and child.

- ○ Provide consistent care to the child.

- ○ Avoid asking the child probing questions.

- ○ Promote self-esteem.

- ○ Assist with alleviating feelings of shame and guilt.

- ○ Assist the child with grieving the loss of parents, if indicated.

- ○ Discharge can begin once legal determination of placement has been decided.

- • Teamwork and Collaboration – Assist with referrals to social services.

APPLICATION EXERCISES

1. A nurse is collecting data from a toddler during a well-child visit. Which of the following findings should the nurse identify as a possible sign of physical neglect?

    A. Lack of hygiene

    B. Recurrent urinary tract infections

    C. Lacerations on the torso

    D. Difficulty walking

2. A nurse is reinforcing teaching with the teacher of a child who has attention-deficit/hyperactivity disorder (ADHD). Which of the following classroom strategies should be included in the teaching? (Select all that apply.)

    _____ A. Eliminate testing.

    _____ B. Allow for regular breaks.

    _____ C. Combine verbal instruction with visual cues.

    _____ D. Establish consistent classroom rules.

    _____ E. Decrease stimuli in the environment.

3. A nurse is reinforcing teaching with a parent about posttraumatic stress disorder (PTSD). Which of the following should be included in the teaching? (Select all that apply.)

    _____ A. Children who have PTSD require psychotherapy.

    _____ B. A clinical manifestation of PTSD is phobias.

    _____ C. Depression is seen within 1 day after the incident.

    _____ D. PTSD develops following a traumatic event.

    _____ E. There are six stages of PTSD.

4. A nurse is reinforcing teaching to the parent of a child who has ADHD. The nurse should include which of the following as a characteristic of impulsivity?

    A. Loses things

    B. Frequently interrupts

    C. Is easily distracted

    D. Talks excessively

5. A nurse is caring for a child who has depression. Which of the following findings are associated with this diagnosis? (Select all that apply.)

_____ A. Prefers being with peers

_____ B. Weight loss

_____ C. Report of low self-esteem

_____ D. Sleeping more than usual

_____ E. Hyperactivity

6. A nurse is assisting with the development of an education program about shaken baby syndrome. Use the ATI Active Learning Template: Basic Concept to complete this item to include at least seven clinical manifestations the nurse should include in the program.

APPLICATION EXERCISES KEY

1. A. **CORRECT:** The nurse should identify lack of hygiene as a possible sign physical neglect.

    B. INCORRECT: The nurse should identify recurrent urinary tract infections as a possible sign of sexual abuse.

    C. INCORRECT: The nurse should identify lacerations on the torso as a possible sign of physical abuse.

    D. INCORRECT: The nurse should identify difficulty walking as a possible sign of sexual abuse.

    Ⓝ NCLEX® Connection: Psychosocial Integrity, Abuse/Neglect

2. A. INCORRECT: Allowing for added time when testing can assist the client who has ADHD to be successful.

    B. **CORRECT:** Allowing for regular breaks will assist the client who has ADHD to focus on the required tasks.

    C. **CORRECT:** Combining verbal instruction with visual cues will assist the client who has ADHD with learning information.

    D. **CORRECT:** Providing consistent classroom rules will assist the client who has ADHD to become successful.

    E. **CORRECT:** Stimuli in the environment distract the client who has ADHD, so they should be decreased.

    Ⓝ NCLEX® Connection: Physiological Adaptations, Alterations in Body Systems

3. A. **CORRECT:** Children who have PTSD should receive psychotherapy to assist with resolution of the traumatic event.

    B. **CORRECT:** The child who is experiencing PTSD often has new phobias that can be related to the traumatic event.

    C. INCORRECT: Depression is a clinical manifestation that is seen approximately 2 weeks following the incident.

    D. **CORRECT:** PTSD develops following a traumatic event such as assault, serious injury, or a life-threatening episode.

    E. INCORRECT: PTSD has three stages: the initial response, second, and third phase.

    Ⓝ NCLEX® Connection: Physiological Adaptations, Alterations in Body Systems

4.   A. INCORRECT: Losing things is a characteristic of inattention.

     B. **CORRECT:** Frequently interrupting is a characteristic of impulsivity.

     C. INCORRECT: Being easily distracted is a characteristic of inattention.

     D. INCORRECT: Talking excessively is a characteristic of hyperactivity.

     Ⓝ NCLEX® Connection: Physiological Adaptations, Basic Pathophysiology

5.   A. INCORRECT: A preference for being alone is a finding associated with depression.

     B. **CORRECT:** Weight loss or gain are findings associated with depression.

     C. **CORRECT:** Low self-esteem is a finding associated with depression.

     D. **CORRECT:** Sleeping more than usual is a finding associated with depression.

     E. INCORRECT: Fatigue is a finding associated with depression.

     Ⓝ NCLEX® Connection: Physiological Adaptations, Basic Pathophysiology

6.   *Using the ATI Active Learning Template: Basic Concept*
   - Clinical Manifestations
     - Vomiting, poor feeding, and listlessness
     - Respiratory distress
     - Bulging fontanels
     - Retinal hemorrhages
     - Seizures
     - Posturing
     - Alterations in LOC
     - Apnea
     - Bradycardia

     Ⓝ NCLEX® Connection: Physiological Adaptations, Basic Pathophysiology

Dudek, S. G. (2010). *Nutrition essentials for nursing practice* (6th ed.). Philadelphia: Lippincott Williams & Wilkins.

Grodner, M., Roth, S. L., & Walkingshaw, B. C. (2012). *Nutrition foundations and clinical applications of nutrition: A nursing approach* (5th ed.). St. Louis, MO: Mosby.

Hockenberry, M. J., & Winkelstein M. L. (2013). *Wong's essentials of pediatric nursing* (9th ed.). St. Louis, MO: Mosby.

Lowdermilk, D. L., Perry, S. E., Cahsion, M. C., & Aldean, K. R. (2012). *Maternity & women's health care* (10th ed.). St. Louis, MO: Mosby.

Lehne, R. A. (2013). *Pharmacology for nursing care* (8th ed.). St. Louis: Saunders.

Perry, S. E., Hockenberry, M. J., Lowdermilk, D. L., & Wilson, D. (2010). *Maternal child nursing care* (4th ed.). St. Louis, MO: Mosby Elsevier.

Pillitteri, A. (2010). *Maternal and child health nursing: Care of the childbearing and childrearing family* (6th ed.). Philadelphia: Lippincott Williams & Wilkins.

Wilson, B. A., Shannon, M. T., & Shields, K. M. (2013). *Pearson nurse's drug guide 2013*. Upper Saddle River, NJ: Prentice Hall.

Varcarolis, E. M., Carson, V. B., & Shoemaker, N. C. (2010). *Foundations of psychiatric mental health nursing: A clinical approach* (6th ed.). St. Louis, MO: Saunders.

Appendix

CONTENT_____ REVIEW MODULE CHAPTER _____

TOPIC DESCRIPTOR_____

Related Content (e.g. delegation, levels of prevention, advance directives)	Underlying Principles	Nursing Interventions
		› Who?
		› When?
		› Why?
		› How?

Appendix

CONTENT _____ REVIEW MODULE CHAPTER _____

TOPIC DESCRIPTOR_____

DESCRIPTION OF PROCEDURE:

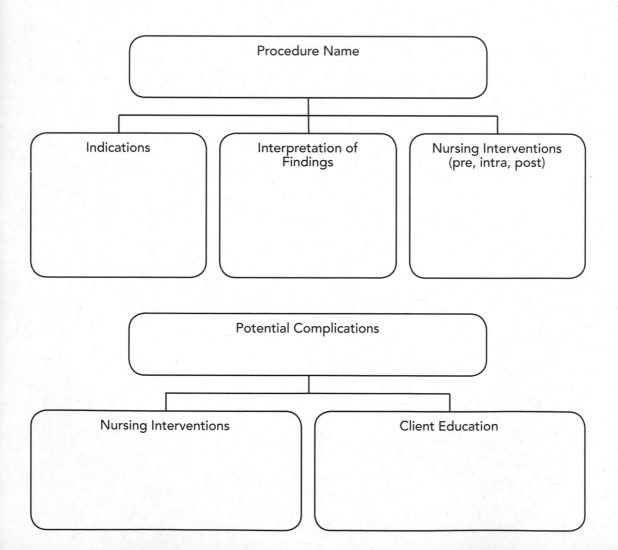

Appendix

CONTENT _____ REVIEW MODULE CHAPTER _____

TOPIC DESCRIPTOR _____

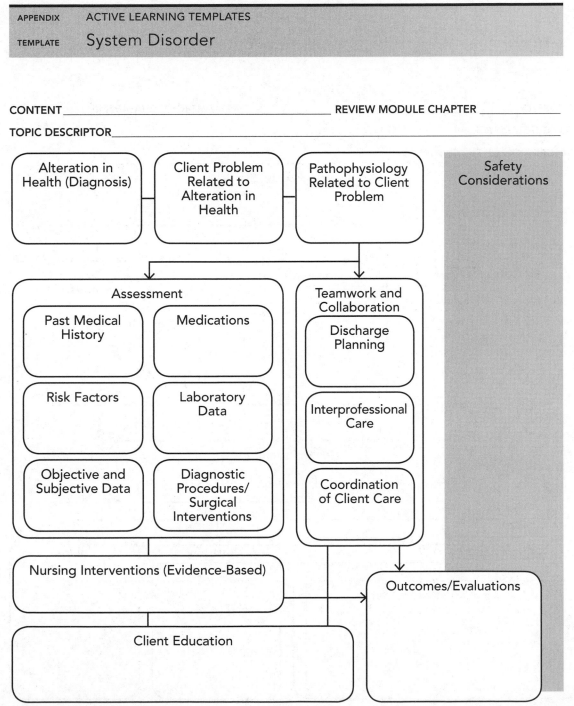

Appendix

CONTENT _____ **REVIEW MODULE CHAPTER** _____

TOPIC DESCRIPTOR _____

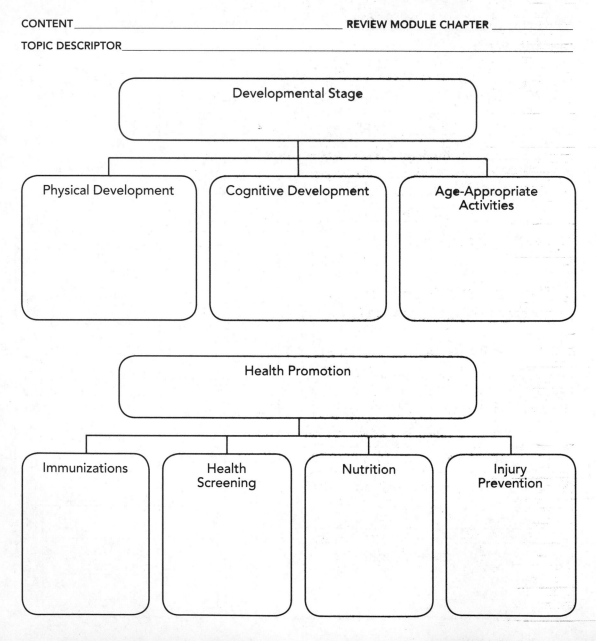

APPENDIX	ACTIVE LEARNING TEMPLATES
TEMPLATE	Medication

CONTENT _____ REVIEW MODULE CHAPTER _____

TOPIC DESCRIPTOR_____

MEDICATION _____

EXPECTED PHARMALOGICAL ACTION:

```
                        ┌─────────────────────────────────┐
                        │       Therapeutic Uses          │
                        │                                 │
                        └─────────────────────────────────┘
        ┌───────────────────────────┐       ┌───────────────────────────┐
        │     Adverse Effects        │       │   Nursing Interventions    │
        │                            │       │                            │
        └───────────────────────────┘       └───────────────────────────┘
        ┌───────────────────────────┐       
        │    Contraindications       │       
        │                            │       ┌───────────────────────────┐
        └───────────────────────────┘       │     Client Education       │
        ┌───────────────────────────┐       │                            │
        │ Medication/Food Interactions│      └───────────────────────────┘
        │                            │       
        └───────────────────────────┘       
        ┌───────────────────────────┐   ┌───────────────────────────┐
        │  Medication Administration │   │  Evaluation of Medication  │
        │                            │   │       Effectiveness        │
        └───────────────────────────┘   └───────────────────────────┘
```

Appendix

CONTENT _____ REVIEW MODULE CHAPTER _____

TOPIC DESCRIPTOR _____

DESCRIPTION OF SKILL:

Procedure Name

Indications

Nursing Interventions
(pre, intra, post)

Outcomes/Evaluations

Potential Complications

Nursing Interventions

Client Education

Appendix

CONTENT _____ REVIEW MODULE CHAPTER _____

TOPIC DESCRIPTOR_____

DESCRIPTION OF PROCEDURE:

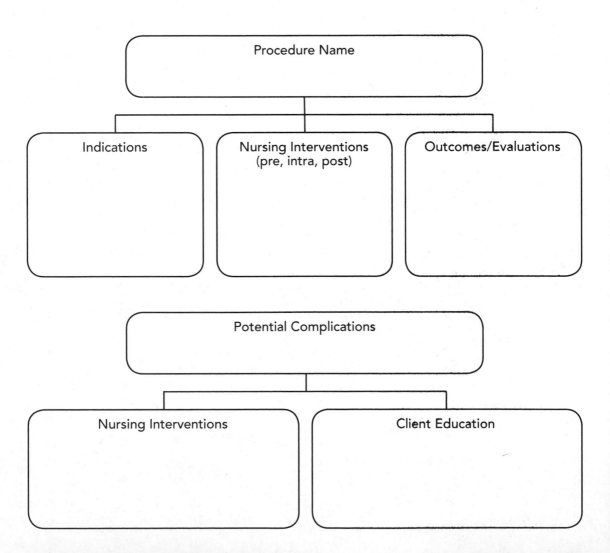

Procedure Name

Indications

Nursing Interventions
(pre, intra, post)

Outcomes/Evaluations

Potential Complications

Nursing Interventions

Client Education